A More Excellent Way

1 Corinthians 12:31

♦ ♦ ♦

A Teaching on the
Spiritual Roots of Disease

♦ ♦ ♦

The Ministry of

Pastor Henry Wright

ORDER FROM:
LAKE HAMILTON BIBLE CAMP
P. O. BOX 21516
HOT SPRINGS, AR 71903
(501) 525-8204

Pastor Henry Wright originally taught this material at a seminar given to Wycliffe members at the JAARS Center in Waxhaw, North Carolina, in July 1998. This manuscript is an edited transcription of that seminar.

First Edition printed in Anchorage, Alaska, May 1999.
Second Edition printed in Anchorage, Alaska, June 1999.
Third Edition printed in Anchorage, Alaska, July 1999.
Fourth Edition published in Thomaston, Georgia, December 1999.
Fifth Edition/Second Printing published in Thomaston, Georgia, September, 2001.

Pastor Henry Wright
Pleasant Valley Church, Inc.
1519 Pleasant Valley Road
Molena, GA 30258
1-706-646-2074 ♦ 1-800-453-5775
Fax: 1-706-646-2865 ♦ e-mail: pvcm3@alltel.net

Dedication

This book is dedicated to my mother, Norma Anne Wilson Wright, who went to be with the LORD, Thanksgiving Day, 1977. When I was in her womb she was dying with cancer, the type of cancer was fibro sarcoma cancer, fast-growing and fatal. This cancer was wrapped around her jugular vein and had spread to large areas in her neck and up into the base of her brain. In this condition, paralyzed, wasting away and dying, she was present at a church service in Hatfield's Point, New Brunswick, Canada, about 2 months after I was born. At this service God touched her and she was instantly healed. Her doctors were unable to find any trace of the masses of cancer that they had observed prior. The cancer was gone. No medical treatment had been given. She lived for 34 more years and was probably the only place of peace I ever had growing up. Her faith and her example and the testimony of her life continues to set an example for me, and not only me, but others that I can touch because of her steadfast faith in God. Her healing sets a standard within me against the enemy, for of a truth, God is no respecter of persons and what He has done for one, He will do for another.

Acknowledgments

My thanks to Art Mathias and Linda Follett for transcribing a live teaching into printed material that set the stage for this book. My thanks also to Bob Reed for his editorial assistance and layout design in the initial stages of this book. To the editing and publication team of Pleasant Valley Church, my thank you is as follows: thanks to Anita Hill for her diligence in researching the medical information; to Marcia Fisher for her thoughtful participation in medical research and pertinent observations; to Karen Kelly, Pat Koralewski and Marcia Fisher who read every word out loud in the editing stage; to Lu Malcolm for creating an index for the book and all the volunteers who edited it for this edition; to Nellie Lower for her contribution in scripture proofing and scripture content; also thanks to Tom Kelly and Ed Kelly for their diligence in verifying the accuracy of all scriptures; my thanks to Beverly McLaughlin for her part in content flow; also my thanks to Pat Koralewski and Karen Kelly for their expertise in grammar and sentence structure; also thanks to Leigh Barnard for her part in proofreading of the original transcript; my thanks to Dianne Kelly for her excellent work in manuscript formatting, design and the actual typing of the book; and also thanks to my wife Donna for loaning me to you, the reader, and also for her thoughtful contribution to the "spirit" of the book. The patient understanding of all these precious people has made the production of this book a joy.

Preface

This book is designed to sow seed of knowledge into your hearts about a big problem. The problem is spiritual, psychological and biological disease and what can we do about it and where is God in it today.

I ask for much grace and mercy in the reading because this teaching is not designed to be a theological dissertation but designed to be an insight into a problem and its solution: disease prevention and eradication. You will find this material to be scripturally accurate as well as medically and scientifically observable.

I find myself on the cutting edge of a problem and its solution. I do not have all the answers and I am still learning more every day. I reserve the right to revise this information as God increases the depth of my understanding.

One of my desires is to better equip the Church with respect to defeating spiritual, psychological and biological diseases. Also one of my goals is to take away the mystery of disease and to be able to show from God's perspective why mankind has disease.

Over the years God has shown me many insights into why mankind has disease. It is not that God cannot heal or that He doesn't want to: the problem is that man doesn't understand disease. We have gone into captivity and are perishing because of either lack of knowledge or just no knowledge at all. My investigation over the years, from the Scriptures and by practical discernment, has unearthed many spiritual roots and blocks to healing. In fact, the basic principles that, when applied, will move the hand of God to heal, are the same that, when applied, will prevent disease.

God's perfect will is not to heal you, His perfect will is that you don't get sick. Today I and this church/ministries stand 100% for disease eradication and prevention, not disease management, and on a regular basis if at all possible. To this end, I and this church are dedicated.

I don't want this book to become a method or a science or a formula or a quick-fix to take the place of relationship with God. One of the main themes of this book is the connection between sin and disease. Another theme in the book is the consequences of separation from God, His Word, His love; separation from ourselves; and separation from others.

One of the things that concerns me for those that will use this book to try to help others is that they will make it into a science or, at worst, use the knowledge in a legalistic manner to condemn others. A heart of compassion is the key to using this book.

The Authorized King James Version of the Bible is the foundation for this teaching. Please do not change the King James Version as a scriptural foundation as this teaching will lose the integrity and intent of its meaning.

Contents

Art Mathias' Testimony

My sister introduced me to Pastor Wright's teaching ministry in November 1998. She is a member of Wycliffe and attended the seminar in Waxhaw, North Carolina, in July 1998. After studying Scripture and applying the principles that were taught in the seminar, previously diagnosed tumors disappeared in her body.

In February 1997, I injured my neck in an accident. I had severe pain in my right arm and shoulder that began about 5 days after the accident. I went to a doctor and did physical therapy for a couple weeks and the pain went away. However, throughout that summer my arm was not right. It seemed weak at times and my balance was off.

In October 1997, the severe pain and muscle cramps returned in my right arm and shoulder. I went back to the doctor, tried more physical therapy and had no success. From October through December I went to several doctors and tried every therapy you could imagine, including acupuncture. In early December, a surgeon sent me for an MRI on my shoulder; it was negative. He gave me some pain pills and told me to come back in 6 weeks if it still hurt. However, he was too busy to deal with me at the end of the year rush.

The pain continued and atrophy began in my arm and shoulder. I was really getting scared. I tried to get an appointment with several local neurosurgeons, but was told there was at least a one-month backlog of patients. One of the receptionists suggested that I see a neurologist who could do an electrical conduction test to find nerve damage.

I was desperate and willing to do anything. I needed a referral, so I lied and gave the name of a doctor that I had seen previously for this problem. The doctor did the test and found that the nerve from the 7th cervical vertebrae was damaged.

She sent me for a MRI on my neck. It showed that I had 3 disc that were ruptured or fragmented and were putting severe pressure on my spinal cord and on a nerve going down my right arm. I was lucky not to be paralyzed.

Now, what would do I do? To say the least I was very scared. The doctor recommended surgery to remove the disc. Which surgeon should I choose? What were the long-term side effects from this kind of surgery?

I started to try to get appointments and talk to several doctors. In the meantime my arm was getting weaker and the atrophy more pronounced every day. The specialist told me that I would never regain the full use of my right arm.

My fears continued to grow. Believe me when I say there are quacks that call themselves doctors. You need to be very careful.

I was prayed for and was anointed by the elders in my local church, but I was not healed.

On January 21, 1998, I had the recommended surgery. The surgeon removed the three damaged disc and fused the vertebrae with bone taken from my hip. I was in the hospital for three days.

When I got home I found that I could not sit in my easy chair. It seemed to make me nervous and I hurt every place that touched the chair. As time went on, my fingers and toes would burn. The muscles in my hands and arms and feet and legs would cramp. I lost feeling in the tips of my fingers, my feet would get numb, and the sides of my legs would also get numb. I went back to the surgeon. He examined me, and took more x-rays, but could not find anything wrong. In April I had another MRI on my neck. The surgeon again could not find anything that would cause my symptoms.

I seemed to be getting worse. I got more scared when we could not find out what was happening to me. I could not sleep because of fear and pain. The doctor's only help was to give me drugs to dull the pain and to cover up the problems. When I read about the side effects from the drugs, I quit taking them. I have never been so sick and so scared.

One doctor thought I had something called arachnoiditis. A couple days before surgery I underwent a myelogram where a contrast dye was injected into the spinal cord, and then x-rays and a CAT scan were done. The dye can cause arachnoiditis. Arachnoiditis is the inflammation of the arachnoid layer that surrounds the spinal cord. Basically a person becomes paralyzed from the point of inflammation. My fear level again multiplied.

In late April I went to a neurologist. She examined me and told me that I probably had something called peripheral neuropathy, and ordered a bunch of tests. I made the mistake of looking up peripheral neuropathy on the Internet. The symptoms and prognosis are very similar to MS. Needless to say my fear factor again increased and I felt worse.

A friend took me to her pastor where they laid hands on me and prayed, but again I was not healed.

In early June 1998, I went to the Mayo Clinic in Arizona. After 3 days of very painful and expensive testing they confirmed what they called small fiber neuropathy. The small nerves in my hands and feet were dying, but they were not able to determine the cause. Their only treatment involved more drugs with horrible side effects.

I was scared and willing to try anything, so I began to see alternative doctors and practitioners. I tried many different remedies and treatments.

In August, I began to notice that sometimes the pain in my feet would stop at the top of my socks. So I started to buy different socks. I must have bought 50 different pairs, but it did not help. I started to look at what they were made of, and the only common fabric was nylon. I had myself tested to see if I was allergic to it. I was. This started me down the road of learning that I was allergic to almost 100 different foods and fabrics. I was even allergic to my own saliva. It was these allergies that were causing the numbness, the cramping, the stomachaches, and the nerve damage.

I was relieved to know about the allergies, but wondered what was causing them. Medical doctors' only answer for allergies is to avoid the allergen; they do not know the cause. I live in Alaska and it is cold. How do I avoid almost every fabric and so many foods and still stay alive? It is also very difficult to identify what you are allergic to. Allergies become complex as combinations of foods or fabrics become new allergens.

Naturopathic doctors and other alternative health practitioners have allergy elimination treatments that do help. However, after learning the true cause of allergies from Pastor Wright's teachings, I understand that while these treatments do help, they are not the answer. They do not deal with the true root of the problem, which is spiritual rather than physical.

In early December 1998, I received the tapes that have been transcribed into this teaching. The profile for Multiple Chemical Sensitivity/Environmental Illness taught by Pastor Wright described me to the proverbial "tee."

As I studied through the material, my eyes were opened to the true cause of my disease. My eyes were opened to a God who does truly love me. My earthly father is much too busy and self-centered to have time for me. I have tried very hard over the years to gain his acceptance and love with little or no success. I have related to my Heavenly Father in much the same way. My eyes were opened to what unforgiveness, bitterness, fear, and stress did to my body. My eyes were opened to what God really wants for me in this life. I have been a Christian all of my life, and yet this was a new teaching for me.

As I write this, in mid-March, 1999, I have taken back all of my foods; I can eat anything. I have taken back all of my clothes; I can wear anything. God has healed me! As I learned to conquer fear and to trust God, and as I learned to forgive others, and myself, God has healed me!

There are several reasons that I have transcribed and edited these tapes. First, Pastor Wright does not have written material at this time to disseminate. He has been too busy with his ministry to stop and turn his teachings into a book. Second, his teachings have been of tremendous healing value to me and I know they will change other's lives also.

I pray that you will be blessed as I have been blessed as you study this material.

May God Bless You!

Art Mathias

Art Mathias' Note: Pastor Wright is speaking at a seminar, and this transcription was made from that seminar's audio tapes. There will be some repetition of material, as Pastor Wright frequently reviewed a prior session at the beginning of a new one. Some of those redundancies have been left in this document, as it was felt that they added to the overall understanding of the teaching that was given. Pastor Wright's teaching style also includes repetition because of Isaiah 28.

> [9]**Whom shall he teach knowledge? and whom shall he make to understand doctrine?** *them that are* **weaned from the milk,** *and* **drawn from the breasts.** [10]**For precept** *must be* **upon precept, precept upon precept; line upon line, line upon line; here a little,** *and* **there a little:** [11]**For with stammering lips and another tongue will he speak to this people.** [12]**To whom he said, This** *is* **the rest** *wherewith* **ye may cause the weary to rest; and this** *is* **the refreshing: yet they would not hear.** [13]**But the word of the** LORD **was unto them precept upon precept, precept upon precept; line upon line, line upon line; here a little,** *and* **there a little; that they might go, and fall backward, and be broken, and snared, and taken.** Isaiah 28:9-13

Introduction

When I began in ministry in the early 1980's, I was part of a church that believed that God did get involved in people's lives, and that there was something happening between conversion and heaven. But even in that church of over 1500 people, coming week after week, the elders anointing them with oil, praying the prayer of faith, fasting and prayer, and standing on the Word, people were not getting well from incurable diseases.

I observed that as I crossed America, regardless of denomination, regardless of the Church, less than 5% of all of God's people (forget about the world) were getting healed of their diseases. It is even worse than that today. I don't know if you have ever been prayed for because of a disease and didn't get well. If you went before God and believed Him, believed that He loved you and He would heal you and it didn't happen, that is a staggering attack on your faith and your trust in the living God.

Scripture tells us that God loves us, that He came and died for us in the person of the Lord Jesus. He healed the people of their diseases and cast out their evil spirits. The disciples did it, the 70 did it, and the early church did it. Then we entered into a Dark Age of time from which I don't think we have ever recovered.

When I began in ministry, I wanted to know why God said in Psalm 103:3 that He not only forgives us of all our iniquities but He heals us of all our diseases.

> **³Who forgiveth all thine iniquities; who healeth all thy diseases;** Psalm 103:3

In the Old Testament, people were raised from the dead, people were healed, and many other miracles were done. In the New Testament, I found that we had a new and better covenant. In 3 John 2 it says – dearly beloved I wish above all things that you prosper and be in good health even as your soul prospers.

> **²Beloved, I wish above all things that thou mayest prosper and be in health, even as thy soul prospereth.** 3 John 1:2

In 1 Thessalonians 5:23, we're told—may the God of Peace sanctify you **wholly** in **spirit**, in **soul**, and in **body**.

> **²³And the very God of peace sanctify you wholly; and *I pray God* your whole spirit and soul and body be preserved blameless unto the coming of our Lord Jesus Christ.** 1 Thes. 5:23

Well, I didn't see much sanctification of the body, I didn't see much sanctification of the soul and I found a need for sanctification in God's people in holiness. You know, I am sure everyone in here is holy by faith but I have found that God's people struggle with the things of life. Paul did. Read Romans 7:14 to the end of the chapter.

> **¹⁴For we know that the law is spiritual: but I am carnal, sold under sin. ¹⁵For that which I do I allow not: for what I would, that do I not; but what I hate, that do I. ¹⁶If then I do that which I would not, I consent unto the law that**

> *it is* **good. [17]Now then it is no more I that do it, but sin that dwelleth in me. [18]For I know that in me (that is, in my flesh,) dwelleth no good thing: for to will is present with me; but *how* to perform that which is good I find not. [19]For the good that I would I do not: but the evil which I would not, that I do. [20]Now if I do that I would not, it is no more I that do it, but sin that dwelleth in me. [21]I find then a law, that, when I would do good, evil is present with me. [22]For I delight in the law of God after the inward man: [23]But I see another law in my members, warring against the law of my mind, and bringing me into captivity to the law of sin which is in my members. [24]O wretched man that I am! who shall deliver me from the body of this death? [25]I thank God through Jesus Christ our Lord. So then with the mind I myself serve the law of God; but with the flesh the law of sin.** Romans 7:14-25

You'll find he had a major struggle with his own spirituality. In fact, he said he had **sin that dwelt within him**.

When I began to become involved with people, getting involved in their lives, I prayed for people, and I believed God would heal them. Less than 5% of anyone I prayed for got well. I preached a gospel that got people saved and got them to heaven, but left them stranded between conversion and heaven. Would that be the gospel I would preach? Would I come up with a doctrine that would establish it? It would be easy to say, "Sorry, no help for you, no hope for you." But in my heart, the scriptures I read seemed to indicate differently.

I went to God one day and I said, "You'd better talk to me, Boss, because if you have called me to represent You to Your people, and to those yet unsaved, You'd better show me a little more fruit. If it's not happening, You'd better tell me why or else I'm going to go back into sales and marketing. I'll go to church, I'll love you, I'll be a good Christian, I might even be a deacon, but you can forget about me speaking. I'm not speaking for You if my words are not being honored, because that is fraud."

In James 1:5, the Bible says – if any man lack wisdom, let him ask of God and God will give it to him liberally – and upbraid him not because he has the audacity to ask God for a little information.

> **[5]If any of you lack wisdom, let him ask of God, that giveth to all *men* liberally, and upbraideth not; and it shall be given him.** James 1:5

I went before God in the early 1980's and God began to show me His truth about disease from the Scriptures. It wasn't that He *could not* heal. It was that we had to become sanctified in certain areas of our lives before He *would* heal. **Diseases in our lives can be the result of a separation from Him and His Word in specific areas of our lives.** God would have to become double minded, would have to become evil in condoning evil, in order to bless us in our sins. Except for those times when He would – have mercy on whom He would have mercy – disease was an issue to do with circumcision of the heart.

¹⁹And he said, I will make all my goodness pass before thee, and I will proclaim the name of the LORD before thee; and will be gracious to whom I will be gracious, and will shew mercy on whom I will shew mercy. Exodus 33:19

¹⁵For he saith to Moses, I will have mercy on whom I will have mercy, and I will have compassion on whom I will have compassion. Romans 9:15

A lot of people struggle with the supposed "gaps" between the Gospels, the book of Acts and the other Epistles. After Acts, there is little further discussion about healing and deliverance. Thus some have said, "Well, it passed away because you don't find it." "Healing was only for Christ or the disciples and not for us." I struggled with that. I'll be honest with you.

One day my eyes were opened and I saw something and I have never looked back from the ministry God set before me.

The Lord came and He demonstrated the love of God and power over the devil and disease in spite of sin. He demonstrated it in Matthew, Mark, Luke, and John; His disciples and the early church also demonstrated it in Acts. Then, from Romans all the way through Jude, you will find the Scriptures teaching us about sanctification. You can't have Matthew, Mark, Luke, John, and Acts until you have dealt with Romans to Jude. You cannot expect God to bless us if we are separated from Him in an area that needs to be dealt with. I like to say it this way, **"We have been taught so much about God's promises and not much about His Spirit of discernment and the consequence of sin."**

As a pastor, if somebody came to me with simple arthritis, and asked me to pray for them, I would say, "No, I'm not going to do it." If they said, "But the Word says to come before the elders and be anointed with oil and be prayed for," I would respond, "No, I've been there, done that!" Do you know how many times I've prayed for people with arthritis in the past? None of them were healed. I quit praying for them; it was a waste of my time.

But one day God opened my heart. I was ministering in 1985, when 5 ladies came up to me. Each of them had arthritis. Two of the ladies had gnarly disfiguration. I said to them, "You know there is sometimes a responsibility before God for healing."

I want to tell you, healing, and things you get from God, to a degree, are conditional to your obedience. I am not into legalism. I'm into grace and mercy. **But I want to tell you that with freedom comes a degree of responsibility.**

As you study through this teaching, I'm going to touch the very fabric of your lives. If you're interested in your lives and your families' lives, this is a good time to listen. I'm going to sow seed. Just as the rain comes down and waters the crops and returns to the clouds, the Bible says the Word does not return void (Isaiah 55:11).

¹¹So shall my word be that goeth forth out of my mouth: it shall not return unto me void, but it shall accomplish that which I please, and it shall prosper *in the thing* whereto I sent it. Isaiah 55:11

I'm going to seed (plant) **knowledge** into your life.

The knowledge I have is not only accurate scripturally, but it's also accurate medically. Coast to coast in America, I deal with disease. Even doctors contact our ministry regarding their own lives. There are doctors in America that call and discuss with me the implications of their patient's disease. I have doctors who refer their patients to me to discuss the spiritual roots of disease.

I sense the tide shifting across broad denominational lines. Our ministry is a trans-denominational ministry. What is a trans-denominational ministry? It is one that believes that in spite of denominations, God is still on the throne. The Lord Jesus is still the Word that came in the flesh, and the Holy Spirit is still on the earth today—One Faith, One Lord, and One Baptism, until we come into the unity of faith (Ephesians 4:5, 13).

> ⁵**One Lord, one faith, one baptism,** Ephes. 4:5

> ¹³**Till we all come in the unity of the faith, and of the knowledge of the Son of God, unto a perfect man, unto the measure of the stature of the fulness of Christ:** Ephes. 4:13

That is what I mean by trans-denominational.

If I stumble over your sacred cows of theology, I'm sorry. It's not in my heart to do that even unintentionally. I ask you to thoughtfully listen to what I have to say. You'll find that what I have to say may bear witness and answer a lot of your questions.

I told the 5 ladies with arthritis *that there would be a condition to their healing*. I asked them to think about the people who had injured each of them in their lifetime, either through word or deed—someone who didn't treat them right, victimized them, lied about them, abused them, either emotionally, physically, verbally, or maybe even sexually.

I asked them, "When you think of their name, or their face, whether they're living or dead, what do you feel? Do any of you have that high-octane ping going off inside?" They all said, "Yes, there is somebody I have not had resolution with." There was bitterness and unforgiveness. I told them that in exchange for their healing, they would have to get that right with God, right then, or else we were wasting our time. They were going to have to forgive that person.

The Scriptures say:

> ¹⁵**But if ye forgive not men their trespasses, neither will your Father forgive your trespasses.** Matthew 6:15

Have you ever read that scripture? Do you think it is there just for the fun of it? Do you think it is a situational scripture that only applies to some and not to all?

People ask me, "Pastor, does God forgive all manner of sin?" Yes and no. He wants to; that's His nature. He said He does:

⁹**If we confess our sins, he is faithful and just to forgive us *our* sins, and to cleanse us from all unrighteousness.** 1 John 1:9

But after conversion, there is an absolute requirement and responsibility to forgive others as mentioned in Matthew 6:14-15.

¹⁴**For if ye forgive men their trespasses, your heavenly Father will also forgive you:** ¹⁵**But if ye forgive not men their trespasses, neither will your Father forgive your trespasses.** Matthew 6:14-15

How, then, do you resolve this scripture in 1 John 1 with the one in Matthew that says, "If you from your heart do not forgive your brother his trespass, your Father which is in heaven will not forgive you yours"?

⁸**For by grace are ye saved through faith; and that not of yourselves: *it is* the gift of God:** ⁹**Not of works, lest any man should boast.** Ephes. 2:8-9

When you take a good look at these scriptures you'll find that, yes, you can go to heaven with sin because it is by faith we're saved, not by works. But the consequences of unforgiveness may bind you to a disease that is the result of this sin of bitterness and unforgiveness.

Christians, for the most part, believe we are saved by grace and by faith. But just because you are born again and your spirit has become alive in God, it does not mean you have resolved the consequences of the sin issue in your life. Otherwise, we wouldn't need sanctification, would we?

I told the 5 ladies that an exchange would happen for their obedience. I said, "If you, from your heart, will forgive that person of their trespasses, sincerely, whether you feel like it or not, I'm going to ask God to heal you. But, if you just do it because you want the healing for selfish reasons and you are using this kind of like a mechanism, or a system, or a mantra, we're still wasting our time." The Bible says, "If you, from your heart" … from your spirit, forgive.

⁶**Not with eyeservice, as menpleasers; but as the servants of Christ, doing the will of God from the heart;** Ephes. 6:6

³⁵**So likewise shall my heavenly Father do also unto you, if ye from your hearts forgive not every one his brother their trespasses.** Matthew 18:35

Your head might still be pitching a fit about what they did to you because that's in your memory. The Bible says – as many who are led by the Spirit of God, they are the sons of God.

¹⁴**For as many as are led by the Spirit of God, they are the sons of God.** Romans 8:14

Are you being led by your psychology (soul) or is the Spirit of God leading you? Who lives within your human spirit and makes you sons and daughters of God? Are you being led by the Spirit of God or by the intellect and other thoughts? I ask the question because it's an important question.

I led them into a prayer of repentance and forgiveness. I am here to tell you that when I finished the prayer, I looked up to them and said, "How's your arthritis doing?" All of a sudden it dawned on them that they had no more pain. Fingers had straightened, the pain was gone, and all 5 ladies stood there totally freed from crippling arthritis and its pain. *I never ministered healing one time.*

When they met the conditions of *His* nature, He was there to heal. That's the reason I am not too impressed by (and I say this carefully) healing crusades that don't take into account that disease may be a result of sin that has not been dealt with.

I don't know if you are aware of this but **fear is a sin**. Fear is a sin. Fear is the #1 plague of America, and it's the #1 plague of the world—fear of tomorrow, fear of death, fear of man, fear of dying, fear of disease, fear of mothers-in-law, fear of your neighbor, fear of yourself. We are a people of God who are in bondage. We're paying an incredibly high price. God's people are being sent back in the world for help, when the answer is waiting in His Word to set you free.

I am more interested in getting you into a better life, not just getting you into heaven. The Lord's Prayer says – thy will be done, in earth as it is in heaven.

> ⁹**...Our Father which art in heaven, Hallowed be thy name. ¹⁰Thy kingdom come. Thy will be done in earth, as *it is* in heaven.** Matthew 6:9-10

When I read 3 John 2, it was over for me – dearly beloved, I wish above all things that you prosper and be in good health even as your soul prospers.

> ²**Beloved, I wish above all things that thou mayest prosper and be in health, even as thy soul prospereth.** 3 John 1:2

God's perfect will is not to heal you. God's perfect will in the Word is that you don't get sick. In Deuteronomy 28 and Exodus 15, God promised that if we are obedient to Him, that none of the diseases of Egypt will fall upon us.

> ²⁶**And said, If thou wilt diligently hearken to the voice of the Lᴏʀᴅ thy God, and wilt do that which is right in his sight, and wilt give ear to his commandments, and keep all his statutes, I will put none of these diseases upon thee, which I have brought upon the Egyptians: for I *am* the Lᴏʀᴅ that healeth thee.** Exodus 15:26

> ¹**And it shall come to pass, if thou shalt hearken diligently unto the voice of the Lᴏʀᴅ thy God, to observe *and* to do all his commandments which I command thee this day, that the Lᴏʀᴅ thy God will set thee on high above all nations of the earth:** Deut. 28:1

(Also see Deuteronomy 28:1-14.)

Editor's Note: Deuteronomy 28:60 makes mention of the diseases of Egypt coming upon us because of disobedience.

> ⁶⁰**Moreover he will bring upon thee all the diseases of Egypt, which thou wast afraid of; and they shall cleave unto thee.** Deut. 28:60

Newsweek magazine, in an article in 1990 called "The Power To Heal," said: "The fate of the spirit is relegated to religious specialists who have little to say about their followers' physical well being." Many pastors in America today don't understand diseases. They don't understand disease and they don't understand psychological problems. They know how to get you born again. They know how to balance a budget. They know how to visit hospitals, marry people and bury the dead. But they don't know what to do with disease. So they'll send you out into the street to an unregenerated and unrenewed specialist in a disease, and maybe even call them the anointed of God.

In the Old Testament, if somebody had leprosy and later said they were clean, to whom were they sent to determine if they were healed? The priest! The New Testament says, if there be any sick among you, call who? The elders of the church.

[14]Is any sick among you? let him call for the elders of the church; and let them pray over him, anointing him with oil in the name of the Lord: James 5:14

If I have anything to do with it in my lifetime, I intend to bring the pastoral ministry back to where God wanted it from the beginning. That happens when God honors what ministers are teaching by healing diseases as the Word is applied to the lives of the people.

Last year, I taught in a church in Texas. A member of that church had been healed of multiple chemical sensitivity (MCS/EI). She had not been able to go to church for over 20 years. She was isolated, could only eat 2 to 4 foods, suffered from electromagnetic sensitivity, chronic fatigue syndrome, and multiple allergies. God healed her. He healed all the peripheral diseases around MCS/EI. That church is really rocking because she is back singing in the choir every Sunday. They asked me to come and teach on roots of disease, so I went there and taught. I came back again that evening and taught for another 2½ hours on the spiritual roots of disease and the consequences of sin.

The next morning they brought a lady to me privately that had cancer of the lung and cancer of the bone. She had been to all the doctors and had all the bone scans and x-rays. She was the mother of two children. Because I knew the spiritual root of her disease, I just kind of laid it out. This is your disease; this is what I see. It took about 3 seconds and she was bawling like a baby. I had touched her pain. I had touched her spiritual dynamics. God opened her up with discernment and I put my hand right on that thing that had been festering for years, causing eventual destruction of the two sentries of her immune system that protect us from cancer, called anti-oncogenes. When those enzymes are destroyed in our bodies, the cell is compromised and cancer cell mitosis can begin at any time.

I told her, "I don't know what God's going to do but I do know you are going to have to get right with God in this area of your life." She said, "Pastor, I've known that all the time but I just couldn't get to there, I just couldn't get over it." I said, "Would you like to go there and get over it?" She said, "Yes." I led her into a place before the Lord and before the Father, a place of soul searching, a place of repentance, a place of getting right with God. I just ministered to her and broke the power of the spirit of death, that power of cancer, and commanded its power to be broken.

Thirty days later, I got a phone call. She had been back to the doctor and had bone scans and X-rays. There was no evidence of lung cancer or bone cancer.

Her pastor has already sent me 2 letters, asking me to train his deacons, train his teams. He was ready to start learning how, along with members of his congregation, to care for the sheep, **a more excellent way**. He said, "Pastor, thank you for coming and allowing the Lord to speak through you about the connection between sin and disease."

See, we think of sin as robbing banks, we think of sin as maybe prostitution, we think of sin as maybe lying and stealing. Would you consider fear to be sin? Would you consider bitterness to be sin? Would you consider self-hatred to be sin? Would you consider these things to be sin? The Word says it is. I think certain sins have become socially acceptable. We are paying too high a price for these areas of unrecognized sin in the area of disease.

About 30% of all cancers have a spiritually rooted component. I specialize in cancer to some degree, but I don't have all the answers. We are somewhat familiar with uterine, ovarian, breast, and prostate cancers. We have insight into how these cancers develop. In the section on the spiritual roots of disease I will go into this in detail.

About 80% of all the diseases of mankind have a spiritual root with various psychological and biological manifestations. I am not a doctor. I am not a psychologist. I do not mix psychology with ministry. I am a servant of the Father and the Lord Jesus Christ. No man has taught me, but He has taught me.

Spiritually Rooted Disease

Spiritually rooted disease is the result of separation on three levels:

1. Separation from God, His Word and His love.

2. Separation from yourself.

3. Separation from others.

1. Separation from God, His Word and His Love

Mankind is diseased because first of all we are separated from God, His Word, His truth and His love—and that includes members of His church. Do you know how many of the wonderful, believing saints I talk to are not sure God loves them? They had an earthly father that did not represent God the Father in their life. God the Father is now guilty by association. He's a mean, bad dude.

Religion teaches that God the Father is sitting on the throne with lightning bolts waiting to strike you dead if you're bad today. That's not what I read in scripture. Our God is a loving God who says, "…God is love"

> **16And we have known and believed the love that God hath to us. God is love; and he that dwelleth in love dwelleth in God, and God in him.** 1 John 4:16

and "For God so loved the world that He gave…"

> **16For God so loved the world, that he gave his only begotten Son, that whosoever believeth in him should not perish, but have everlasting life.** John 3:16

Jesus said – you've seen Me, you've seen the Father.

> **19Then answered Jesus and said unto them, Verily, verily, I say unto you, The Son can do nothing of himself, but what he seeth the Father do: for what things soever he doeth, these also doeth the Son likewise.** John 5:19

> **28Then said Jesus unto them, When ye have lifted up the Son of man, then shall ye know that I am *he,* and *that* I do nothing of myself; but as my Father hath taught me, I speak these things.** John 8:28

> **9Jesus saith unto him, Have I been so long time with you, and yet hast thou not known me, Philip? he that hath seen me hath seen the Father; and how sayest thou *then,* Shew us the Father?** John 14:9

I like to have a little fun with religion. I love relationship, but to me religion is a killer. I try to bring people into that place of healing—that place of receiving. You see, healing doesn't ultimately come from Jesus. It comes from the Father. Jesus said, "I only do the things I saw My Father doing. I only say the things I heard My Father saying."

> **38I speak that which I have seen with my Father: and ye do that which ye have seen with your father.** John 8:38

> **30I can of mine own self do nothing: as I hear, I judge: and my judgment is just; because I seek not mine own will, but the will of the Father which hath sent me.** John 5:30

James 1:17 says—all good things come down from the Father of lights where there is
no variableness of turning.

> [17]Every good gift and every perfect gift is from above, and cometh down
> from the Father of lights, with whom is no variableness, neither shadow of
> turning. James 1:17

Psalm 68:19 says – blessed be the Lord, who daily loads us with benefits…the LORD
of our salvation.

> [19]Blessed *be* the Lord, *who* daily loadeth us *with benefits, even* the God of
> our salvation. Selah. Psalm 68:19

I get a real kick out of these "Jesus is Lord" signs on churches. I wonder what
happened to the Father. He's not Lord? The Lord's prayer says: "Our Father who art
in heaven…" (Matthew 6:9-13):

> [9]After this manner therefore pray ye: Our Father which art in heaven,
> Hallowed be thy name. [10]Thy kingdom come. Thy will be done in earth, as *it is*
> in heaven. [11]Give us this day our daily bread. [12]And forgive us our debts, as we
> forgive our debtors. [13]And lead us not into temptation, but deliver us from evil:
> For thine is the kingdom, and the power, and the glory, for ever. Amen.
> Matthew 6:9-13

Jesus said in John 16:23 – in that day you will ask Me nothing, but you will pray the
Father in My name and He shall give you what you ask.

> [23]And in that day ye shall ask me nothing. Verily, verily, I say unto you,
> Whatsoever ye shall ask the Father in my name, he will give *it* you. John 16:23

I like to see these "Jesus is Lord" signs, but I'd like to see "Father is Lord" just above
it. Jesus said – My Father and I are One….but He is greater than I (John 14:28).

> [30]I and *my* Father are one. John 10:30

> [28]Ye have heard how I said unto you, I go away, and come *again* unto you.
> If ye loved me, ye would rejoice, because I said, I go unto the Father: for my
> Father is greater than I. John 14:28

The order of the Godhead and the government of God is first, the Father; second, the
Word that came in the flesh as Jesus; and third, the Holy Spirit.

2. Separation from Yourself

Do you know how many people do not like themselves? Do you know how many
people struggle with self-hatred, lack of self-esteem and guilt? It's a massive plague.
How can you not love yourself if God loves you? He's greater than you are. He who
is greatest and holiest of all, God the Father, says He loves you. Under what gospel do
we have the audacity to say we do not love ourselves? If we do, we make ourselves in
opposition to God. We make ourselves a god unto ourselves, deny His statement of
love, and open ourselves up to the enemy to agree with us. Instead of hearing God
speaking to you, by His Word and by the Holy Spirit, telling you that you are loved

and that you are "OK," you are going to hear this voice coming into your mind telling you how rotten, or stupid, or worthless you are.

In this ministry, we deal with many autoimmune diseases: lupus, Crohn's, diabetes, rheumatoid arthritis, and MS, to name a few. All autoimmune diseases have a spiritual root of self-hatred, self-bitterness, and guilt. Diabetes can be defeated. Lupus or rheumatoid arthritis can be defeated. All autoimmune diseases can be defeated and/or prevented.

Do you know what really irritates me? When somebody says, "That's incurable, they are just going to die anyway." Do you know what that does in my spirit? I am so grieved. That means to me that person believes that Satan and death are greater than God and the Lord Jesus and His Word. I do not agree.

Do you think God needs a disease to get you to heaven? Do you think that God needs to torment you so you can get over the great divide? Why have we become so acclimated to this kind of thinking that we have to die and move into Glory because of a disease? I think we've been had! I think we've been bewitched! I think we're following another gospel! Where did euthanasia come from, anyway?

In Psalm 90, God, through Moses, prophesied that your lifetime should be 70 to 80 years. Anything less than that is a curse.

> [10]**The days of our years *are* threescore years and ten; and if by reason of strength *they be* fourscore years, yet *is* their strength labour and sorrow; for it is soon cut off, and we fly away. [11]Who knoweth the power of thine anger? even according to thy fear, *so is* thy wrath. [12]So teach *us* to number our days, that we may apply *our* hearts unto wisdom. Psalm 90:10-12**

Where did this term "retirement" come from? Moses was 80 years of age before he even started his ministry.

3. Separation from Others

Separation opens the door to spiritually rooted diseases. Unforgiveness, or bitterness toward others, contributes to separation.

When you think of someone who has wronged you, do you feel it in the pit of your stomach? We need to start looking at those high-octane pings. You will always remember that individual and what they did to you, but you do not have to carry the thoughts of hate, or bitterness. If you have truly forgiven them from your heart, these thoughts will be gone. You will still have the memory, but God will heal the pain so you can have victory over the situation. It doesn't need to ruin your life.

We are not only into healing, but we are into disease prevention. Would you like to avoid certain diseases in your lifetime? *Newsweek* magazine (Sept. 24, 1990) says,

> The future of medicine does not lie in the treatment of illness but in preventing it. Throughout the 20th century, medicine has advanced primary care by improving curative care. Curative care has its limits. Psychoimmunology (the

science that deals with the mind's role in helping the immune system to fight disease) will become a vitally important clinical field in the 21st century. Perhaps this will be the most important medical field, supplanting our present emphasis on oncology and cardiology. Healthy thinking may eventually become an integral aspect of treatment for everything from allergies to liver transplants and prevention of disease.

The future of medicine does not lie in the treatment of illness but in preventing it.

Family trees are a very important diagnostic tool. Behavior and health problems tend to repeat themselves. We see patterns that repeat from mothers and fathers to their children. This is true in both biological and spiritual disease. Exodus 20 teaches about the sins of the father being passed on to the third and fourth generation. Psychologists also have observed certain personality characteristics and behaviors, such as rage, anger, or molestation, that can roll over to the next generation(s).

> ⁵Thou shalt not bow down thyself to them, nor serve them: for I the LORD thy God *am* a jealous God, visiting the iniquity of the fathers upon the children unto the third and fourth *generation* of them that hate me; Exodus 20:5

> ⁹Thou shalt not bow down thyself unto them, nor serve them: for I the LORD thy God *am* a jealous God, visiting the iniquity of the fathers upon the children unto the third and fourth *generation* of them that hate me, Deut. 5:9

Would you like to prevent disease in your children? Do you think it's possible? That would be **a more excellent way**.

When I get involved with people who are about to be married, I look at the family trees from both sides to see what they are bringing into this family package. If we don't deal with what's happened in the family tree, and if you don't deal with what's in your personal lives, your children will inherit your curses.

If we want to do something for our children, let's go before God and get our lives straightened out, so that we can break the power of sin, so that genetically inherited diseases no longer exist. In our ministry, nationally, we have documented evidence of genetic code changes. When a disease was diagnosed through the genetic investigation by an oncologist, after ministry and healing, the genetic pattern had changed and this person could no longer have that specific disease again. Do you think that's possible?

Are we just going to go on this toboggan ride from generation to generation and do nothing about it? Look into your families and you will see some of the same diseases, personality traits, and characteristics of relationships repeating: mothers and daughters not getting along, fathers and sons fighting with each other. Broken relationships of some kind are passed along until someone decides "Enough" and breaks the cycle.

In an article in *USA Today*, a number of women were asked: "Where do you go when you are sick? Who do you talk to?" About half of all women said that their primary care doctor is their main source of health care information. The other half reported as follows:

- 24% of all women learn about their problems and solutions from magazines and newspapers

- 7% from TV and radio

- 5% from a relative or a friend

- 5% from self-help books

- 4% from school courses

- 2% from a pharmacist.

Not even in a fraction of a percentage is a pastor, church, Bible or God ever mentioned. Yet God is the Creator. He is our Savior. He is our healer and He is our deliverer—if He created us, He knows what's wrong with us! Would we dare go there and ask Him to reveal that to His children? I have. I'm just foolish enough to believe He will answer me—or smart enough.

I am not against doctors, but I believe, in our ignorance and our separation from God, that we've asked the medical community to do something they are not qualified to do—that is to pastor us and deal with spiritual issues. I don't find anywhere in Scripture, especially in Ephesians 4, where a doctor and a psychologist are considered to be a gift from the Lord Jesus in leadership to us.

> **⁸Wherefore he saith, When he ascended up on high, he led captivity captive, and gave gifts unto men.** Ephes. 4:8

> **¹¹And he gave some, apostles; and some, prophets; and some, evangelists; and some, pastors and teachers;** Ephes. 4:11

I have found the five-fold ministry mentioned which includes apostles, prophets, evangelists, pastors and teachers are a gift to the body, but I did not find doctors or psychologists.

> **²⁷Now ye are the body of Christ, and members in particular. ²⁸And God hath set some in the church, first apostles, secondarily prophets, thirdly teachers, after that miracles, then gifts of healings, helps, governments, diversities of tongues.** 1 Cor. 12:27-28

These two professions are many times the result of the failure of the Christian Church and its leadership to execute its scriptural mandate in pastoral care.

Psychologists have become the pastors of America, and God has not ordained them to be such. We have asked our medical community to be our healers of spiritually rooted diseases, and they are not qualified. That's why allopathic medicine is failing. The medical community does not know the etiology of over 80% of all diseases. If they don't know the cause, how can they cure the disease? They can't. The best they can do is a little management of the disease often with drugs that have terrible side effects.

Because the Church has failed in this area, people are running to alternative and New Age modalities of disease management. But these too are failing, because again they only offer "management" of the disease. People are beginning to come back to the Church and the Church should have the answers.

> [10]To the intent that now unto the principalities and powers in heavenly *places* might be known by the church the manifold wisdom of God, Ephes. 3:10

I head up a ministry that has people coming for help from coast to coast and around the world—45% of the people seeking help are unchurched and unsaved. I have them coming in the back door asking, "Pastor, can you help?" The world is turning the corner, coming back to God, but the Church is turning the corner away from God. *I think it is time to let God be God in our midst with understanding and discernment.*

In our Ministry Brochure there is a statement that is worth repeating:

> *The true etiology of many diseases reveals an often overlooked, spiritual dimension. This dimension, more often than not, goes unaddressed by the afflicted, their health care providers, and even their spiritual leaders.*

My Purpose and Insight

Disease Prevention, Not Disease Management, Is My Goal

My parents were ministers. I'm a third generation spiritual leader. I grew up with the knowledge that God heals because of my mother's miraculous healing.

My mother was dying with fibro sarcoma cancer, fast growing and fatal, which had wrapped around her jugular vein. Just two months after my birth, she was dying. She was paralyzed. Masses of cancer had grown around her jugular vein and up into the base of her brain—up and down her whole neck area. She made a Hannah-type covenant that if God would heal her, she would raise me, Henry, in the knowledge of God.

In this private moment of prayer while others were praying for her, God healed her instantly. When checked by the doctors, they were amazed to find no evidence of cancer. No medical treatment had been given, and yet the masses of cancer were gone, evaporated. Even more remarkable, *her healing broke a pattern,* a genetic curse from her past. You see, her mother had died of cancer within 2 months of giving birth to her. With this curse defeated, my mother lived another 33 years.

In my later years, you noticed I said, "Later years...," I dedicated my life to God and the study of the Scriptures. The Bible says to teach a child in the way he should go and when he is old, he shall not depart from it.

> **⁶Train up a child in the way he should go: and when he is old, he will not depart from it.** Proverbs 22:6

The Scriptures seemed to indicate that the LORD wanted to heal *all* of our diseases.

> **³Who forgiveth all thine iniquities; who healeth all thy diseases;** Psalm 103:3

Yet I observed that only a small percentage of people have ever defeated incurable diseases, including those that looked to churches for their healing.

I understood the frustration of Carl Jung as he observed his minister father preach a gospel that offered no solutions for the diseases of the soul and the body. Today's psychology is, in part, the fruit of that frustration as an attempt to manage the diseases of the soul through therapy and drugs. I observed the Church, religions, alternative medicine, spiritual groups, allopathic medicine, chiropractic, and eastern mysticism, trying to decrease the effects of disease through various methods. **In the end, all I really ever saw was disease management.**

I want to say something to you; the best you have going for you in American medicine are HMO's. The insurance industry recognizes that disease is on the increase and they're going to cut their cost, cut their risk for the benefit of the stockholders, and you're going to pay the price. They are going to pay what they want to pay for your medical care, and no more. I suggest that there is **a more excellent way.**

I did a seminar in New York City, held in an off-Broadway theater that was donated to our ministry for two days. In my audience was a doctor from New York, and at the end of two days he came up to me and said,

> Pastor, I am a member of the medical community here in NYC. I have been here listening to you for two days. When you say that disease management is the best that the medical community can offer, you have been very generous to our industry. *The best we could only hope to achieve is disease management.* It would be good if we could do that.

National statistics from the past two years show that with all modalities of treatment for cancer, including surgery, chemotherapy, vitamins, supplements, and all the various types of therapies, the average life extension was only one year. That one year of prolonged life came at great expense and with tremendous pain and suffering.

I don't know about you, but when I read Psalm 103:3, it says the LORD not only forgives us of all our iniquities but He heals us of all our diseases. It doesn't say: "He helps us manage all our diseases."

³Who forgiveth all thine iniquities; who healeth all thy diseases; Psalm 103:3

Let me say something to you: I couldn't heal a fly with a toothache. I don't have any powers, I'm just a sheepherder. I'm not a healer, I'm just a guy. I know He Who is God, and I know His Word. As a minister, I cannot teach a gospel that makes God less than *omnipotent*; I have to hold out for that. I also have to hold out that God is *omniscient*—He knows everything: past, present and future. I also have to hold out that He is *omnipresent*—He's available world wide, all the time, everywhere.

The fourth area that I have to hold out for is something you have probably not heard a lot about; **God is also omnificent**, all creative, ever able to fix that which needs to be fixed. *Being omnificent makes Him magnificent*—King of kings and LORD of all lords. He is God of all gods. He is the Creator of all flesh. He is the sustainer of all of mankind. He is in love with you, and I am in love with Him. I hope you are too!

Over the years, God has shown me many insights into why mankind has disease. **It is not that God cannot heal you, or that He doesn't want to. The problem is that man does not understand disease.** We have gone into captivity and are perishing, either because of lack of knowledge or just no knowledge at all. In Isaiah 5:13, God said to the prophet Isaiah—My people are gone into captivity, because they have no knowledge. Hell hath enlarged itself and swallowed them up and all of their fame into the depths of hell.

> **¹³Therefore my people are gone into captivity, because *they have* no knowledge: and their honourable men *are* famished, and their multitude dried up with thirst. ¹⁴Therefore hell hath enlarged herself, and opened her mouth without measure: and their glory, and their multitude, and their pomp, and he that rejoiceth, shall descend into it.** Isaiah 5:13-14

He is not talking about unsaved Gentiles. He's talking about MY PEOPLE, called by My Name, set aside by My covenant. My people in the earth are going into captivity because they have no knowledge. In Hosea 4:6, the prophet says—My people perish because of lack of knowledge.

> **⁶My people are destroyed for lack of knowledge: because thou hast rejected knowledge, I will also reject thee, that thou shalt be no priest to me: seeing thou hast forgotten the law of thy God, I will also forget thy children.** Hosea 4:6

So whether it's lack of knowledge or no knowledge,

> **⁶All we like sheep have gone astray; we have turned every one to his own way...**Isaiah 53:6

I would like to make sure we change that, if we can.

My investigation over the years from the Scriptures, practical discernment and review of scientific and medical evidence, has unearthed many spiritual roots and blocks to healing. **In fact, the basic principles that, when applied, will move the hand of God to heal, are the same principles that, when applied, will prevent disease.**

The very same principles that you can apply in your life to move the hand of God to sustain you, to heal you, and to deliver you—if you start applying them now in your life (even if you don't have a disease)—may keep you from getting that disease in your lifetime.

Remember Deuteronomy 28 and Exodus 15:26—because of our obedience to God in His Word and our fellowship with Him in the covenant, He will put none of the diseases of Egypt upon us.

> **²⁶And said, If thou wilt diligently hearken to the voice of the LORD thy God, and wilt do that which is right in his sight, and wilt give ear to his commandments, and keep all his statutes, I will put none of these diseases upon thee, which I have brought upon the Egyptians: for I *am* the LORD that healeth thee.** Exodus 15:26

That is a valid promise even today. Now, either we are going to continue in promise or we're going to teach bondage.

God's Perfect Will is Not to Heal You; His Perfect Will is That You Don't Get Sick

Today, I stand 100% not for disease management but for disease eradication and prevention on a regular basis, if at all possible.

> **¹⁴Turn, O backsliding children, saith the LORD; for I am married unto you: and I will take you one of a city, and two of a family, and I will bring you to Zion: ¹⁵And I will give you pastors according to mine heart, which shall feed you with knowledge and understanding.** Jeremiah 3:14-15

It is my prayer that you will and could receive this. As a pastor, I consider this to be my ministry, and a gift to you. I desire to feed you with knowledge and understanding.

2 Timothy 2:24-26 says:

> **²⁴And the servant of the Lord must not strive; but be gentle unto all *men*, apt to teach, patient, ²⁵In meekness instructing those that oppose themselves; if God peradventure will give them repentance to the acknowledging of the truth; ²⁶And *that* they may recover themselves out of the snare of the devil, who are taken captive by him at his [the devil's] will.** 2 Tim. 2:24-26

In this teaching I can give you enough information and enough knowledge that you will be able to come before God, so that the work of sanctification, healing and deliverance can begin for you and your loved ones, your friends or your families. *Remember, I told you that my purpose is to sow seed*—to leave behind a foundation for God, by His Spirit, according to the Word of God and according to knowledge that's available both from the scientific and medical communities and from the Word. My purpose is to bring you to a place where you may recover yourself from the snare of the devil.

The other day someone said, "Pastor, I believe God gave me my disease. I'm closer to Him because of it." I had someone else say, "Well, I just believe my disease is from God—it just teaches me how to be humble. It's my thorn in the flesh, but His grace is sufficient for me."

Could be, but I asked him if he was going to a doctor.

He said, "Oh, yes."

I asked, "Why are you going to a doctor?"

He said, "So I can get well."

I said, "You hypocrite! How dare you interfere with God's will in your life by going to a doctor?"

I was ministering in a Church of Christ in southern Maine many years ago, and the head deacon came up to me after the service. It had been a powerful service that lasted 3½ hours. This deacon had injured himself. He was moaning, groaning, and complaining, so I said, "Would you mind if I pray for you? Maybe God would heal you of that pain." He said, "Oh no, brother, I don't want any prayer, this pain reminds me of the sufferings of Christ, what He did for me on the cross. It is a constant reminder of what He did for me." I looked at him and said, "Suffer on brother!"

I think that sometimes we create theologies based on our lack of knowledge. **The beginning of all healing of spiritually rooted diseases begins when you make your peace with God, and accept His love once and for all, accepting yourself and accepting others**. In Deuteronomy 6:5 it says—and thou shalt love the LORD thy God with all thine heart, and with all thy soul, and with all thy might.

> **⁵And thou shalt love the LORD thy God with all thine heart, and with all thy soul, and with all thy might.** Deut. 6:5

Leviticus 19:18 says— …but thou shalt love thy neighbor as thyself: I am the LORD.

¹⁸Thou shalt not avenge, nor bear any grudge against the children of thy people, but thou shalt love thy neighbour as thyself: I *am* the LORD. Leviticus 19:18

And then again it says in Matthew 22:37-40:

³⁷Jesus said unto him, Thou shalt love the Lord thy God with all thy heart, and with all thy soul, and with all thy mind. ³⁸This is the first and great commandment. ³⁹And the second *is* like unto it, Thou shalt love thy neighbour as thyself. ⁴⁰On these two commandments hang all the law and the prophets. Matthew 22:37-40

If you do not love yourself, you cannot love your neighbor. You may pretend you do. If you do not love yourself, then you cannot love your neighbor, because you are unable to receive their love.

People's inability to give and receive love today is a tragedy. If somebody were to come up to you, give you a big hug, give you a million dollars, and say you were the best thing since peanut butter, could you receive that? Could you receive it without feeling guilty?

We have been so tragically victimized in the family that it is amazing we are even here today. **The failure in all family problems begins with the man.** The salvation of the whole family should begin with the salvation of the father and husband of the home. God did not create woman to be the spiritual leader of the home; He created the man. The Bible says the head of the woman is the man. The head of the man is Christ and the head of Christ is the Father.

²²Wives, submit yourselves unto your own husbands, as unto the Lord. ²³For the husband is the head of the wife, even as Christ is the head of the church: and he is the saviour of the body. ²⁴Therefore as the church is subject unto Christ, so *let* the wives *be* to their own husbands in every thing. Ephes. 5:22-24

Many women today are having real problems. Eighty-five to ninety percent of my caseload nationally is female. God has used me to heal more females than you can imagine. God's first ministry is to the fatherless and the widows, not to how many scriptures you can read in your Bible today (even though it is important to be in the Word to build your faith). James 1:27 says:

²⁷Pure religion and undefiled before God and the Father is this, To visit the fatherless and widows in their affliction, *and* to keep himself unspotted from the world. James 1:27

That is sanctification. Pure religion is when you begin taking care of the fatherless, taking care of the widows and keeping yourself unspotted from the world.

I deal with many people whose fathers are still alive, but they are fatherless. I deal with many women whose husbands or ex-husbands are still alive, and yet they are spiritual widows. The fallout and the diseases that have come upon us because of these sins are of great magnitude.

I think the world will come to a well church faster than it will come to a sick church. There's more to salvation than saving your proverbial butt from hell. The gospel message includes day by day blessings. I believe that it's God's will that He blesses people.

Faith vs. Fear

Many people struggle with faith. Maybe you're sick, you have a disease and you have been told you don't have enough faith. Maybe you have been listening to some of these people teach that you need to do something to get more faith.

The Bible says in Romans 12:3—to every man and woman has been given a measure of faith.

> ³...**through the grace given unto me, to every man that is among you...but to think soberly, according as God hath dealt to every man the measure of faith.** Romans 12:3

You have enough faith. You could always pray, "Lord, increase my faith," however, you have enough if you only believe. You are going to have to determine the difference as to whether you're following God from your head or your heart.

If we follow God out of our head, we're all in trouble. My poor head pitches a fit most of the time. If I didn't have the Word of God down in my spirit, mixed with faith by the Holy Spirit that lives within me, my life would be a wasteland. My poor head pitches a fit with the Word of God sometimes.

We need to be continually renewed by the washing of the water of the Word (2 Corinthians 4:16; Ephesians 5:26; 4:23; Colossians 3:10).

> ²⁶**That he might sanctify and cleanse it with the washing of water by the word,** Ephes. 5:26

> ²³**And be renewed in the spirit of your mind;** Ephes. 4:23

> ¹⁶**For which cause we faint not; but though our outward man perish, yet the inward** *man* **is renewed day by day.** 2 Cor. 4:16

> ¹⁰**And have put on the new** *man,* **which is renewed in knowledge after the image of him that created him:** Col. 3:10

Romans 10:17 says—faith comes by hearing and hearing by the word of God.

> ¹⁷**So then faith** *cometh* **by hearing, and hearing by the word of God.** Romans 10:17

In Hebrews 11:1 we're told—faith is the substance of things hoped for, the evidence of things not yet seen.

> ¹¹:¹**Now faith is the substance of things hoped for, the evidence of things not seen.** Hebrews 11:1

Do you have hopes? Is everybody here hopeless? Do you have something burning on the inside that represents hope about something in your life, about you or somebody else? Do you? Then you have faith, because faith is the substance of things hoped for, the evidence of things not yet seen. If it's already come to pass, do you need hope? Do you need faith?

I was hungry this morning; I am no longer hungry. I ate. I no longer need hope or faith regarding my lunch. I am dreaming about dinner.

Fear is the substance of things *not* hoped for, the evidence *not* yet seen. Do you know how many of God's people are in "fear faith," not real faith? You may be in fear faith and think it's real faith but if you were in real faith, you wouldn't have the problem, unless you didn't understand why you had the problem. I deal with fears such as phobias, paranoia, delusions, projections, anxiety, panic, panic attacks, phobic realities, agoraphobia, claustrophobia, and mother-in-law phobia.

Fear projects into the future. Faith also projects into the future, does it not? Fear involves projection, number one, and then displacement, which is avoidance. God has taught you in the Word, from the Old Testament all the way through the New Testament, that you do *not* run from an enemy. When you study the warfare garments in Ephesians 6:11-20, there isn't anything for your backside! You don't run from an enemy in your life, and you don't hide from your mother-in-law. You don't hide from your enemy. You don't hide from fear of disease. You don't hide from your disease. You don't go disappear down inside.

It's time for you to come up and take your place in the land of the living once and for all. What's the worst that can happen to you anyway? You can die and go to heaven, so what's your problem? What are you afraid of?

In the Church, we sometimes attack each other too. That's an autoimmune disease! The sign out in front of your church, the one you see as you walk in the front door, says, "Hallelujah, Love One Another." You'll know them because of the love they have one for another.

> [20]**Wherefore by their fruits ye shall know them.** Matthew 7:20

> [34]**A new commandment I give unto you, That ye love one another; as I have loved you, that ye also love one another. [35]By this shall all *men* know that ye are my disciples, if ye have love one to another.** John 13:34-35

In Isaiah 58:1-4, the people of God were saying—Hallelujah, LORD, we love you. You are our Father and You have redeemed us from Egypt. Yet they were destroying each other and God would not protect them or hear them.

> [58:1]**Cry aloud, spare not, lift up thy voice like a trumpet, and shew my people their transgression, and the house of Jacob their sins. [2]Yet they seek me daily, and delight to know my ways, as a nation that did righteousness, and forsook not the ordinance of their God: they ask of me the ordinances of justice; they take delight in approaching to God. [3]Wherefore have we fasted, *say they,* and thou seest not? *wherefore* have we afflicted our soul, and thou takest no knowledge? Behold, in the day of your fast ye find pleasure, and exact all your labours. [4]Behold, ye fast for strife and debate, and to smite with the fist of wickedness: ye shall not fast as *ye do this* day, to make your voice to be heard on high.** Isaiah 58:1-4

Yes, we come and we worship You with the songs of David, and we come before You, and yes, You are our LORD, our God, and we love to come, we love to pray, we love to fast, we love the law, we love, love, love but, why haven't You healed us? That's the question of God's people in Isaiah 58. Do you know what God said? "Yea, I've watched you fasting and praying, but you pray for strife and eat each other alive. I have caused My ears to become deaf to you."

What is Isaiah saying? God is saying: you want My blessings but you don't want My friends; you don't want My sons and daughters.

I was talking with somebody the other day that was kind of chewing about somebody …you know, gossiping. I looked at them and I said, "How dare you say that about a friend of Jesus. Do you realize that person is a friend of Jesus? What do you think Jesus thinks about you talking that way about His friend?"

Do you think Jesus is our friend? Do you think I have a scripture to stand on? He said, "I no longer call you servants, I call you friends" (John 15:15 among many others).

> [15]**Henceforth I call you not servants; for the servant knoweth not what his lord doeth: but I have called you friends; for all things that I have heard of my Father I have made known unto you.** John 15:15

Friends don't talk about each other. Friends build each other up. Friends cover with love—perfect love covers a multitude of sins (1 Peter 4:8).

> [8]**And above all things have fervent charity among yourselves: for charity shall cover the multitude of sins.** 1 Peter 4:8

In Gal 6:1, we're told—if a brother be overtaken in a fault, those of you who consider yourselves spiritual, restore such a one—not to stone them by sundown. Restore such a one in a spirit of meekness and consider yourself also, lest you be tempted in like manner and fall away in the same type of bondage. Verse 2, Bear you one another's burdens and so you thus fulfill the law of Christ.

> [1]**Brethren, if a man be overtaken in a fault, ye which are spiritual, restore such an one in the spirit of meekness; considering thyself, lest thou also be tempted.** [2]**Bear ye one another's burdens, and so fulfil the law of Christ.** Galatians 6:1-2

My purpose is to sow seed into your hearts. Whether God gives the increase or not, I don't know. I don't know you. I don't live inside your body, you do. I don't know if you're going to get lost in the desert between Egypt and Promise or not. I'm sure going to lay some stuff on you—I'm going to bring you some insight and I'm going to bring you some discernment.

I promise you I have the fruit to prove, nationally, that God has honored this teaching. Many times I know disease, even when I don't know the person and don't know the circumstances, I know what's behind the disease spiritually. I was able last evening to tell a person the secret parts of their heart. Why? So they could recover themselves into right standing with God and be healed. That's the fruit of this ministry.

2 Timothy 2:24-26 says—And the servant of the Lord must not strive; but be gentle unto all men, apt to teach, patient, In meekness instructing those that oppose

themselves; if God peradventure will give them repentance to the acknowledging of the truth; And that they may recover themselves out of the snare of the devil, who are taken captive by him at his [the devil's] will.

When a person is in captivity by the devil, they don't know it. They don't understand. Why? Nobody has told them. Read 2 Timothy 2:23 to the end of the chapter in the majority text (otherwise known as the King James):

> **[23]But foolish and unlearned questions avoid, knowing that they do gender strifes. [24]And the servant of the Lord must not strive; but be gentle unto all men, apt to teach, patient, [25]In meekness instructing those that oppose themselves; if God peradventure will give them repentance to the acknowledging of the truth; [26]And that they may recover themselves out of the snare of the devil, who are taken captive by him at his [the devil's] will. 2Tim 2:23-26**

Promise Without Discernment is Still Bondage

Jeremiah 3:14:

> **[14]Turn, O backsliding children, saith the LORD; for I am married unto you: and I will take you one of a city, and two of a family, and I will bring you to Zion: [15]And I will give you pastors according to mine heart, which shall feed you with knowledge and understanding. Jeremiah 3:14-15**

He gave them pastors according to His own heart to teach them with knowledge and understanding. What am I doing with you? Giving you knowledge and understanding and discernment. Say this with me:

"Promise without discernment is still bondage."

Go to Hebrews 5, the last verse, with me—one who is able to handle strong meat is one who, by reason of exercise of his senses, is able to *discern both good and evil.*

> **[14]But strong meat belongeth to them that are of full age, *even* those who by reason of use have their senses exercised to discern both good and evil. Hebrews 5:14**

I think, ladies and gentlemen, we have been so God-conscious that we have forgotten discernment concerning evil. A sign of maturity is not just knowing good, it's knowing evil as well, so that you know what is of God and what is not. That's a sign of maturity.

I'm not into sin consciousness. That produces condemnation. I am into conviction, and that requires discernment. *All condemnation is of the devil. All conviction is of God.* They both say the same thing but there is a wrong spirit behind one and a right spirit behind the other. If you're in condemnation, you are trying to hide from the problem. If you're in conviction, you're running to face the problem. Have you been there? Have you done that?

Conflict Resolution

Let me tell you something with great authority: *you do not have to resolve one issue with somebody that has victimized you in order for God to heal you* providing you have resolved that issue between you and God concerning them.

If you are waiting for resolution between them and you before you can be well, you've bought the biggest lie you've ever bought. That would be tying you back to the tragedy, back to the victimization, back to the breakdown.

You stand alone before God and alone you shall be in your salvation, in your healing, in your deliverance, and in your judgment. All of us shall stand before God one day and we can't tote a bunch of people with us and say, "They made me do it. They made me do it." You will stand alone.

Remember 2 Timothy 1:7—God has not given us the spirit of fear but of power, love, and a sound mind.

> **[7]For God hath not given us the spirit of fear; but of power, and of love, and of a sound mind.** 2 Timothy 1:7

The antidote to fear is the Godhead. The antidote to fear is trusting the Godhead. All three members of the eternal Godhead are found in this scripture as follows: power is the Holy Ghost; love is God the Father; and a sound mind is God the Word. John 3:16 says—for God so loved the world that He gave His only begotten Son. Who gave the only begotten Son? The Father.

> **[16]For God so loved the world, that he gave his only begotten Son...** John 3:16

Jesus said—you've seen Me, you've seen the Father. I only do the things I saw My Father doing, I only say the things I heard My Father saying (John 14:9).

> **[9]Jesus saith unto him, Have I been so long time with you, and yet hast thou not known me, Philip? he that hath seen me hath seen the Father; and how sayest thou *then*, Shew us the Father?** John 14:9

> **[19]Then answered Jesus and said unto them, Verily, verily, I say unto you, The Son can do nothing of himself, but what he seeth the Father do: for what things soever he doeth, these also doeth the Son likewise.** John 5:19

> **[28]Then said Jesus unto them, When ye have lifted up the Son of man, then shall ye know that I am *he*, and *that* I do nothing of myself; but as my Father hath taught me, I speak these things.** John 8:28

> **[38]I speak that which I have seen with my Father: and ye do that which ye have seen with your father.** John 8:38

> **[30]I can of mine own self do nothing: as I hear, I judge: and my judgment is just; because I seek not mine own will, but the will of the Father which hath sent me.** John 5:30

The Father is Love, but the sound mind comes from which other member of the Godhead? *Jesus, who is God, the Word.*

You have God the Father, God the Word who came in the flesh, and you have God the Holy Spirit. The eternal Godhead. God in three Persons. In Deuteronomy 6:4, it says—hear, O Israel, the LORD our God is one LORD. That word "one" is the Hebrew word *echad,* which translated means *plural unity.* Right there in the Torah (in Deuteronomy) you find the Godhead. You also find it other places, such as Genesis 1:26 and Isaiah 48:16-17.

> [26]**And God said, Let us make man in our image, after our likeness: and let them have dominion over the fish of the sea, and over the fowl of the air, and over the cattle, and over all the earth, and over every creeping thing that creepeth upon the earth.** Genesis 1:26

> [16]**Come ye near unto me, hear ye this; I have not spoken in secret from the beginning; from the time that it was, there** *am* **I: and now the Lord GOD, and his Spirit, hath sent me.** [17]**Thus saith the LORD, thy Redeemer, the Holy One of Israel; I** *am* **the LORD thy God which teacheth thee to profit, which leadeth thee by the way** *that* **thou shouldest go.** Isaiah 48:16-17

From that standpoint, the antidote to fear is fellowship with the Godhead. I'll tell you what I think: if I threw a $1,000,000 bill out here, you'd be scrambling for it because it would be your prize. I think we have lost our first love. *I think it's time to get hot for God again.* I think it's time to fall in love with Who He is, all over again.

Communion

In dealing with autoimmune disease, 1 Corinthians 11:29-31 is an example of a block, not a root, but a block to healing:

> [29]**For he that eateth and drinketh unworthily, eateth and drinketh damnation to himself, not discerning the Lord's body.** [30]**For this cause many** *are* **weak and sickly among you, and many sleep.** [31]**For if we would judge ourselves, we should not be judged.** 1 Cor. 11:29-31

Many of God's people were weak. Could that be like Chronic Fatigue Syndrome? A little exhaustion?

When we get into the fear, anxiety and stress teaching in a later chapter, I will show you where exhaustion comes from in the human body, other than from a hard day's work. We'll talk about potassium depletion, ionic base, about what the medical community knows about exhaustion tied to Multiple Chemical Sensitivity/Environmental Illness, and also Chronic Fatigue Syndrome.

"Some people are sick"—some are sickly. Does the word "sickly" to you mean "sick"? What about, "and many sleep"? It doesn't mean they sleep in church; it means they die premature deaths. Why? Because they do not rightly discern the Lord's body.

There are two levels. The first area of the Lord's Supper or Communion because people are sick and weak and die premature deaths, is because we have eliminated one half of communion.

I may bump into some of your theology, but if I do, I sure do love you, and I hope you love me too!

It splits right down the middle—those who believe God heals today and those who don't believe God heals today. It's a dispensational issue.

Communion or the Lord's Supper represents two realities: the shed blood, which is the cup, and the bread, which is His broken body. *Christ's broken body is not* *for forgiveness of sin.* The Bible says—without the shedding of blood there is no forgiveness of sins.

> **²²And almost all things are by the law purged with blood; and without shedding of blood is no remission.** Hebrews 9:22

> **¹¹For the life of the flesh *is* in the blood: and I have given it to you upon the altar to make an atonement for your souls: for it *is* the blood *that* maketh an atonement for the soul.** Leviticus 17:11

So His shed blood makes it possible, because He was the sacrificial lamb that allows us to appropriate forgiveness from God our Father. It's by His shed blood that we have the penalty paid for sin.

Many people are appropriating the blood for the curse. However, it's Jesus' broken body that paid the penalty for the curse to fulfill the law that says—cursed is he that hangeth on a tree (Gal. 3:13).

> **²³His body shall not remain all night upon the tree, but thou shalt in any wise bury him that day; (for he that is hanged *is* accursed of God;) that thy land be not defiled, which the LORD thy God giveth thee *for* an inheritance.** Deut. 21:23

> **¹³Christ hath redeemed us from the curse of the law, being made a curse for us: for it is written, Cursed *is* every one that hangeth on a tree:** Galatians 3:13

It was by His stripes that we were healed and we appropriate that today to our lives (Isaiah 53:5, 1 Peter 2:24).

> **⁵But he *was* wounded for our transgressions, *he was* bruised for our iniquities: the chastisement of our peace *was* upon him; and with his stripes we are healed.** Isaiah 53:5

> **²⁴Who his own self bare our sins in his own body on the tree, that we, being dead to sins, should live unto righteousness: by whose stripes ye were healed.** 1 Peter 2:24

If we come to a Communion service, and partake of the cup and the bread, but we deny healing and deliverance as part of the atonement today, we eliminate the provision of God in our lives as a human being apart from salvation and eternal life in that day. For that reason, because we eliminate the broken body, but we celebrate it, and we don't believe it, then we cannot partake. For that reason many of us are filled with disease and insanity today because we have said in our heart that it passed away two thousand years ago yet we still participate in the sacrament of Communion which represents its reality for today. If you don't believe it, you don't have to worry about it happening. But be careful, ignorance is a form of knowledge and so is unbelief.

If you don't believe God heals today, don't worry about it; He won't. If you don't believe that God heals today then He will not. According to your faith be it unto you! (Matthew 9:29).

> **²⁹Then touched he their eyes, saying, According to your faith be it unto you.** Matthew 9:29

Let every man be fully persuaded in his own mind (Romans 14:5).

> **⁵One man esteemeth one day above another: another esteemeth every day** *alike.* **Let every man be fully persuaded in his own mind.** Romans 14:5

I've taken this position: that many times we have disease among God's people *because we have eliminated one half of the provision of the Communion and the sacrament of Communion, the Lord's Supper.*

Now, the other aspect of 1 Corinthians 11:29-31 has to do with us eating each other alive. This is "not discerning the Lord's body." Who was the Lord's body apart from what He did at the cross? Who else, if not the Lord's body in the earth today—the Church? We are the body of Christ. When we go to Isaiah 58:1 it says:

> **⁵⁸:¹Cry aloud, spare not, lift up thy voice like a trumpet, and shew my people their transgression, and the house of Jacob their sins.** Isaiah 58:1

This has to do with God's people, the Old Testament Church. He's not talking about the heathen; he's not talking about Gentiles. He's talking about God's people, and ladies and gentlemen, God's people blow it and sin. We fall short of the glory of God continually in some areas of our lives. The Bible says in Hebrews 12:15:

> **¹⁵Looking diligently lest any man fail of the grace of God; lest any root of bitterness springing up trouble** *you,* **and thereby many be defiled;** Hebrews 12:15

When you are around someone who falls short of the glory of God, it means they have spiritually pooped all over you. They have defiled you, they have violated you, and they have demonstrated part of their old nature.

What are you going to do with it? Eye for eye, tooth for tooth? That passed away! Jesus did away with eye for eye and tooth for tooth and said, "You're going to love them" (Matthew 5:38-44).

> **³⁸Ye have heard that it hath been said, An eye for an eye, and a tooth for a tooth: ³⁹But I say unto you, That ye resist not evil: but whosoever shall smite thee on thy right cheek, turn to him the other also...⁴⁴But I say unto you, Love your enemies, bless them that curse you, do good to them that hate you, and pray for them which despitefully use you, and persecute you;** Matthew 5:38-44

If we have bitterness, if we have rejection, if we have unloving spirits, if we have hatred, it's ping-pong time and then slam-dunk, right? Many times our lives are like a massive ping-pong game; I'm going to get you before you get me. That root of bitterness will keep you from the blessings of God.

In Isaiah 58:2-3, God speaking by the prophet Isaiah, says:

> **²Yet they seek me daily, and delight to know my ways, as a nation that did righteousness, and forsook not the ordinance of their God: they ask of me the ordinances of justice; they take delight in approaching to God. ³Wherefore have we fasted,** *say they,* **and thou seest not?** *wherefore* **have we afflicted our soul, and thou takest no knowledge? Behold, in the day of your fast ye find pleasure, and exact all your labours.** Isaiah 58:2-3

This is a conversation from God's people to Him. We've been fasting and praying. We need some help. Help God! It looks like the heavens are brass; You're not listening. You're not listening. You're not answering our prayers. We have been fasting, we have afflicted our soul and *You don't even pay attention.* You take no knowledge.

God said in Isaiah 58:4:

'**Behold, ye fast for strife and debate, and to smite with the fist of wickedness: ye shall not fast as *ye do this* day, to make your voice to be heard on high.** Isaiah 58:4

God goes on and talks about the fast that He's called us to—it's not absence of food and water. Many people quote verse 6 in Isaiah 58 out of context to try and prove that fasting and prayer will move God's hand to heal and deliver you.

'*Is* **not this the fast that I have chosen? to loose the bands of wickedness, to undo the heavy burdens, and to let the oppressed go free, and that ye break every yoke?** Isaiah 58:6

I don't find it scripturally. I don't find it there; quite the opposite. In fact, in verses 7-12 of Isaiah 58, the fast that God has called us to is that of service to others in love.

Could it be that we have mixed up *fellowship* with *petition*? Could it be that we misunderstand that God is not just interested in being our provider, He's interested in being our Father? The Lord is interested in being our Savior, our spiritual husband forever. That's why we are called the bride of Christ, you know. There's a marriage supper; do you all teach that in your church?

Medication Insight

I have my PDR manual on drugs. Almost everybody in any seminar that I do dealing with disease is on a wide variety of drugs. That's what you've got going for you in today's world, and with every drug you're taking there is a component called "side effects."

One of the things that I do in ministry is that before you receive ministry from me, my staff does a general intake and a medical intake. In the medical intake, we want to know all the medicine and drugs you are on. Each of those drugs has side effects and you may be struggling with what seems to be a disease and instead it may be a side effect of a drug.

I tell you I cannot minister to side effects. I tried years ago and found out I was wasting my time. We're very careful in determining in a person's life that what they are dealing with is actually the root problem disease, and not the side effects from a drug that they're taking. Do you know how many pastors are trying to get people free of diseases and are in effect ministering to the side effects of drugs and wonder why God is not healing the problem? There is no healing for the side effects of a drug.

USA Today (April 24, 1998) contained an article about deadly drugs. "Why Are So Many Drugs Killing So Many Patients?" "Adverse reactions to prescription drugs are the fourth-largest cause of death nationally." It's a Pandora's Box of hell. We will teach you on *pharmakeia* and sorcery.

Now if you are taking prescription drugs, don't let me condemn you. If that's where you're at, that's where you're at.

Would You Be Interested in *A More Excellent Way*?

Through this ministry, there are now many people in America today that no longer need drugs of any type and who are living normal lives. Would you consider that to be a viable option for your life? We are on the "cutting edge" of medicine in America, and it's awesome to be involved as a pastor. Isn't the "cutting edge of medicine" a funny place for a pastor to be?

The article in April 24, 1998, *USA Today* about deadly drugs continues: the #1 killer in America is Heart Disease. #2 is Cancer, #3 is Strokes, #4 is Adverse Drug Reactions to prescription drugs, #5 is Pulmonary Disease, and #6 is Accidents of all classes. Is that a sobering statistic?

Let's look at the antidepressant drug, Prozac. Prozac is the drug of choice today. It sometimes is being prescribed by doctors without any thought of the consequences, doctors who don't have any understanding as to what it even involves. Prozac is sometimes given to people who have anxiety, yet one of the first principle side effects of Prozac is anxiety. Do you know what another side effect of Prozac is? Loss of libido. Do you know what loss of libido is? Loss of sex drive. The guy is depressed and anxious, and now his wife wonders why he's lost all interest and he's not chasing her. Galatians 5:20, in the majority text (KJV), calls it *witchcraft*. We'll study what Paul has to say about that subject later.

I operate in various gifts of the Holy Spirit. I don't make a big deal of it. It's there when it needs to be there. I don't know if you believe in the gifts of the Holy Spirit found in 1 Corinthians 12 or not. They are there and they are there for a reason. If I didn't believe in them, I wouldn't be teaching about spiritual healing. I wouldn't be teaching about disease. I wouldn't have any basis to do it. To teach about disease and teach about healing and get no one healed is kind of ridiculous.

I am reminded of the Scriptures—you say you have faith, I'll show you my faith by my works (James 2:18). Faith without works is dead (James 2:17). There is another scripture that is a little tougher, it says, They who say, 'Yea Lord' but deny the power thereof, from such turn away (2 Tim. 3:5). When the Lord comes, will He find faith in the earth? (Luke 18:8).

> [18]**Yea, a man may say, Thou hast faith, and I have works: shew me thy faith without thy works, and I will shew thee my faith by my works.** James 2:18

> [17]**Even so faith, if it hath not works, is dead, being alone.** James 2:17

> [5]**Having a form of godliness, but denying the power thereof: from such turn away.** 2 Tim. 3:5

> **⁸I tell you that he will avenge them speedily. Nevertheless when the Son of man cometh, shall he find faith on the earth?** Luke 18:8

In Hebrews 4, we learn that the children of Israel did not enter into the land of promise because they did not mix the gospel they had heard and received with faith.

> **¹⁹So we see that they could not enter in because of unbelief. ⁴:¹Let us therefore fear, lest, a promise being left *us* of entering into his rest, any of you should seem to come short of it. ²For unto us was the gospel preached, as well as unto them: but the word preached did not profit them, not being mixed with faith in them that heard *it*.** Hebrews 3:19-4:2

That is the first reason; the second reason they did not enter into their rest (as God entered into His rest in creation the 7th day He rested) is because they did not cease from their own labors.

> **⁹There remaineth therefore a rest to the people of God. ¹⁰For he that is entered into his rest, he also hath ceased from his own works, as God *did* from his.** Hebrews 4:9-10

Do you know that when you start truly believing God you cease to perform as if you were God? Do you know there are so many people trying to be a God to themselves *that they truly are the author and finisher of their own life?*

Do you know how many people I deal with who are driven to succeed, to leave a million dollars for their children, even when they know that their children are going to blow it on nothing?

> **¹⁸Yea, I hated all my labour which I had taken under the sun: because I should leave it unto the man that shall be after me. ¹⁹And who knoweth whether he shall be a wise *man* or a fool? yet shall he have rule over all my labour wherein I have laboured, and wherein I have shewed myself wise under the sun. This *is* also vanity.** Eccles. 2:18-19

So, can this be called vanity? (Ecclesiastes) Do you know how many people are driven?

Have you not heard the scripture, in the "book of whoever" that says that as many as are *driven* by the Spirit of God are the sons of God? Does it say that? In the "book of whoever" it does. But it does not say that in the Word of God, does it? What does the Scripture say? For as many as are *led* by the Spirit of God, they are the sons of God (Romans 8:14).

> **¹⁴For as many as are led by the Spirit of God, they are the sons of God.** Romans 8:14

The devil drives and God leads. That's why the Lord is called the Shepherd that leads us into green pastures (Psalm 23).

> **²³:¹A Psalm of David.The LORD *is* my shepherd; I shall not want. ²He maketh me to lie down in green pastures: he leadeth me beside the still waters.** Psalm 23:1-2

We Cannot Bypass the Penalty of Sin in Our Lives

I would say that probably 70 to 80 percent of all disease in America and in the world that is considered incurable, with the name *syndrome* or *incurable* attached to it, has a spiritual root.

I'm not against nutritionists; in fact we have two nutritionists who are part of our ministry. I believe in a good balanced diet; I believe that you've got to take care of the temple. I believe if you get your rest, drink enough water, eat the proper foods and so on, you'll have overall good health on that basis. *However, good nutrition, rest and water in themselves do not heal the defects that come from separation from God and His Word, or deal with sanctification and sin and the resultant diseases.*

I want to say something to you. *Nutrition does not replace repentance.* I am reminded of the Lord when He was ministering to someone. He had just healed them and He made this incredible statement—go your way and sin no more lest a worse thing come upon you (John 5:14).

> **14Afterward Jesus findeth him in the temple, and said unto him, Behold, thou art made whole: sin no more, lest a worse thing come unto thee.** John 5:14

Why did He say that? Because the Lord, Himself, your Savior, my Savior, my Boss, directly tied the lack of sanctification to disease.

There are many people today trying to bypass the penalty of the curse of disobedience by various modalities and they are getting nowhere. Allopathic medicine has its place. We need doctors, we need people who understand the human body and the human soul, but there aren't many practitioners for the human spirit. That is our next topic.

God Wants to Heal Us

In my investigation, in getting involved in people's lives, I've found that God wanted to heal us. He said that in Psalm 103:3—I am the Lord that forgiveth thee of all thine iniquities and healeth thee of all of thy diseases.

> **3Who forgiveth all thine iniquities; who healeth all thy diseases;** Psalm 103:3

I also found it in 3 John 2: Beloved, I wish above all things that thou mayest prosper and be in health, even as thy soul prospereth.

> **2Beloved, I wish above all things that thou mayest prosper and be in health, even as thy soul prospereth.** 3 John 1:2

And I read in I Thessalonians 5:23—may the God of peace sanctify you **wholly** in spirit, in soul and in body.

> **23And the very God of peace sanctify you wholly; and *I pray God* your whole spirit and soul and body be preserved blameless unto the coming of our Lord Jesus Christ.** 1 Thes. 5:23

I believe God wants to work with us. I believe He is a loving Father. I believe also that we have become separate from God in our understanding of disease. We would like to take a shot at correcting that.

In understanding disease—spiritual, psychological, and biological—we'll find that the Bible has a lot to say about the subject. I'm privileged to be on the "cutting edge" of medicine from coast to coast because of this Biblical understanding of disease. There are doctors who consult with me across America, as well as therapists, psychologists, pastors, and individuals.

It's a funny thing to be a pastor and be on the "cutting edge" of medicine. It's an enigma to the medical community. As one doctor said, "What is a pastor from Georgia doing messing around with disease?" Well, I'm messing around with it because my Boss is the Great Physician. I'm messing around in it because the Creator of all flesh is the One who knows what's wrong with us. I'm messing around with it because God ordained it. I'll show it to you in scripture that the pastor is to be responsible for all the affairs of God's people.

I think, and I say this very carefully, that God is just about ticked off at the psychologists being the pastors of America. If there are any psychologists reading this, I love you man, I love you woman. But I do think you have taken some things away from the pastors that are rightfully theirs to deal with. Under Old Testament law, if anyone had leprosy, in order to be considered cured, who did they go show themselves to? The priest. In the New Testament, it goes a little further. James 5:14-15 says:

> **[14]Is any sick among you? let him call for the elders of the church; and let them pray over him, anointing him with oil in the name of the Lord: [15]And the prayer of faith shall save the sick, and the Lord shall raise him up; and if he have committed sins, they shall be forgiven him.** James 5:14-15

Right here in these verses we see the lack of sanctification in a believer's life and the consequence, which shows us the relationship of sin to disease.

As I began to serve God in ministry, I believed God could heal. I saw it in the Word, and I saw it in life. As I mentioned before, I'd pray for people but less than 5% ever got well. The same thing happened in the church I was in, and in other churches across America. In my prayer time, I went to God and asked Him about this dilemma: I saw just as many Christians in doctors' offices as non-believers. I saw the same number of people in psychiatrists' offices, saint or sinner. Both were there with psychological and biological problems. I didn't see any difference between saint and sinner when it came to any other of the pathologies of mankind: drug use, divorce, alcohol, etc. I said, "God, my name is Henry. I feel Your call on my life and if You want me to help mankind, You had better solve this dilemma of what happens between salvation and heaven."

I began to search the Scriptures and give my heart to God. The Bible says—if any of you lack wisdom, let him ask of God, that giveth to all men liberally, and upbraideth not [because he had the audacity to ask God something]; and it shall be given him (James 1:5).

⁵If any of you lack wisdom, let him ask of God, that giveth to all *men* liberally, and upbraideth not; and it shall be given him. James 1:5

Then I ran across another scripture — you have not because you ask not (James 4:2, 1 John 5:15).

²Ye lust, and have not: ye kill, and desire to have, and cannot obtain: ye fight and war, yet ye have not, because ye ask not. James 4:2

¹⁵And if we know that he hear us, whatsoever we ask, we know that we have the petitions that we desired of him. 1 John 5:15

I just figured I'd ask. Gradually and surely I began to understand.

It wasn't that God could not heal, it was that He couldn't without denying His own holiness and giving us a leavened gospel that would say we could keep our sin and receive His blessings.

The Doctrine of Balaam

I bumped into the very reality of the doctrine of Balaam (Numbers 22-24, 31; II Peter 2:15; Jude 11; Revelation 2:14). I really believe that the doctrine of Balaam is in the church today. This is not an indictment, it is an observation. What is the doctrine of Balaam? You know who Balaam and Balak were? Balaam was the seer; Balak was the heathen king. Balak wanted the children of Israel destroyed. He didn't like them—they were in his country, and he wanted them out. But they were blessed. He called for Balaam, the seer to find a way to curse God's people. The first thing Balaam should have done was stay home. But he didn't. The Bible says that Balaam taught Balak how to get God's people cursed. Here's the deal. Balak came to Balaam and said, "I want them cursed." Balaam said, "I can't do it. They are a blessed people. God is their Father. He's bringing them out of Egypt. They are in covenant; they have the law. I cannot curse them, for they are blessed."

Balak had this incredible thought. "What would happen if I could get them to sin?" He came up with the idea of tempting the girls of Israel with the boys from his country, and tempting the boys with the girls in his country. He tempted them to worship the pagan idols. The first thing you know, Israel was sinning. Guess what came? *The curse came, and there was no longer any provision for safety, and 24,000 Israelites died in the plague that came as the result of their sin.*

I think the Church has come to a place where they have overplayed grace and mercy to the point that they say "Because you are in covenant, you can sin like the devil and there are no consequences." I disagree.

I'll tell you why I disagree. I have had to get sanctified and still am under the pressure of the Holy Spirit every single day. I used to be so afraid that I would shake like a leaf when someone came to the door. If I talked to you, I would never look you in the eye. I'd look at your nose, your toes, or the ceiling. Now people wish I would stop looking them in the eye. I used to be a walking hypochondriac. I'd be in the doctor's office 6 months out of the year. I'd have strep throat 4 or 5 times a year and miss from 2 to 3 months of work because of massive infections. God healed me of all of it. My immune system was healed. How and why was I healed? I had to confess sin in my life. I had to get sanctified. I'm working out my own salvation every single day now with fear and trembling. I don't mind repenting to God.

I heard somebody teaching the other day say, "You never have to repent again, once you are saved." I disagree! If I blow it, if I sin against you, I'm going to repent to you. If I sin against you and I injure you knowingly or unknowingly and I'm aware of it, I will repent to you and ask you to forgive me. I will do that with every single person on this planet that I have known, do know, or ever will know.

The Bible says—if you have ought against your brother, go to your brother alone.

> **[22]But I say unto you, That whosoever is angry with his brother without a cause shall be in danger of the judgment: and whosoever shall say to his brother, Raca, shall be in danger of the council: but whosoever shall say, Thou fool, shall be in danger of hell fire. [23]Therefore if thou bring thy gift to the altar, and there rememberest that thy brother hath ought against thee; [24]Leave there thy gift before the altar, and go thy way; first be reconciled to thy brother, and then come and offer thy gift.** Matthew 5:22-24

If that's the condition between us and one another, *how much more should it be with us and our Heavenly Father?* But if we walk in the light, as he is in the light, we have fellowship one with another (1 John 1:7).

> **[7]But if we walk in the light, as he is in the light, we have fellowship one with another...** 1 John 1:7a

And if we don't, the blood of Jesus Christ His Son cleanseth us from all unrighteousness.

> **[7]...and the blood of Jesus Christ his Son cleanseth us from all sin.** 1 John 1:7b

Scripture tells us that *we must ask* for forgiveness (1 John 1:9-10).

> **[9]If we confess our sins, he is faithful and just to forgive us *our* sins, and to cleanse us from all unrighteousness. [10]If we say that we have not sinned, we make him a liar, and his word is not in us.** 1 John 1:9-10

These scriptures are addressed to the Church, not to the unchurched.

In 2 Corinthians 7:1 it says—dearly beloved, let us cleanse ourselves from all filthiness of the flesh and spirit.

> **[7:1]Having therefore these promises, dearly beloved, let us cleanse ourselves from all filthiness of the flesh and spirit, perfecting holiness in the fear of God.** 2 Cor. 7:1

He is speaking to the saints, not to the heathen.

I want to tell you something: the principles you apply to your life that will move the hand of God to heal you in covenant are the same principles that, if you apply them to your life, will prevent disease in your life.

Spirit of Fear

Earlier I quoted from an article in *Newsweek* magazine, entitled "Greater Expectations," that said **"the future of medicine lies not in treating illness but in preventing it."** This was written 9 years ago.

It continues:

> **Throughout the 20th century, medicine has advanced primarily by improving curative care...but curative care has its limits... Accompanying the use of more refined technology to prevent and treat illness, psychoimmunology** *[the name has since been changed to psychoneuroimmunology],* **the science that deals with the mind's role in helping the immune system to fight disease, will become a vitally important clinical field—perhaps the most important medical field in the 21st century—supplanting our present emphasis on oncology and cardiology. Healthy thinking may eventually become an integral aspect of treatment for everything from allergies to liver transplants.**

2 Timothy 1:7 says, "For God hath not given us the spirit of fear; but of power, and of love, and of a sound mind."

All three members of the Godhead are present in this scripture:

- Power—Who is the power of God? God, the Holy Spirit.

- Love—Who is the Love factor? God, the Father.

For God the Father so loved the world that He gave His only begotten Son (the Lord Jesus) that whosoever believeth on Him shall not perish but have everlasting life.

> **[16]For God so loved the world, that he gave his only begotten Son, that whosoever believeth in him should not perish, but have everlasting life.** John 3:16

1 John 4 says that God is love.

> **[8]...for God is love.** 1 John 4:8

Talking about the Father. Psalm 68:19-20—He (the Father) daily loadeth us with benefits even the Elohim of our salvation who is the Lord Jesus. The Father is Love and also is our Provider. Ezekiel 18, the last verse—Adonay Yehovih (the Father)—it is not the Father's will that any man should perish but all should be saved.

> **[32]For I have no pleasure in the death of him that dieth, saith the Lord God: wherefore turn *yourselves,* and live ye.** Ezekiel 18:32

That's what it says in the Old Testament in the Hebrew, and in the New Testament, the Greek says the same thing in harmony with the Old. The Father's intention is to save and to preserve, because of love.

- A sound mind—the third part of the Godhead is the *antidote to fear*.

How do we get a sound mind? We are renewed by the washing of the water of the Word. Who is the Word? Jesus is the Word. John 1:1 tells us:

¹:¹In the beginning was the Word, and the Word was with God, and the Word was God. John 1:1

In v. 14, we learn—and the Word became flesh

¹⁴And the Word was made flesh, and dwelt among us, (and we beheld his glory, the glory as of the only begotten of the Father,) full of grace and truth. John 1:14

Revelation 19:11-14 says—One comes on the white horse, and the saints with Him, and His name is the Word of God. Jesus Christ is the Living Word.

¹¹And I saw heaven opened, and behold a white horse; and he that sat upon him *was* called Faithful and True, and in righteousness he doth judge and make war. ¹²His eyes *were* as a flame of fire, and on his head *were* many crowns; and he had a name written, that no man knew, but he himself. ¹³And he *was* clothed with a vesture dipped in blood: and his name is called The Word of God. ¹⁴And the armies *which were* in heaven followed him upon white horses, clothed in fine linen, white and clean. Rev. 19:11-14

What is the antidote to fear? A relationship with the whole Godhead: fellowship with the Father, fellowship with Jesus, Who is the Word, and fellowship with the Holy Spirit as He indwells you. You won't have any fear then. You will be hanging out with God.

The people coming out of Egypt under Moses did not enter into promise, first, because of their *unbelief,* and, second, because they *did not cease from their own labors.*

¹⁹So we see that they could not enter in because of unbelief. ⁴:¹Let us therefore fear, lest, a promise being left *us* of entering into his rest, any of you should seem to come short of it. ²For unto us was the gospel preached, as well as unto them: but the word preached did not profit them, not being mixed with faith in them that heard *it.....* ⁹There remaineth therefore a rest to the people of God. ¹⁰For he that is entered into his rest, he also hath ceased from his own works, as God *did* from his. ¹¹Let us labour therefore to enter into that rest, lest any man fall after the same example of unbelief. Hebrews 3:19-4:2, 9-11

Do you know that man is trying to become his own healer? How much money have you spent trying to heal yourself and how much money have you spent on physicians? I know of one person with Multiple Chemical Sensitivity/Environmental Illness who spent over $500,000 trying to get well.

The Lord and I didn't charge her one cent! The father of another person who was healed of MCS/EI had spent $400,000. She's well today, and it didn't cost her a cent.

Don't you think that is a more excellent way?

It's free, a free gift. Just like salvation is a free gift, God's love and His knowledge and His understanding is a free gift. The Bible says in Proverbs 25:2 that it is the glory of God to conceal a thing: but the honour of kings is to search out a matter.

²*It is* the glory of God to conceal a thing: but the honour of kings *is* to search out a matter. Proverbs 25:2

When I minister to someone and they are not healed, what do you think we ought to do? Make up a theology that God doesn't heal today? Make up a theology that that person didn't have enough faith? What do you think we ought to do?

I will tell you what I do; I go to work. I go back to God and say, "Why not? You better talk to me, Boss. Why weren't they healed?" Do you know what? Many times there is a reason that healing didn't happen.

2 Timothy 2:24-26 says:

> **[24] And the servant of the Lord must not strive; but be gentle unto all men, apt to teach, patient, [25] In meekness *instructing those that oppose themselves*; if God peradventure will give them repentance to the acknowledging of the truth; [26] And that they may recover themselves out of the snare of the devil, who are taken captive by him at his [the devil's] will.** 2 Timothy 2:24-26

Now what are we doing giving God the glory for disease when it was the devil who put it on us to begin with? I said this the other day to someone and they said, "Well, Pastor, I believe God gave me this disease; it's from Him, it's my thorn, and His grace is sufficient for me. I believe this disease is God working me over. It's His chastening."

I said, "Are you going to a doctor about it?"

He said, "Well, of course, yes."

I asked him, "Why?"

He said, "Because I want to get well."

I said, "You old hypocrite, what are you doing interfering in God's will for your life?"

It's amazing to me to hear people giving God the glory for a disease and then go to a doctor trying to get healed. If that's the case, if disease is from God, then Jesus Christ of Nazareth was the biggest rebel against His Father that I have ever seen. The Bible says that He healed everyone that came to Him and cast out all their devils. Not one time did He say, "This disease is from God so enjoy it."

> **[38] How God anointed Jesus of Nazareth with the Holy Ghost and with power: who went about doing good, and healing all that were oppressed of the devil; for God was with him.** Acts 10:38

> **[8] ....For this purpose the Son of God was manifested, that he might destroy the works of the devil.** 1 John 3:8

Now I don't know whose Lord you follow, but that's the Lord I see; that's my Boss. That's the gospel I preach. If someone is not healed, there is a spiritual root and there is a block that has to be dealt with. There's a root problem which gives the devil a right to your life. Go before God and just lay it out. When you get the root figured out, we'll check and see if any blocks to healing exist.

I have documented from Scripture over 30 blocks that will prevent God from healing you. You know that's why we get so disillusioned when people go to healing seminars, listen to television evangelists, or go to church healing services. They sincerely pray for God to heal them. What happens when they don't get healed? What do you do then?

I'll tell you what I do; I go and find out why they aren't being healed. We are finding the reasons every day.

Do you think fear is sin? I deal with allergies, simple and multiple. I tell people with allergies this: "When the spies came into promise, what was the land filled with? Dairy products, sugar, and wheat."

> [27]And they told him, and said, We came unto the land whither thou sentest us, and surely it floweth with milk and honey; and this *is* the fruit of it. Numbers 13:27

It's time to take back your dairy products, your sugar, and your wheat (grains). The Word of God tells us in 1 Timothy 4:3-5 that there is nothing evil in itself (including food), but all things taken with thanksgiving are sanctified with prayer and the word of God. There is nothing evil in itself.

> [14]I know, and am persuaded by the Lord Jesus, that *there is* nothing unclean of itself: but to him that esteemeth any thing to be unclean, to him *it is* unclean. Romans 14:14

> [4:1]Now the Spirit speaketh expressly, that in the latter times some shall depart from the faith, giving heed to seducing spirits, and doctrines of devils; [2]Speaking lies in hypocrisy; having their conscience seared with a hot iron; [3]Forbidding to marry, *and commanding* to abstain from meats, which God hath created to be received with thanksgiving of them which believe and know the truth. [4]For every creature of God *is* good, and nothing to be refused, if it be received with thanksgiving: [5]For it is sanctified by the word of God and prayer. 1 Tim. 4:1-5

When I read Genesis 1:31, it said that God created all things. He didn't say that His creation was "good." He said it was "very good."

> [31]And God saw every thing that he had made, and, behold, *it was* very good.... Genesis 1:31

Do you think I am going to tell my Father in Heaven and the LORD Jesus that what they created in food was bad?

There are many people who were allergic to food that are eating it normally today without any reactions or problems and who are now living normal lives. **Would that be a more excellent way?**

Proverbs 17:22 says:

> [22]A merry heart doeth good *like* a medicine.... Proverbs 17:22

Our success rate with MCS/EI in America today is phenomenal in almost 10 years of ministry in that one disease. Our success rate with Chronic Fatigue Syndrome is equally incredible after 8 years in that one disease.

Our success rate in certain diseases is so phenomenal that it defies imagination. I get calls and letters frequently from people who have listened to my tapes. The lights go on. Remember 2 Timothy 2; God meets them, and heals them. They walk out of diseases.

When we don't get a healing, what do we do? Will we go into unbelief, go into doubt, make a new doctrine, rewrite the Bible, go hide, and become atheists? No! We'll go back to God, and ask Him why the devil still holds us captive at his will. That's what 2 Timothy seems to indicate. We need to find the strongholds in our lives that are keeping us from receiving God's healing.

In Isaiah 42:22 it says,

> **²²But this *is* a people robbed and spoiled; *they are* all of them snared in holes, and they are hid in prison houses: they are for a prey, and none delivereth; for a spoil, and none saith, Restore.** Isaiah 42:22

I say **restore**! I stand boldly before God, and all men, and I say restore those who are in prison houses and are a prey to the beast of the field. I take a stand, I put my foot down and I say let's go for the win.

God is still on the throne, He still answers prayer, He still talks to His people and gives them knowledge and understanding that He may show Himself strong. His eyes still rove to and fro throughout the earth. His ears are still open to their cries and He is looking to see if there be any who do seek after Him, so that He may show Himself on their behalf.

> **⁹For the eyes of the LORD run to and fro throughout the whole earth, to shew himself strong in the behalf of *them* whose heart *is* perfect toward him...** 2 Chron. 16:9

I believe that!

In Jeremiah 2:8, we read—the priests said not, Where is the LORD?

> **⁸The priests said not, Where *is* the LORD? and they that handle the law knew me not: the pastors also transgressed against me, and the prophets prophesied by Baal, and walked after *things that* do not profit.** Jeremiah 2:8

In the case of diseases in God's people in the Christian Church, not many pastors are saying today, "Where is the LORD?"

We taught earlier from 1 Corinthians 11 about communion, the Lord's supper, and why Scripture tells us that many are sick, many are weak and many die premature deaths. They did not rightly discern the body of Christ. Do you think that is an indictment or do you think that is a challenging statement of discernment?

In Jeremiah 2:8 it is very clear the priests did not say, "Where is the LORD?" and they that handled the law did not know me and the pastors also transgressed against me and the prophets prophesied by Baal and walked after things that do not profit.

Look at Jeremiah 6:13-14 concerning the spiritual condition of the Old Testament Church and its leadership:

> [13]**For from the least of them even unto the greatest of them every one** *is*
> **given to covetousness; and from the prophet even unto the priest every one**
> **dealeth falsely.** [14]**They have healed also the hurt** *of the daughter* **of my people**
> **slightly, saying, Peace, peace; when** *there is* **no peace.** Jeremiah 6:13-14

Today there are many sermons about God being our peace and Jesus being made peace unto us. But the evidence of that is missing. There is little peace.

There are as many believers on Prozac as there are unbelievers. I know because I talk to them every week. Prozac is a cheap substitute for the Holy Spirit, Who is called the Comforter by the Lord.

Jeremiah picks up the theme again later on in chapter 8 that says the same thing all over again. Back in Jeremiah 3:14-15 it says—turn, oh backsliding children, saith the LORD, for I am married unto you.

> [14]**Turn, O backsliding children, saith the** LORD**; for I am married unto**
> **you: and I will take you one of a city, and two of a family, and I will bring you**
> **to Zion:** [15]**And I will give you pastors according to mine heart, which shall feed**
> **you with knowledge and understanding.** Jeremiah 3:14-15

> [5]**For thy Maker** *is* **thine husband; the** LORD **of hosts** *is* **his name; and thy Redeemer**
> **the Holy One of Israel; The God of the whole earth shall he be called.** Isaiah 54:5

The Lord is your spiritual husband. You guys have a husband, not in the carnal, human standpoint, but in the mystical standpoint of Him being our Master forever. The Lord is my husband and I want to be a good helpmate. We're going to have a marriage supper of the Lamb.

> [7]**Let us be glad and rejoice, and give honour to him: for the marriage of**
> **the Lamb is come, and his wife hath made herself ready.** Rev. 19:7

> [17]**And the Spirit and the bride say, Come. And let him that heareth say,**
> **Come. And let him that is athirst come. And whosoever will, let him take the**
> **water of life freely.** Rev. 22:17

We are all called the bride of Christ. Do you believe that? I believe it. Where the Lamb goes, I go. Where He's been, I'm going. What He's done, I want to do. What He's said, I want to say. Because He said, "I only do and say the things I heard My Father saying" (John 14:9-10; 5:19; 8:28).

If it pleased Jesus to do and say the things the Father said, then I ought to be obedient and follow Him and my Father, and say the same things, think the same things, and do the same things. We would be a better Church.

There are always some that claim to have a new special revelation, and are seeking followers. When you have mastered Genesis to Revelation we'll talk about new revelations. "Turn away oh backsliding children saith the LORD, for I am married unto you..." (Jeremiah 3:14). If you're ever struggling with your identity problem, you ought to take this scripture and stick it in the face of the enemy and say, "My husband is the LORD, I am married to Him."

Take that lack of self-esteem and that self-hatred and that guilt and tell it to hit the road, Jack! I am the LORD's and He loves me, He has called me, and the Father has given me to the LORD forever. You are no accident in God's heart. "I will take you one of a city and two of a family and I'll bring you to Zion and I will give you pastors according to my heart which shall feed you with knowledge and understanding."

¹⁴"Turn, O backsliding children, saith the LORD; for I am married unto you: and I will take you one of a city, and two of a family, and I will bring you to Zion: ¹⁵And I will give you pastors according to mine heart, which shall feed you with knowledge and understanding. Jeremiah 3:14-15

I'll not say peace, peace when there isn't any. Nor am I going to send you to Prozac. We are going to come before God, find where the bondage is, where the roots are, where the blocks are, and get right before God, so that the Scriptures can be fulfilled.

Christ said—peace I leave with you, my peace I give unto you: not as the world giveth, give I unto you.

²⁷Peace I leave with you, my peace I give unto you: not as the world giveth, give I unto you. Let not your heart be troubled, neither let it be afraid. John 14:27

Would you be interested in that kind of peace? The peace that passeth all understanding. Do you believe that's a rare commodity or can it be reclaimed? I'm here to tell you that we're reclaiming it all over America with God's help. Jesus also said—come unto Me all you who are heavy laden and I will give you rest.

I was asked to sit down with the leadership of a large denomination in America in a spiritual think-tank workshop. They are staggering under the revelation of what I'm teaching. There are people in their churches being healed all over the country. Their hearts are open to **a more excellent way** of the Lord's blessing and grace as they deal with sanctification and the healing that is coming into their people. I've been asked to present ideas that will lead this denomination into healing and deliverance as a way of life. I think it is about time.

Whether it be Lutheran, Baptist, Nazarene, Episcopal, Independent Baptist, Free Will Baptist, whatever the denomination is, from coast to coast, the truth of God's Word is true for each one.

²⁰Knowing this first, that no prophecy of the scripture is of any private interpretation. 2 Peter 1:20

I had the wonderful opportunity of sitting down with the head of a Christian denomination in America recently. Many of their pastors and their people are in contact with our ministry, and their hearts are open **to a more excellent way.** I told the leader that the worst thing that can happen to them is to become another dead church. Don't go there! Let me challenge you; don't throw the baby out with the bath water. Love the people, hate the sin, but separate the people from their sin so that the love of God might possibly flow into them through you regardless of denomination or theological positioning.

> [13]**Therefore my people are gone into captivity, because** *they have* **no knowledge: and their honourable men** *are* **famished, and their multitude dried up with thirst.** [14]**Therefore hell hath enlarged herself, and opened her mouth without measure: and their glory, and their multitude, and their pomp, and he that rejoiceth, shall descend into it.** Isaiah 5:13-14

> [6]**My people are destroyed for lack of knowledge: because thou hast rejected knowledge, I will also reject thee, that thou shalt be no priest to me: seeing thou hast forgotten the law of thy God, I will also forget thy children.** Hosea 4:6

Ignorance is a form of knowledge but it can be dangerous to our health. God loves people even when they are in error. Were you ever in error? Have you ever been ignorant? Were you ever lost in your sins? Have you ever had to change your theology? I have had to change mine. Do you think it is possible to change your thinking? God said—I'll give you pastors according to My own heart.

> [15]**And I will give you pastors according to mine heart, which shall feed you with knowledge and understanding.** Jeremiah 3:15

Go to Jeremiah 32:17-18:

> [17]**Ah Lord God! behold, thou hast made the heaven and the earth by thy great power and stretched out arm,** *and* **there is nothing too hard for thee:** [18]**Thou shewest lovingkindness unto thousands, and recompensest the iniquity of the fathers into the bosom of their children after them...** Jeremiah 32:17-18

Genetically Inherited Disease

Manic depression is an inherited mental disease, caused by a continual underproduction of serotonin as a result of a defect in the 27th lower right-hand side of the X chromosome. It is a recessive gene passed through the mother and the only way to defeat it is to reorder the genetics in the Lord to make it work properly again.

If God created an X chromosome perfect from the foundation of the world and if the devil, because of the generations of sin, mixed up the amino acid base that changed the genetics, God can change it back the way it was. *The devil is not more powerful than God is.* If Satan can mess up genetics, Who do you think can fix it? Would we dare believe that? I'm willing to give it a shot. I think we should say, "God, change the genetics," and expect Him to do it. He did.

But what if we don't ask? What if we had withdrawn with unbelief, doubt and fear? Do you think we would get that kind of a healing? No, I want to be just like a kid. "Daddy, I want a lollipop." What does the Bible say? Except ye be converted, and become as little children, ye shall not enter into the kingdom of heaven.

> [3]**And said, Verily I say unto you, Except ye be converted, and become as little children, ye shall not enter into the kingdom of heaven.** Matthew 18:3

Have we become so sophisticated in our religiosity that we have forgotten how to simply trust the living God for our lives? Have we turned the immortal, invisible God into an intellectual concept? *Do we serve God with our heads or do we serve God with our hearts?*

Jeremiah 32:19 says that He is great in counsel, and mighty in works.

> **[19]Great in counsel, and mighty in work: for thine eyes *are* open upon all the ways of the sons of men: to give every one according to his ways, and according to the fruit of his doings:** Jeremiah 32:19

We choose what we shall have daily, blessings or curses, life or death.

> **[19]I call heaven and earth to record this day against you, *that* I have set before you life and death, blessing and cursing: therefore choose life, that both thou and thy seed may live:** Deut. 30:19

As for me and my house, we will serve the LORD.

> **[15]And if it seem evil unto you to serve the LORD, choose you this day whom ye will serve; whether the gods which your fathers served that *were* on the other side of the flood, or the gods of the Amorites, in whose land ye dwell: but as for me and my house, we will serve the LORD.** Joshua 24:15

If I step outside the parameters, I'm going to get back in the parameters.

Spiritually Rooted Diseases

What would you think if I asked you to take responsibility for a spiritual root in exchange for healing? Would it be worth it? Would you dare believe that that could happen? I want to tell you that God's Word says that He watches over His Word to perform it.

> **[12]Then said the LORD unto me, Thou hast well seen: for I will hasten my word to perform it.** Jeremiah 1:12

> **[106]I have sworn, and I will perform *it,* that I will keep thy righteous judgments.** Psalm 119:106

In the New Testament Mark says that the disciples went everywhere and preached the gospel and the Lord in Heaven worked with them, confirming the Word with signs and wonders following.

> **[15]And he said unto them, Go ye into all the world, and preach the gospel to every creature.** Mark 16:15

> **[20]And they went forth, and preached every where, the Lord working with *them,* and confirming the word with signs following. Amen.** Mark 16:20

I don't chase signs and wonders but I have discovered signs and wonders follow them that believe. If you don't believe, don't worry about it because it will never happen, but leave the rest of us alone who are believing.

I learned something about God: He has created us with a free will and He's not going to force you to come to Him. He's not going to force you to become born again. He's not going to force you to go to heaven. He's going to deal with you, but you're going to have to do the responding.

Do you know people don't get born again against their will? We are just like a stubborn mule. You couldn't make us do something if you tried. I can't make you do anything against your will. You'd thrash me; you wouldn't put up with it. God can't make you do it either.

If I could sow seed in your lives that God could use sometime in the eternal future to give you a better life, would it be worth it? Later in this teaching, I will break down many diseases, and tell you why people have that disease and what it's going to take to move the hand of God to get healed.

A Jewish lady from New Jersey was healed before she was saved. Do you think God can heal people who are not born again? Do you have to become born again before He will heal you? I've found God will heal people who are not born again. But when they got healed they sure got born again fast!

Another wonderful Jewish lady also came down from New Jersey who had Chronic Fatigue Syndrome, Electromagnetic Field Sensitivity, and Environmental Illness. She could not even live in her home. She was allergic to heat, electricity, couldn't read a book, and couldn't have a light bulb on. She had learned of someone who had been healed and called me and said, "Pastor, I want to come down to Georgia and I want you to heal me."

I said, "Oh, I don't heal anybody, God does."

Well, that brought up another subject. "Do you have to talk about Jesus if I come down there?"

I said, "No, we don't have to talk about Jesus."

She said, "Well, you're a Christian."

I said, "You are Jewish, so I'll talk about the God of Abraham, Isaac and Jacob. Will that be OK?"

She said, "Well, sure!"

I said, "He is the same one you know. I will talk about the God of Abraham, Isaac and Jacob and I'll pray for you in the name of the God of Abraham, Isaac, and Jacob. Could I pray for you in the name of the LORD? Could you handle that?"

She said, "That sounds pretty good, but do I have to accept this Jesus? You said that you don't heal anybody and if I'm healed and it's this Jesus who did it, do I have to accept Him if He heals me?"

I said, "No, but it would be a good thing to consider it because He is going to be the One who does it."

For four months we never discussed her disease. She got so mad at me. She came into my office, "What are we going to talk about today, Pastor?" I would say, "The God of Abraham, Isaac and Jacob. Let's go to the Torah, let's go to Isaiah, let's go to Jeremiah." For four months, I revealed to her the identity of the National God of Israel who came in the flesh to die for her, the promised Messiah. She would take stuff back to her husband

and her rabbi, and they would try to prove me wrong. They couldn't do it. I showed them the Godhead in the Old Testament Torah, in Isaiah, in Psalms—the plural unity of God, the Echad of Deuteronomy 6:4, the One, the plural unity.

'Hear, O Israel: The LORD our God *is* one LORD: Deut. 6:4

They couldn't prove me wrong.

Finally one day she came back after four months and said, "Pastor, I'm only 90% convinced that Jesus is the Promised Messiah but I am 100% convinced that He is God that came in the flesh and I am ready to receive Him as My Savior and My Lord." I led her in the sinner's prayer. We had a happy time. She is a wonderful lady and within 60 days, she was well. After six months of being at our retreat center receiving ministry she went home. She is well today, marvelously healed by her Creator, her Savior, her God and the Father who sent Him who loved her from the foundation of the world with an everlasting love.

There was another Jewish lady in New Jersey, 60 years of age, who had advanced osteoporosis. She contacted our ministry through our National Ministry Line. There is osteoporosis from estrogen deficiency because of menopause and there is osteoporosis that is non-menopausal, which comes from a spiritual root. Do you know what the Bible says the spiritual root is for non-menopausal osteoporosis? I'll give it to you—envy and jealousy are the cause of rotting of the bones:

[30]A sound heart *is* the life of the flesh: but envy the rottenness of the bones.
Proverbs 14:30

Do you think there is a connection and a spiritual root?

When we cracked Environmental Illness in 1990, seven words in the Bible that have been there for 3,000 years were the insight God gave me to unravel this bizarre disease. Today, our ministry is nationally recognized in the healing of MCS/EI because I took God at His word. Our success in the healing of this disease coast to coast and worldwide is second-to-none. I don't mean to be presumptuous. No, I'm just letting you know how our wonderful God has done this.

I was flying across America to see someone who had MCS/EI. I didn't know anything about the disease at that time. This person told me that pesticides had destroyed their immune system, then allergies developed. I didn't know; I thought it could possibly be true. I was sitting in that airplane, talking to God, with my Bible.

I said, "God, talk to me. Here I am, flying across America to see somebody who doesn't know me, I don't know them, and they are expecting You to heal them from a disease that I know nothing about." I had told this individual, "I'll give you ten days of my life to see what God will do. I'll drop what I'm doing. I'll fly across America. I'll come see what God will do." As I was browsing in my Bible, in Proverbs 17:22 was the answer from God for the healing of MCS/EI.

[22]A merry heart doeth good *like* a medicine: but a broken spirit drieth the bones. Proverbs 17:22

Do you know that laughter can strengthen the immune system? It has been documented that laughter causes the body to manufacture T cells and killer cells.

"A merry heart doeth good like a medicine: but a broken spirit drieth the bones." I stared at that verse in Proverbs 17:22 and all of a sudden the lights went on. I went, "Wait a minute, a broken spirit drieth up bones!" Bones, bones, what's in bones? Couldn't be osteoporosis, too young, not diagnosed. Bones, drying up of bones. Immune system. It started to click!

In college I was a premed student, majored in biology with a minor in psychology and so I had a little background in medicine. Wait a minute, the immune system. This person told me their immune system had been compromised by pesticides, but this verse in the Bible didn't say it was pesticides that destroyed that immune system, but it was a broken spirit that dried the bones or destroyed that immune system.

When I got to the person's home, this individual asked, "Has God showed you anything about my disease?" I said, "I'm not sure but I need to ask you a question. I wonder who broke your heart. I wonder who damaged you on the inside so severely that now you have a compromised immune system. I have a feeling the pesticide and the allergies are just a by-product."

Today we have found it to be true. It is not chemicals or odors that causes MCS/EI. *The immune system is compromised because of fear and anxiety coming out of a broken heart.* When you have a compromised immune system, you automatically have allergies.

The lady with osteoporosis in New Jersey didn't know God. Though she was Jewish, she was separated from God. Because we were able to be involved in her life, we knew that she had envy and jealousy coupled with some bitterness coming out of some tragic circumstances of life.

My staff dealt with her over the phone. I have never met her in my life; my staff has never met her. For a long time a large number of people have gotten well in America through our telephone ministry or by applying the principles in our teaching material.

Did you know there is no distance in the Spirit? In the story about the centurion, Jesus said: "I'll come and heal your servant."

He said, "No, no, I'm a man of authority, I tell my servants to go here, do this, do that. I perceive you are a man of authority. Simply speak the word and my servant shall be healed."

When the centurion got back to his hometown, he inquired, and the man was well. What hour was it? It was the same hour that Jesus had spoken.

> [5]And when Jesus was entered into Capernaum, there came unto him a centurion, beseeching him, [6]And saying, Lord, my servant lieth at home sick of the palsy, grievously tormented. [7]And Jesus saith unto him, I will come and heal him. [8]The centurion answered and said, Lord, I am not worthy that thou shouldest come under my roof: but speak the word only, and my servant shall be healed. [9]For I am a man under authority, having soldiers under me: and I

say to this *man,* **Go, and he goeth; and to another, Come, and he cometh; and to my servant, Do this, and he doeth** *it.* [10]**When Jesus heard** *it,* **he marvelled, and said to them that followed, Verily I say unto you, I have not found so great faith, no, not in Israel.** [11]**And I say unto you, That many shall come from the east and west, and shall sit down with Abraham, and Isaac, and Jacob, in the kingdom of heaven.** [12]**But the children of the kingdom shall be cast out into outer darkness: there shall be weeping and gnashing of teeth.** [13]**And Jesus said unto the centurion, Go thy way; and as thou hast believed, so be it done unto thee. And his servant was healed in the selfsame hour.** Matthew 8:5-13

What did that show to me when I was growing up in the Lord? There is no distance in the Spirit. I can minister over the telephone as well as I can in person, most of the time, but not always. Isn't that amazing?

What makes this testimony so incredibly significant is that she was on prednisone. You don't have any chance of defeating osteoporosis while you are on prednisone because it prevents bone density increases as a side effect. She was still taking the drug when she went back to her doctor to have her annual tests. I have in my files the documentation by her doctor of this healing. This is a documented healing by the medical community. She was 60, with progressive osteoporosis. She'd contracted this disease in her 30's and by her early 40's she was in the advanced stages of osteoporosis. They did the bone scans and the tests. And when she went for her results, her doctor told her this: "I don't know what has happened to you. I've been in this business for years. I've been your doctor for years, but all osteoporosis has been halted and not only has it been halted but in all bone scan areas of your bones, structure-wide, you have an average bone density increase of 15% to 18%. *You have the bones of a 30-year-old woman.*" In Psalms it says He will renew our youth like the eagle's.

[5]***...so that* thy youth is renewed like the eagle's.** Psalm 103:5

It happened to her.

That's what God did when she lined up with the principles. You can't have strong bones and have the spiritual root not dealt with. Remember, I just read that to you from Jeremiah. If we follow after the opposite of God and His precepts, then we shall bring to ourselves the opposite of the blessings. The opposite of the blessing is a curse.

Blessings and Curses

In Deuteronomy 28 (read the whole chapter) there is a whole section on blessings and curses. God said: **If** you do this, **then** I'll do this, **but**, if you don't, then all these curses shall come upon you.

[26]**And said, If thou wilt diligently hearken to the voice of the** LORD **thy God, and wilt do that which is right in his sight, and wilt give ear to his commandments, and keep all his statutes, I will put none of these diseases upon thee, which I have brought upon the Egyptians: for I** *am* **the** LORD **that healeth thee.** Exodus 15:26

(It is important to note that the curses do not come from God. They come from Satan.)

> **[13]Let no man say when he is tempted, I am tempted of God: for God cannot be tempted with evil, neither tempteth he any man:** James 1:13

On the cursing side is all manner of disease (Deuteronomy 28:15-68).

On the blessing side it says this:

> **[28:1]And it shall come to pass, if thou shalt hearken diligently unto the voice of the LORD thy God, to observe *and* to do all his commandments which I command thee this day, that the LORD thy God will set thee on high above all nations of the earth: [2]And all these blessings shall come on thee, and overtake thee, if thou shalt hearken unto the voice of the LORD thy God.** Deut. 28:1-2

There are conditions to healing. You don't just get it by barging in and making demands. The condition is obedience to God. Obedience is better than sacrifice.

> **[22]And Samuel said, Hath the LORD *as great* delight in burnt offerings and sacrifices, as in obeying the voice of the LORD? Behold, to obey *is* better than sacrifice, *and* to hearken than the fat of rams. [23]For rebellion *is as* the sin of witchcraft, and stubbornness *is as* iniquity and idolatry. Because thou hast rejected the word of the LORD, he hath also rejected thee from *being* king.** 1 Samuel 15:22-23

I am not into legalism. I'm into something much deeper than legalism. I'm into something called "heart change."

I want to tell you something; I don't serve God because I have to. I serve God because I want to. I don't love God because I have to. I love God just because I love Him. I'm not obedient to God because I am afraid of scorching my butt in hell. I serve God because I want to be an obedient son. I've been a rebel too many years. I'm a sinner saved by the grace of God and I am worthy of death but God chose otherwise. I am a grateful prodigal and I'm a grateful son and I know what I've been saved from. I am not going back. You can go back if you want but I am not going back with you. I just came from there. I know what it's like. I'm not going back into cursings; I'm going on into blessings.

Choose this day what you shall have, blessing or cursing, life or death.

> **[19]I call heaven and earth to record this day against you, *that* I have set before you life and death, blessing and cursing: therefore choose life, that both thou and thy seed may live: [20]That thou mayest love the LORD thy God, *and* that thou mayest obey his voice, and that thou mayest cleave unto him: for he *is* thy life, and the length of thy days: that thou mayest dwell in the land which the LORD sware unto thy fathers, to Abraham, to Isaac, and to Jacob, to give them.** Deut. 30:19-20

It's your choice. In Deuteronomy 28, you will find the 3 key words in Scripture; they are "**IF**," "**THEN**" and "**BUT**." I've said one day I'm going to teach a sermon called, "If, Then and But." *Freedom requires responsibility.* There is a required action on our part in order to receive God's blessings. *You cannot have your sin and also have your blessings (remember the doctrine of Balaam).*

I want to teach you something, if you have ears to hear. In Scripture, when the children of God were coming across Jordan, Joshua separated God's people around two mountains, **Mount Gerizim and Mount Ebal.** Mount Gerizim was the Mount of Blessings; Mount Ebal was the Mount of Curses.

From Deuteronomy 11:26-29 it says,

> **[26]Behold, I set before you this day a blessing and a curse; [27]A blessing, if ye obey the commandments of the LORD your God, which I command you this day: [28]And a curse, if ye will not obey the commandments of the LORD your God, but turn aside out of the way which I command you this day, to go after other gods, which ye have not known. [29]And it shall come to pass, when the LORD thy God hath brought thee in unto the land whither thou goest to possess it, that thou shalt put the blessing upon mount Gerizim, and the curse upon mount Ebal.** Deut. 11:26-29

As God's people came into promise, they were brought into a place of *discernment* immediately. What was the discernment? *Choice!* You are going to choose what you're going to believe. You are going to choose which path you shall follow.

God was bringing a very powerful truth to His people—in your obedience to Me and My commandments, which is best for you, the blessings are immediate and close by. However, if you are disobedient, the curse shall surely come. God built into this a type and shadow, the fact that in His grace and mercy, He would build into our lives time for reflection, time for conviction, and time to work it out. So I'm building into your consciousness today, precepts, concepts, the theology of God to bring you to a place of focus to recover yourself from the snare of the devil, not only for the healing of disease but for the prevention of it.

In Deuteronomy 28, there are a bunch of blessings and then there are a bunch of curses. In the two categories, *under curses are all manners of disease* and then it says and other diseases not written shall come upon you.

> **[61]Also every sickness, and every plague, which *is* not written in the book of this law, them will the LORD bring upon thee, until thou be destroyed.** Deut. 28:61

For every disease allopathic medicine thinks they have cured, five more pop up brand new. Did you realize that?

This is a mess. This little Merck Manual I have here is getting thicker every year, because there are more and more new plagues that are surfacing. *The study of disease is bigger than my Bible.* The book on Pathophysiology, The Biologic Basis for Disease in Children and Adults by Kathryn L. McCance and Sue E. Huether, St. Louis, MO: Mosby-Yearbook-Inc., 2nd edition, ©1994, is thicker than my Bible. The PDR (Physician's Desk Reference) on drugs and the side effects is bigger than my Bible. I think we need to pay attention.

On the blessing side of Deuteronomy 28 not one disease is mentioned. Do you consider disease to be a blessing or a curse? I consider all disease to be a curse. Why?

Because the Bible says so. *It says that when there's blessing, there's no disease (and when there is a curse, all manner of disease is listed).*

You say, "Pastor, I thought we were freed from the power of sin and death at the cross. I thought that Christ said, 'It is finished.' " If it was finished, and the penalty of the curse is paid, and you call yourself a believer, and you have a disease, you must not be born again. Because I don't find one Christian that does not have some type of disease in their life in America today to some degree, if it's finished then how come we have disease?

I teach something, and this may not be your position, but I teach something called *appropriation* of what was done at the cross. It's the only thing that makes any sense. It's called appropriation, and it was granted when Christ died. He died for all the sins of the world. Did He do that? Did He pay for all sins once and for all? Is everyone saved? But it was finished. If it was finished, then why isn't everyone saved? *Because you have to appropriate it by faith.*

It's the same way with healing. Just because it says by His stripes we were healed and He bore the penalty of the curse, does not mean that you get to keep your sin and get your freedom.

> **⁵But he *was* wounded for our transgressions, *he was* bruised for our iniquities: the chastisement of our peace *was* upon him; and with his stripes we are healed. Isaiah 53:5**

If we were totally free at conversion, then why would we need to be sanctified and why would we listen to Paul tell us about circumcision of the heart? *Why would Paul say to cleanse ourselves from all filthiness of the flesh and spirit?*

> **⁷:¹Having therefore these promises, dearly beloved, let us cleanse ourselves from all filthiness of the flesh and spirit, perfecting holiness in the fear of God.** 2 Cor. 7:1

I just raise the question. I don't know what your walk with God is, but I have learned that I am working out my own salvation daily with fear and trembling by appropriating His grace and mercy in His Word and the circumcision of my heart, which is an ongoing process. God is continually cutting away the part of me and my nature that He didn't create from the beginning.

Here in Deuteronomy 28 it talks about barrenness, it talks about divorce, losing your cow and your goats, and in verse 58 it says "If thou wilt not observe to do all the words of this law that are written in this book ..." How do we know when we are under the law? Do you think that God's nature has ever changed? Does He say, "I change not"?

> **⁶For I *am* the LORD, I change not; therefore ye sons of Jacob are not consumed.** Malachi 3:6

Did Christ come and change certain aspects of the law? Yes, He did. He rewrote certain aspects of the law concerning dietary rules, concerning Sabbath, concerning an eye for eye and tooth for tooth. Why could He do that? **Because He is the Word**. He is the One that gave the commandments on Mt. Sinai so why can't He write it again to bring to us a greater freedom, not because we're forced to do it, but because we want to do it. Are you with me?

Deuteronomy 28:58-63, 66-67:

> [58]**If thou wilt not observe to do all the words of this law that are written in this book, that thou mayest fear this glorious and fearful name, THE LORD THY GOD;** [59]**Then the LORD will make thy plagues wonderful, and the plagues of thy seed,** *even* **great plagues, and of long continuance, and sore sicknesses, and of long continuance.** [60]**Moreover he will bring upon thee all the diseases of Egypt, which thou wast afraid of; and they shall cleave unto thee.** [61]**Also every sickness, and every plague, which** *is* **not written in the book of this law, them will the LORD bring upon thee, until thou be destroyed.** [62]**And ye shall be left few in number, whereas ye were as the stars of heaven for multitude; because thou wouldest not obey the voice of the LORD thy God.** [63]**And it shall come to pass,** *that* **as the LORD rejoiced over you to do you good, and to multiply you; so the LORD will rejoice over you to destroy you, and to bring you to nought; and ye shall be plucked from off the land whither thou goest to possess it.** Deut. 28:58-63

> [66]**And thy life shall hang in doubt before thee; and thou shalt fear day and night, and shalt have none assurance of thy life:** [67]**In the morning thou shalt say, Would God it were even! and at even thou shalt say, Would God it were morning! for the fear of thine heart wherewith thou shalt fear, and for the sight of thine eyes which thou shalt see.** Deut. 28:66-67

That's pretty scary.

Looking back at vs. 66 and 67, it talks about our life hanging in doubt before us; and we shall fear day and night, and we shall have no assurance of our life. Verse 67. In the mornings we find ourselves saying, "Would to God it were evening." In the evenings we will say, "Would to God it were morning." The fear of our heart and fear coming from what our eyes see rules our life. That's pretty scary.

All Disease is a Result of Separation on Three Levels

What do you think the solution is? Removing the separation. These three root **"causes of disease"** are:

1. Separation from God and His Word, His person and His love.

2. Separation from you, from yourself—not accepting yourself, not loving yourself, guilt and condemnation.

3. Separation from others—breaches in relationships, hatred, bitterness, envy, jealousy, competition, performance, drivenness, lack of nurturing, lack of love, and on and on the list goes.

I have found that all disease that has a spiritual root has a breakdown on these three levels.

The Beginning of All Healing of Spiritually Related Diseases Begins With:

1. Your coming back in alignment with God, His Word, His person, His nature, His precepts and what He planned on this planet for you from the beginning. The solution is restoration.

2. Accepting YOURSELF in your relationship with God; getting rid of your self-hatred, getting rid of your self-bitterness, getting rid of your guilt and coming back on line with who you are in the Father through Jesus Christ.

3. Making peace with your brother, your sister and all others, if at all possible.

So, *the beginning of all healing is restoration.*

The Bible says this about relationships in Matthew 22:37-40, that you shall love the Lord thy God with all of thy heart, with all of thy soul, and all of thy mind and you shall love your neighbour as yourself.

> **[37]Jesus said unto him, Thou shalt love the Lord thy God with all thy heart, and with all thy soul, and with all thy mind. [38]This is the first and great commandment. [39]And the second *is* like unto it, Thou shalt love thy neighbour as thyself. [40]On these two commandments hang all the law and the prophets.** Matthew 22:37-40

You cannot love your neighbor if you do not love yourself. It is not possible. If you say you do, you are kidding yourself. It's not possible. You bring the strength of God into your life and then you bring the strength of God into others' lives, in that order.

Any breakdown in that sequence long term produces many, many diseases. Why? Because God commanded that you shall love your neighbor as yourself.

When I started to get involved with disease, I found that disease was a result of separation from God, first and foremost. It was right there in Deuteronomy 28. I said to God, "OK, you're telling me something. We have curses and blessings, what does that mean to me? Blessings and Curses, so we either blew it or we didn't blow it." God led me to Proverbs 26:2 in my sequence of thinking when He said the curse without a cause does not come.

> **[2]As the bird by wandering, as the swallow by flying, so the curse causeless shall not come.** Proverbs 26:2

I went, "Hmm, what are you telling me God?" In my understanding and in my mind I felt God was saying this, *"If you see any disease, Mr. Henry Wright, you see a curse and if you see a curse, there is a reason for it.* Did you get the point, son?"

Cause and effect, *"if, then and but."* "Are you telling me God that if I see a disease, it's like a bird that has landed and a swallow that has landed but it had a right to?" He said, "That's what I said over in 2 Timothy 2:24-26."

> **[24]And the servant of the Lord must not strive; but be gentle unto all *men*, apt to teach, patient, [25]In meekness instructing those that oppose themselves; if God peradventure will give them repentance to the acknowledging of the**

truth; [26]And *that* they may recover themselves out of the snare of the devil, who are taken captive by him at his [the devil's] will. 2 Tim. 2:24-26

In order to get the disease removed, I must get the cause removed. That's being sanctified. God said that's what I've called my people to. A people who are sanctified without spot or blemish.

> [26]That he might sanctify and cleanse it with the washing of water by the word, [27]That he might present it to himself a glorious church, not having spot, or wrinkle, or any such thing; but that it should be holy and without blemish. Ephes. 5:26-27

> [7]Let us be glad and rejoice, and give honour to him: for the marriage of the Lamb is come, and his wife hath made herself ready. [8]And to her was granted that she should be arrayed in fine linen, clean and white: for the fine linen is the righteousness of saints. [9]And he saith unto me, Write, Blessed *are* they which are called unto the marriage supper of the Lamb. And he saith unto me, These are the true sayings of God. [10]And I fell at his feet to worship him. And he said unto me, See *thou do it* not: I am thy fellowservant, and of thy brethren that have the testimony of Jesus: worship God: for the testimony of Jesus is the spirit of prophecy. [11]And I saw heaven opened, and behold a white horse; and he that sat upon him *was* called Faithful and True, and in righteousness he doth judge and make war. [12]His eyes *were* as a flame of fire, and on his head *were* many crowns; and he had a name written, that no man knew, but he himself. [13]And he *was* clothed with a vesture dipped in blood: and his name is called The Word of God. [14]And the armies *which were* in heaven followed him upon white horses, clothed in fine linen, white and clean. [15]And out of his mouth goeth a sharp sword, that with it he should smite the nations: and he shall rule them with a rod of iron: and he treadeth the winepress of the fierceness and wrath of Almighty God. [16]And he hath on *his* vesture and on his thigh a name written, KING OF KINGS, AND LORD OF LORDS. [17]And I saw an angel standing in the sun; and he cried with a loud voice, saying to all the fowls that fly in the midst of heaven, Come and gather yourselves together unto the supper of the great God; [18]That ye may eat the flesh of kings, and the flesh of captains, and the flesh of mighty men, and the flesh of horses, and of them that sit on them, and the flesh of all *men, both* free and bond, both small and great. [19]And I saw the beast, and the kings of the earth, and their armies, gathered together to make war against him that sat on the horse, and against his army. Rev. 19:7-19

I've called them to holiness.

> [7]For God hath not called us unto uncleanness, but unto holiness. 1 Thes. 4:7

I've called them to walk before Me because I am their God

> [17]And as for thee, if thou wilt walk before me, as David thy father walked, and do according to all that I have commanded thee, and shalt observe my statutes and my judgments; 2 Chron. 7:17

and I've called them to be cleansed.

> [7:1]Having therefore these promises, dearly beloved, let us cleanse ourselves from all filthiness of the flesh and spirit, perfecting holiness in the fear of God. 2 Cor. 7:1

The curse without a cause does not come (Proverbs 26:2).

When I find any evidence of disease today, what am I looking for? *The cause.* I go to the Word to find it, and I go to the medical community to find out what they know. I'm teaching pastors in America, "Pastors, you need more than Vines, Ungers, Strongs and a Bible. Instead of getting 14 translations, why don't you buy a Merck Manual, a pathophysiology manual, and an anatomy and physiology book and why don't you do a little laymen's study on disease?" Fibromyalgia for example, is anyone interested in that?

Let me read you something: *Fibromyalgia* is what the medical community calls pain in fibrous tissues, muscles, tendons, ligaments, and other connective tissue. Do you know why it is there? I'll tell you why. You ladies have not been nurtured. You are paying a high price for your insecurities and your fears. Let me read this thing here, "The condition occurs mainly in females, Primary Fibromyalgia Syndrome (PFS) is particularly likely to occur in healthy young women who tend to be stressed, tense, depressed, anxious, striving, and driven" (Merck Manual, 16th edition, pp. 1369-1370).

As a pastor, how long did it take me to get into position against this disease? As long as it took for me to read what I just read! Immediately I came back on the fly. Okay, *fibromyalgia: the result of fear, anxiety and stress;* unresolved conflict and stresses, and you know that it's true. When the anxieties and the insecurities issues are dealt with, many times the fibromyalgia goes away. Similarly, when I deal with bitterness, the arthritis many times goes away. When I deal with self-hatred and guilt, many times lupus and other autoimmune diseases go away. When I deal with a broken heart and those wounds, many times allergies go away.

I want to conclude this teaching today with a mandate. The mandate comes out of Ezekiel chapter 34 with a statement from the Father concerning the shepherds of Israel:

> **34:1And the word of the LORD came unto me, saying, 2Son of man, prophesy against the shepherds of Israel, prophesy, and say unto them, Thus saith the Lord GOD unto the shepherds ... Ezekiel 34:1-2**

Who are the shepherds? Pastors. What am I? I'm a shepherd boy. I take care of sheep; I put salve on their wounds, I go over the cliff all over America, and I pull them up to save their lives.

All over America, I find them abandoned by the Church, abandoned by their leaders, abandoned by their families. I've flown across America to help keep one person from dying more than one time. Multiple times. In fact, we said the other day that we were going to change the name of our ministry to "Over The Cliff Ministries." I'm always "over the cliff" with someone who is dying and separated.

Do you remember what the Lord said about the 99 sheep safe in the fold versus the one who went over the cliff?

> **11For the Son of man is come to save that which was lost. 12How think ye? if a man have an hundred sheep, and one of them be gone astray, doth he not**

leave the ninety and nine, and goeth into the mountains, and seeketh that which is gone astray? [13]And if so be that he find it, verily I say unto you, he rejoiceth more of that *sheep,* than of the ninety and nine which went not astray. [14]Even so it is not the will of your Father which is in heaven, that one of these little ones should perish. Matthew 18:11-14

He placed a great premium on the isolated dying ones, and my mission is to gather them into the fold. My mission is to keep them from going over the cliff to begin with and that should be your mission to mankind. **This is a more excellent way: healing and prevention of disease.**

Ezekiel 34 says, "Son of man, prophesy against the shepherds of Israel, prophesy, and say unto them, Thus saith the Lord GOD unto the shepherds; *Woe be to the shepherds* of Israel that do feed themselves! should not the shepherds feed the flocks? Vs. 3: You eat the fat, you clothe yourself with wool but you kill them that are fed. *You do not feed the flock.* Vs. 4: **The diseased have you not strengthened, neither have you healed that which was sick, neither have you bound up that which was broken, neither have you brought again that which was driven away, neither have you sought that which was lost;** but with force and with cruelty have you ruled them.

Vs. 5: "And they were scattered, because there is no shepherd: and they became meat to all the beasts of the field, when they were scattered. Vs. 6: My sheep wandered through all the mountains, and upon every high hill: yea, my flock was scattered upon all the face of the earth, and none did search or seek after them. Vs. 7: Therefore, ye shepherds, hear the word of the LORD; Vs. 8: As I live, saith the Lord GOD, surely because my flock became a prey, and my flock became meat to every beast of the field, because there was no shepherd, neither did my shepherds search for my flock, but the shepherds fed themselves, and fed not my flock;

Vs. 9: "Therefore, O ye shepherds, hear the word of the LORD; Vs. 10: Thus saith the Lord GOD; Behold, I am against the shepherds; and I will require My flock at their hand, and cause them to cease from feeding the flock; neither shall the shepherds feed themselves any more; for I will deliver my flock from their mouth, that they may not be meat for them.

Vs. 11: "For thus saith the Lord GOD; Behold, I, even I, will both search my sheep and I will seek them out. Vs. 12: As a shepherd seeking out his flock in the day that he is among his sheep that are scattered; so will I seek out My sheep, and I will deliver them out of all the places where they have been scattered in the cloudy and dark day. Vs. 15: I will feed My flock, I will cause them to lie down saith the Lord GOD. Vs. 16: **I will seek that which was lost, and bring again that which was driven away, and I will bind up that which was broken and I will strengthen that which was sick: but I will destroy the fat and the strong; I will feed them with judgment.**"

Isaiah talks about the brokenhearted.

[61:1]**The Spirit of the Lord GOD *is* upon me; because the LORD hath anointed me to preach good tidings unto the meek; he hath sent me to bind up the**

brokenhearted, to proclaim liberty to the captives, and the opening of the prison to *them that are* bound; Isaiah 61:1

The healing of MCS/EI is healing of the broken heart.

²²A merry heart doeth good *like* a medicine: but a broken spirit drieth the bones. Proverbs 17:22

I spend more time healing broken hearts in America than you can imagine.

Eighty-five to ninety percent of my caseload nationally for 15 years has been female. God has used me to heal many females from their abandonment by fathers and husbands, and to get them back in line with their Heavenly Father and the Lord who sought them and bought them.

I want to tell you something; you had better thank God for my intensity because I am a warrior. I am out to destroy the works of the devil and to reclaim God's precious flock from the hands of Satan and re-establish you into praising His glory here and now, not when you get to heaven. Then, when you get to heaven, you can give Him thanks for it. AMEN!

Isaiah continues to talk about God's healing and restoration that has been provided.

⁶¹:¹The Spirit of the Lord God *is* upon me; because the Lord hath anointed me to preach good tidings unto the meek; he hath sent me to bind up the brokenhearted, to proclaim liberty to the captives, and the opening of the prison to *them that are* bound; ²To proclaim the acceptable year of the Lord, and the day of vengeance of our God; to comfort all that mourn; ³To appoint unto them that mourn in Zion, to give unto them beauty for ashes, the oil of joy for mourning, the garment of praise for the spirit of heaviness; that they might be called trees of righteousness, the planting of the Lord, that he might be glorified. Isaiah 61:1-3

Isaiah 61:4 is generational in nature and provides for the healing of generations. This is the breaking of inherited genetic curses. This is breaking inherited familiar spirits from your family trees, the rollovers, specifically meaning spiritually, psychologically and biologically inherited diseases.

⁴And they shall build the old wastes, they shall raise up the former desolations, and they shall repair the waste cities, the desolations of many generations. Isaiah 61:4

I'm going to tell you that there is a revival coming to this planet, and there is a revival coming to this nation, but it will not be the type of revival that you may think it is.

The revival coming is one of *sanctification and purification*. I will tell you with all the authority of my heart that I can know, that the only way that it will be ushered in is the same way it was ushered in the first time: by the Lord when He came. The healing of diseases, the casting out of evil spirits, and the establishment of His grace and His mercy—you can go and read about it from Romans to Jude.

A lot of people struggle with this: how come we didn't see healing of diseases and the great teaching of healing of diseases and casting out of evil spirits after Acts? The reason for that is this: Matthew, Mark, Luke and John are the Lord showing us God's love in spite of sin. John demonstrated God's power through Christ over evil in spite of sin—all to demonstrate God's love for us.

Acts demonstrated the early Church's power over the same thing.

After the demonstration was done, it's sanctification from Romans to Jude. Without sanctification, you can't have Matthew, Mark, Luke, John and the book of Acts happening at all. It is not gonna happen.

When you have Romans to Jude in your life the blessings will come; the showers of blessing will come. Then the knowledge of God will flow *because God's not going to bless disobedient children long term.*

I have had to learn this the hard way. Would it be a fair exchange, obedience for disease? Would it be a fair exchange, sanctification for disease? Would it be a fair exchange, obedience for insanity? Would it be a fair exchange, trust in God for fear and anxiety? Would it be a fair exchange to believe and receive God's love versus an unloving, unclean spirit of self-hatred? Would it be a fair exchange to forgive your brother in exchange for the healing of cancer? Would it be a fair exchange to deal with fear and anger in exchange for a heart attack?

This is a more excellent way!

You know what the Word says, don't you, about fear and heart attacks?

> [26]**Men's hearts failing them for fear, and for looking after those things which are coming on the earth: for the powers of heaven shall be shaken.** Luke 21:26

That's what it says.

I can go to a pathophysiology text and find one of the basic causes for most heart attacks is *fear and anxiety.* How about *aneurysms, strokes, hemorrhoids, varicose veins?* Do you know what the cause is for these? *Anger and rage.*

Do you want to prevent *aneurysms* and *strokes* in your life? Get anger and rage out of your life as fast as you can. Rage, anger and hostility and that deep root of bitterness need to be dealt with, because you're going to explode at some point. *As you are exploding spiritually, your body will respond in your lifetime.*

Some people teach that there were certain spiritual attacks in Scripture that God didn't remove, such as the attack on Job and Paul's thorn in the flesh. Proverbs teaches us that there is a reason (Proverbs 26:2). Let's take a look.

Job had spiritual problems. Job's first spiritual problem—he told us himself about his fear:

> [25]**For the thing which I greatly feared is come upon me, and that which I was afraid of is come unto me.** Job 3:25

The second thing that Job feared was evidenced when he became preoccupied with the spiritual safety of his children.

> **⁴And his sons went and feasted *in their* houses, every one his day; and sent and called for their three sisters to eat and to drink with them. ⁵And it was so, when the days of *their* feasting were gone about, that Job sent and sanctified them, and rose up early in the morning, and offered burnt offerings *according* to the number of them all: for Job said, It may be that my sons have sinned, and cursed God in their hearts. Thus did Job continually.** Job 1:4-5

That was an open door for fear. Then, in Job 40 and 41, when we look at the characteristics of Behemoth and Leviathan, we find that Job had pride and spiritual arrogance (behemoth).

> **¹⁹He *is* the chief of the ways of God: he that made him can make his sword to approach *unto him*.** Job 40:19

> **³⁴He beholdeth all high *things:* he *is* a king over all the children of pride.** Job 41:34

In his great discourse with God about his own righteousness as he saw it, God cut him back down to size (Job 40:1-14). When Job prayed for his friends, God removed the power of Satan and restored to him twice what he had previously (Job 42:7-17).

In the case of Paul's thorn in the flesh, we're not exactly sure that it was a disease. The word "flesh" is a Greek word, but the word "flesh" as found in Romans 7 also has to do with our spiritual nature. It could also mean our human body. Greek is a very limited language as opposed to Hebrew. In fact, in Greek, you'll find one word having more than one meaning.

In the Old Testament, there are almost 9000 different Hebrew words that were used. The Greek Scriptures used a little over 5500 in the writing of the New Testament. The reason for that is that the Jews, in the Hebrew, have a word for just about every meaning. This is not the case with the Greeks. Even in the English language, we sometimes have a word that has more than one meaning.

The teachings of Paul on the *flesh* have to do with the carnal nature; that part that is unrenewed within us called "the flesh." However, the word *flesh* can also mean your human body. Paul's thorn in the flesh may not necessarily have been a biological disease.

In Romans 7:15, Paul is talking about a spiritual battle he is having or has had. The good that I want to do, I don't do it and the evil that I don't like doing, that's what I do. And so in the day that I want to do good and I don't do it, and the evil that I wish I would not do, I do it. The day that I do the evil, it is no longer I that am doing the evil, but sin that dwelleth in me (is doing it).

> **¹⁵For that which I do I allow not: for what I would, that do I not; but what I hate, that do I. ¹⁶If then I do that which I would not, I consent unto the law that *it is* good. ¹⁷Now then it is no more I that do it, but sin that dwelleth in me. ¹⁸For I know that in me (that is, in my flesh,) dwelleth no good thing: for to will**

is present with me; but *how* to perform that which is good I find not. [19]For the good that I would I do not: but the evil which I would not, that I do. [20]Now if I do that I would not, it is no more I that do it, but sin that dwelleth in me. [21]I find then a law, that, when I would do good, evil is present with me. [22]For I delight in the law of God after the inward man: [23]But I see another law in my members, warring against the law of my mind, and bringing me into captivity to the law of sin which is in my members. Romans 7:15-23

This is an apostle, 20 plus years an apostle, saying that he had the indwelling presence of sin. In fact, he went on in that chapter and said there is a war, a kingdom at work within him that wars against the law of God, bringing him into captivity to the law of sin (as a believer).

It would seem to be, if we looked at Paul's discourse in Romans 7, that his thorn in the flesh may not have been a biological disease; it may have been an area of his carnal nature that he just never got under control.

He did say it was a "Messenger of Satan," and that it was not removed. The Word tells us why it wasn't removed. Because there was a chance that Paul might be overexalted in pride, because Paul was a Pharisee. He was a "Pharisee of Pharisees" and the chance of Paul having spiritual pride would have been very good. I don't have a specific answer. We do know that it was a messenger from Satan.

[7]And lest I should be exalted above measure through the abundance of the revelations, there was given to me a thorn in the flesh, the messenger of Satan to buffet me, lest I should be exalted above measure. 2 Cor. 12:7

We do know that Paul prayed for God to remove it, and that God's answer was that it wasn't removed. But, I only offer this as a possibility: I do, however, consider Paul's discourse in Romans 7 showing us that he had spiritual battles and the indwelling presence of sin.

Peter was a little different. Jesus said to Peter—Satan desires to sift you like wheat and when you have recovered yourself, strengthen the brethren.

[31]And the Lord said, Simon, Simon, behold, Satan hath desired *to have* you, that he may sift *you* as wheat: [32]But I have prayed for thee, that thy faith fail not: and when thou art converted, strengthen thy brethren. Luke 22:31-32

Jesus did nothing to prevent that sifting of Peter by Satan. Why? Because Peter had spiritual problems.

The Chastening of the Lord. I have a particular opinion about the chastening of the Lord. I read in the Bible that when we follow our enemies, God gives us over to the blessings of our enemies, which is a curse (Deuteronomy 28:15ff). When we have had enough, or when the Old Testament saints had finally had enough (the blessings of their enemies which in fact was oppression and bondage), they would cry out to God: they'd repent, He would end their captivity, and He'd bless them. He would release them when they repented and turned back to Him.

Keep this in mind: the Lord is not putting evil on us, but giving us over to the devices of our own heart until we've had enough. When we recognize the spiritual defects of our life through conviction by the Holy Spirit, and through the washing of the Word, the spiritual defect is then purified. Some call it the "Baptism of Fire"—the purging work, the sanctifying work of the Holy Spirit.

God did not give the spiritual defect. How could He put sin into our lives? That would be contrary to His holy nature.

> [13]**Let no man say when he is tempted, I am tempted of God: for God cannot be tempted with evil, neither tempteth he any man:** James 1:13

He wants to purge us from it.

> [8]**He that committeth sin is of the devil; for the devil sinneth from the beginning. For this purpose the Son of God was manifested, that he might destroy the works of the devil.** 1 John 3:8

In Acts 10:38 it says:

> [38]**How God anointed Jesus of Nazareth with the Holy Ghost and with power: who went about doing good, and healing all that were oppressed of the devil; for God was with him.** Acts 10:38

So it is very clear that God wants to destroy the works of the devil and to heal all that are oppressed by the devil.

Depression, Anxiety Attacks and the Use of Prozac and Other Drugs

The side affects of these drugs are incredible. They are serotonin[1] enhancers. When serotonin is released off the dendrite ends in your body, the drugs block the return, thus prolonging the effectiveness of it. It is out there longer, which gives the person a sense of well being.

The key issue that we need to deal with is why do we have a serotonin deficiency?

A serotonin deficiency will cause depression. *Depression*, by clinical definition, is the result of a chemical imbalance in the body, either through the introduction of drugs, uppers and downers, over- or under-production (hyper/hypo) of normal neurotransmitters that are manufactured by our body.

One of the things that I deal with in this ministry is the over- (hyper) or under- (hypo) secretion of neurotransmitters. For example, *manic depression* may be associated with an underproduction of serotonin, caused by a genetic defect producing a wide range of highs and lows, from manic to depressive. Migraines, binge eating, weight problems, obsessive/compulsive behavior (OCD), may also indicate an under-secretion of serotonin. It's non-genetic, and it's not the same as an anxiety disorder.

---

[1]Serotonin is a neurotransmitter that facilitates many body functions, including feeling good about yourself.

Prozac and other drugs used to treat depression are designed to increase your self-esteem. *A lack of self-esteem is the root problem.*

Lack of self-esteem, self-rejection, self-hatred, and guilt are very damaging to the human spirit, and are many times caused by a father although in some cases it can be the mother. Somewhere, there has been a lack of nurturing in childhood. Sometimes it can be inherited because the lack of nurturing has not been there from generation to generation.

The problem with *Prozac* is this: one of the primary side effects of *Prozac* is anxiety and a secondary side effect is reduction of libido and that creates a double problem.

Females taking *Prozac* may lose their libido and that has a negative effect on their sexual relationship with their husbands. Males can lose their sex drive with their wives. That's going to create another problem: more anxiety, more guilt, more rejection, and more conflict. This may result in a further decrease in serotonin levels, and now we've got a bigger problem: a deeper depression. The only way to unravel this thing is to take a look at what may be causing this serotonin deficiency and that is a *spiritual problem*.

Why are some not healed?

Sometimes you can have two people with the same sin and the same identical disease, and **one is healed and the other is not. Why?** God doesn't necessarily judge you in your sin immediately, *He judges you for your heart toward it.* It is hard to teach this because if you are not careful, you'll make sin abound again.

King David was called a man after God's own heart. Yet, David had a man killed, he was an adulterer, etc. What made David different from Saul, his predecessor? Saul never repented. Psalm 51 tells us that David did.

The difference is in our attitude toward sin. Your heart toward God concerning sin is what moves Him. In Isaiah 57:15 it says

> **[15]For thus saith the high and lofty One that inhabiteth eternity, whose name *is* Holy; I dwell in the high and holy *place*, with him also *that is* of a contrite and humble spirit, to revive the spirit of the humble, and to revive the heart of the contrite ones.** Isaiah 57:15

What is the predicator for moving the hand of God? Your sinlessness, or your heart toward sin? I'll be very honest with you, historically and Scripturally, it seems that if you have a hatred for sin, even if you are still in your sin, God judges you according to the righteousness of your heart toward Him. Out of that perfect hatred for sin, God starts to deal with you so that you are better able to resist the sin, and thus removes the torment and that struggle and eventually produces your freedom from that sin.

There are other people who, when confronted with sin, harden their hearts and are not convicted; they don't have a perfect hatred for it. In fact, they either condone it or ignore it. God is going to judge you after the intent of your heart, not to the degree of your sanctification first. In Romans 7:15-17, we saw that the Apostle Paul also struggled with the issue of sin in his life.

I did a teaching some years ago on the *7 Steps to Sin* (James 1:12-16). Temptation is not sin. Having evil thoughts is not sin. If that were the case, we are all deep in sin. Thoughts come and go. The evil one in his kingdom is always out there tempting you. Temptation is not sin. Jesus was tempted in all points such as we are, yet was without sin.

> **[15]For we have not an high priest which cannot be touched with the feeling of our infirmities; but was in all points tempted like as *we are, yet* without sin.** Hebrews 4:15

Many people, because they are tempted, feel that they have sinned. You only have sin when the action of that sin is fulfilled; then it becomes your sin. I know what the Word says about a man lusting in his heart after a woman.

> **[28]But I say unto you, That whosoever looketh on a woman to lust after her hath committed adultery with her already in his heart.** Matthew 5:28

There is a difference between temptation concerning women and fantasy lust. Fantasy lust is a sin because you're committing the act in your mind, not just being tempted with the act. Many men and women fall because of being ignorant at this level. They say, "Well, I'll just go ahead and do it because I've already thought about it. *This is Satan's snare; convincing you that the temptation equals the act.*

The 7 steps to sin are found in James 1:12-16.

> **[12]Blessed *is* the man that endureth temptation: for when he is tried, he shall receive the crown of life, which the Lord hath promised to them that love him. [13]Let no man say when he is tempted, I am tempted of God: for God cannot be tempted with evil, neither tempteth he any man: [14]But every man is tempted, when he is drawn away of his own lust, and enticed. [15]Then when lust hath conceived, it bringeth forth sin: and sin, when it is finished, bringeth forth death. [16]Do not err, my beloved brethren.** James 1:12-16

Temptation is not sin.

How do we correct a wrong when the person is dead?

Many people are bound by disease because of unresolved issues concerning people who have died. Do you know how many people have bitterness against dead people? How can you make it right with a dead person? You can't. The same is true if you don't know where the person is.

I'll tell you how God judges it. *He judges it by your heart.* If you have something from your past and it is not possible for you to make it right with the person, then you make it right with God and it is taken care of; you don't have to carry the guilt any longer.

If someone is holding a sin against you, it is their problem, not yours. They have to get it right before God just like you do. Whether they do or they don't really doesn't have anything to do with you because you are standing alone before God in the integrity of your heart.

You need to stay in freedom, and not in guilt. There may be something in your life such as a breach with someone and they won't even talk to you. They won't make peace with you. Your ability to be free of that situation does not mean that you have to resolve it personally with that person. You can come before God and He'll work with your heart, but you don't have to have it resolved with anyone in order for you to be free. You have to have it resolved before God. Your heart has to make the paradigm shift concerning this issue.

Victimization

How do you honor your parents, or husband, or wife, (or children,) when they constantly "beat you up" in some manner?

There are many people condemned with the scripture—honor your mother and your father.

> [19]**Honour thy father and *thy* mother...** Matthew 19:19

You only have to honor mother or father or anyone to the degree that they honor God. If you have a mother and father who are evil before God, you do not have to honor them in their evil. Now, you can't touch them either. You don't have to go along with their sin. Some people tell me: " I just don't want to talk about what my mother did to me or my father did to me because that's not honoring them." No, that is not about honoring them—it's just defining the evil. You don't have to honor the evil in parents. We cannot afford to preach a gospel that produces a codependency with evil. My definition of codependency is calling evil good in the name of love.

However, the first thing that you must be able to do is separate them from their sin. You must always have a perfect hatred for evil.

> [10]**Ye that love the LORD, hate evil...** Psalm 97:10

The Bible says so—that you're to have a perfect hatred for evil, but you must love the person. That is hard to do.

What happens to us because someone behaves in an evil manner against us? We believe them to be evil. God looked down from heaven when I was evil and He separated me in His mind and in His heart from my sins, and my evil, and He loved me. He looked past my sins, and loved me anyway.

Pure religion, undefiled, is to visit the fatherless, take care of the widows in their afflictions, and keep yourself undefiled from the world.

> [27]**Pure religion and undefiled before God and the Father is this, To visit the fatherless and widows in their affliction, *and* to keep himself unspotted from the world.** James 1:27

If you leave mother and father, brother and sister, houses and lands, for the gospel and what God stands for, God will give to you in this life an hundredfold, mothers and fathers, brothers and sisters, houses and lands, an hundredfold and in the world to come, eternal life.

> **[29]And Jesus answered and said, Verily I say unto you, There is no man that hath left house, or brethren, or sisters, or father, or mother, or wife, or children, or lands, for my sake, and the gospel's, [30]But he shall receive an hundredfold now in this time, houses, and brethren, and sisters, and mothers, and children, and lands, with persecutions; and in the world to come eternal life.** Mark 10:29-30

I'm going to offer you a possibility that if you're around a good body of believers, where there are some good fathers and mothers in the Lord, I pray that God gives them to you quickly. They can fill you up with that love that you need, and you don't have to be violated in your spirit any more, and you do not have to be cursed in it, nor guilty in it.

You can still love your parents, but you do not have to be victimized by the sin through them. God did not ask anybody, anywhere, to be a victim for any reason. Separate from the person and remove yourself if you have to. In a victimization situation, be it children, or husbands, or wives, I call for immediate separation. I'd never send a wife back to an abusive husband. God has called us to peace and He said that if it is at all possible, we are to live peaceably with one another.

> **[18]If it be possible, as much as lieth in you, live peaceably with all men.** Romans 12:18

I will not tolerate victimization on any level. It's time out, it's separation time, time to declare where your treasure is, and get it together in righteousness.

There's no way that God condones victimization under any name or under any title. He's called us to peace. In fact, in Mark it says—when you go out, if you can't leave your peace at the house you've entered into, shake the dust off your feet and go find some place where you can leave your peace.

> **[10]And he said unto them, In what place soever ye enter into an house, there abide till ye depart from that place. [11]And whosoever shall not receive you, nor hear you, when ye depart thence, shake off the dust under your feet for a testimony against them. Verily I say unto you, It shall be more tolerable for Sodom and Gomorrha in the day of judgment, than for that city.** Mark 6:10-11

(I know this scripture pertains to evangelism but the principles remain true.) God has called us to peace not to torment. This has nothing to do with loving your parents; it's following God. You can love someone who has evil but you don't have to be a victim.

Separation from abusive situations is Godly, it's not ungodly. There may be a time, after you've been sanctified and strengthened in the area of your weaknesses, that you can go back into the situation and be all right. You don't have to do that until you are healed, and it may be that God won't ever want you to do that. I don't know. I do know that to go back prematurely to a place where you have been weakened, by abuse, or victimization on any level, is not right. First, you need to get strengthened and healed in yourself. Give those who have wronged you to the Lord; you don't have to fix them.

When I minister to children who have been subjected to victimization, the worst thing I can do is send them back to the abusive parent. My position is that all victims are removed *immediately until somebody decides where their treasure is.*

> **³⁴For where your treasure is, there will your heart be also.** Luke 12:34

This is true whether the victim is the husband, the wife or the child. We are not going to play games with victimization. The tragedy is just too high a price to pay. *If we had taken a stand at this level against victimization a long time ago, we wouldn't have the tragedies it is causing today.* You cannot go back into a victimization situation in the name of love. It's **codependent,** it's further victimization, it's built-in guilt, and you will not be able to have your peace. Nobody is strong enough spiritually to be a doormat for that type of thing and survive it for long. Remember my definition for codependency? Calling evil good in the name of love.

If God made us able to handle evil, then we'd enjoy it. We'd enjoy murder, strife, and jealousy. The reason evil behaviors and situations hurt so bad is because He didn't create us to be victimized. God did not design it to be a part of our life. That's why it's foreign to us, and that's why it hurts so badly.

As a pastor in our church, in dealing with abuse in a marriage, I tell the couple to either get it together or get out of it because everything else is fraud and sin. Be hot, be cold, but don't stay in it if you're only lukewarm. The Lord said about His Church and His relationship with it as His wife:

> **¹⁵I know thy works, that thou art neither cold nor hot: I would thou wert cold or hot. ¹⁶So then because thou art lukewarm, and neither cold nor hot, I will spue thee out of my mouth.** Rev. 3:15-16

This concept brings everybody to a place of decision; it makes each party confess the answer to the question, "Where is your treasure?" Is the wife that man's treasure? If I tell him to get it together or get out of it, he's going to have to make up his mind. The Bible says, "As a man thinketh in his heart, so he is" (Prov. 23:7). It's the same for the wife; either "get it together, or get out of it." I am not condoning divorce; I am also not condoning fraud. I am against fraud. Marriage is a sacramental union, or it is a fraud. God has called us to truth, not to fraudulent relationships.

Many marriages have been saved because I've taken this stand as a pastor. I've had people come to me later and say, "Thank you for taking that stand because we wouldn't have survived it otherwise." Doesn't God bring us to that kind of decision? "Choose what you will have this day; blessings or cursing; life or death" (Deut. 30:19).

I teach the **Ten Commandments of successful relationships**. Your relationship with God and others should be this way:

1.	Communicate	6.	Communicate
2.	Communicate	7.	Communicate
3.	Comunicate	8.	Communicate
4.	Communicate	9.	Communicate
5.	Repent	10.	Repent

If we would do this with God, and with each other, we could turn the world upside down. First, beginning in our own lives, then in our families and then in our churches, in our governments, our societies, and then the world.

I've been involved with many people, helping them in their lives, and I came up with an incredible revelation. In my studies of the Word, in my studies of various things, I have never come up with a more astounding revelation than this in all of my life. It has set a standard for helping other people and it has set a standard in my own life.

I finally discovered **the root problem for misunderstandings**. Would you like to know what it is? This is incredible. The root problem for misunderstandings **is that somebody just didn't understand.**

It seems very simple, and if we could go directly to that level, we would eliminate all misunderstandings. If we try to find out who misunderstood, we end up in a war zone over the misunderstanding. All we need to do is go back and communicate; then, if we need to, repent...and the misunderstanding is resolved. The Word is very clear; do we have a problem with our brother? Go to your brother directly and communicate. If you need to repent about past actions, do so, and then make peace with your brother. That's the Word. I like it, don't you?

> **[22]But I say unto you, That whosoever is angry with his brother without a cause shall be in danger of the judgment: and whosoever shall say to his brother, Raca, shall be in danger of the council: but whosoever shall say, Thou fool, shall be in danger of hell fire. [23]Therefore if thou bring thy gift to the altar, and there rememberest that thy brother hath ought against thee; [24]Leave there thy gift before the altar, and go thy way; first be reconciled to thy brother, and then come and offer thy gift.** Matthew 5:22-24

Promise without discernment is still bondage

The Word says—we see through a glass darkly,

> **[12]For now we see through a glass, darkly; but then face to face: now I know in part; but then shall I know even as also I am known.** 1 Cor. 13:12

and I'd like to turn on a light in that darkness. I want you to have a better life. I want you to have a happier life, a saner life, and a life that's filled with more health because the Word promises it to you.

But there are conditions. *With freedom comes great responsibility.* Freedom comes with a high price; it requires an effort. The Bible says this in James 4:7:

> [7]**Submit yourselves therefore to God. Resist the devil, and he will flee from you.** James 4:7

What does resisting require? An effort! I know that God does the work in us, but He requires our participation. That is an effort. Why does God ask us to have discernment and to put forth an effort in order to obtain freedom? Eziekel 18:32 and 2 Peter 3:9 tell you why.

> [32]**For I have no pleasure in the death of him that dieth, saith the Lord GOD: wherefore turn** *yourselves,* **and live ye.** Ezekiel 18:32

> [9]**The Lord is not slack concerning his promise, as some men count slackness; but is longsuffering to us-ward, not willing that any should perish, but that all should come to repentance.** 2 Peter 3:9

In Ezekiel 18, God is defending the charge made by the people of Israel that He is not fair. 2 Corinthians 7:1 says—Dearly beloved let us therefore cleanse ourselves from all filthiness of the flesh and the spirit."

> [7:1]**Having therefore these promises, dearly beloved, let us cleanse ourselves from all filthiness of the flesh and spirit, perfecting holiness in the fear of God.** 2 Cor. 7:1

In each of these verses an action on our part is required.

Condemnation is of the devil. In the book of Revelation it says, "The accuser of the brethren is cast down, who accused them before God day and night" (Rev. 12:10). Have you ever heard that voice in your head that tells you how rotten you are and that you are a failure and always will be? Condemnation is of the devil.

Conviction is because of God's love for us. The Holy Spirit was sent to the earth some 2,000 years ago to dwell in each individual believer, to seal our spirits for God forever, to lead us into all truth, to be our comforter, our guide, and to raise us up on that day (refer to John 14). Isn't that fantastic?

I hope that you're being nourished in my teaching. I hope you are being edified. I hope you are being built up. I hope I can represent a better life so that 3 John 2 can be fulfilled—dearly beloved I wish above all things that you prosper and be in good health even as your soul prospers.

> [2]**Beloved, I wish above all things that thou mayest prosper and be in health, even as thy soul prospereth.** 3 John 1:2

I am not into *"name it and claim it."* I'm not into being presumptuous; I don't believe that God is a slot machine so put a nickel in and you'll get something out. That is not what Scripture teaches.

God is faithful, and He wants to bless you, and you don't have to pump Him up. He is already pumped up. He came and died for you. He laid His life down, died for us and He wants to bless you. He wants to do more than bless you. He wants you to be like Him. From glory to glory we are being changed into His image.

> **[18]But we all, with open face beholding as in a glass the glory of the Lord, are changed into the same image from glory to glory, *even* as by the Spirit of the Lord.** 2 Cor. 3:18

God, *Elohiym,* said, in Genesis 1:26:

> **[26]And God said, Let us make man in our image, after our likeness: and let them have dominion over the fish of the sea, and over the fowl of the air, and over the cattle, and over all the earth, and over every creeping thing that creepeth upon the earth.** Genesis 1:26

The work of God in the earth today is one of *sanctification.* Often you will not receive healing and deliverance from God without first submitting to God. Why do we call Him "Lord"?

Scripture gives us the answer in Romans 14:11—every knee shall bow, every tongue shall confess that He is Lord (Jesus).

> **[11]For it is written, *As* I live, saith the Lord, every knee shall bow to me, and every tongue shall confess to God.** Romans 14:11

> **[23]I have sworn by myself, the word is gone out of my mouth *in* righteousness, and shall not return, That unto me every knee shall bow, every tongue shall swear.** Isaiah 45:23

I am reminded of another scripture about humbling yourself before God so that He will raise you up in due season.

> **[6]Humble yourselves therefore under the mighty hand of God, that he may exalt you in due time:** 1 Peter 5:6

Also, Matthew 6:33—seek ye first the kingdom of God and His righteousness and then all these things shall be added unto you.

> **[33]But seek ye first the kingdom of God, and his righteousness; and all these things shall be added unto you.** Matthew 6:33

What is the predicator? The action that must come first? Seek God and His righteousness then all things shall be added unto you (Matthew 6:33). Draw nigh to God and He'll draw nigh unto you. Humble yourself before the Lord and He will lift you up.

> **[8]Draw nigh to God, and he will draw nigh to you. Cleanse *your* hands, *ye* sinners; and purify *your* hearts, *ye* double minded. [9]Be afflicted, and mourn, and weep: let your laughter be turned to mourning, and *your* joy to heaviness. [10]Humble yourselves in the sight of the Lord, and he shall lift you up.** James 4:8-10

Peter 5:6-9 says:

> **[6]Humble yourselves therefore under the mighty hand of God, that he may exalt you in due time: [7]Casting all your care upon him; for he careth for you. [8]Be sober, be vigilant; because your adversary the devil, as a roaring lion, walketh about, seeking whom he may devour: [9]Whom resist stedfast in the**

faith, knowing that the same afflictions are accomplished in your brethren that are in the world. 1 Peter 5:6-9

Wow!

I want to remind you that Matthew, Mark, Luke, John, and the book of Acts are a demonstration of God's love through the Lord and through the Apostles in the early church. Then, from Romans to Jude, God deals with our **sanctification**.

Without sanctification, you won't see Matthew, Mark, Luke, John and Acts made manifest in your life. There is little sanctification being taught today, and that is why we don't see many healed or delivered. It wasn't that the Lord did away with miracles, healing and deliverance; it is that long-term He could not perform them unless the Church submitted to Him in holiness. That teaching is given to us in the teachings of Paul.

Manic Depression

Manic Depression is a genetic defect disease. On a wall in my office I have a chart of the chromosomes. In the X chromosome, on the 27th section, you will find Manic Depression/Bipolar Disorder. The specific defective gene that produces it can be identified by science. It is a recessive gene passed down through the mother. This is a rollover of genetic defect. This defect produces a reduction in the secretion of serotonin.

Prozac is a serotonin enhancer. It doesn't increase the secretion of serotonin; it just keeps it out on the end of the dendrite in the nerve synapse longer, which balances the imbalance. It doesn't solve the problem.

Drugs do not solve problems; in fact drugs can interfere with dealing with root problems because they mask the real issues.

I don't tell people to get off their drugs; that would be the stupidest thing I ever said. If you are taking prescription drugs, and you are getting before God and dealing with the issues in your life, under a doctor's supervision, you can get detoxified gradually. Your body will pitch a fit if you try to take away the new chemical reality that's been created by drug therapy. *God created us perfect in Adam. In sin, we have become imperfect.*

As a minister, I hold out for the removal of depression as a spiritual defect. *Depression is the cause of the under-secretion of serotonin.*

There was a wonderful lady in America who called me. Her sister had been helped by our ministry. She said, "Pastor, I've got to have help. I'm a professional and an alcoholic; my marriage is disintegrating; I'm at odds with my family; I'm about to lose my job; I'm on *Prozac,* and I'm coming apart."

In two 30-minute sessions, over the phone, over a two-week period, God delivered her from alcoholism, healed her of a broken heart, and delivered her of the depression and anxiety. I saw her last January; she is happy, her marriage has been restored, she has been restored to fellowship with her family, she's never touched alcohol again, and she was off *Prozac* by the end of the first week after her healing. She's vibrant, she's going to church, she's active in her church body, and is enthusiastically alive. We sat down together and just rejoiced before the Lord, Who had healed her and delivered her.

A more excellent way is not to be artificially maintained. If God wanted you to be artificially maintained, He would have set in motion artificial maintenance programs for His people. He created you perfect. He created you with an immune system, a body that was designed to take care of itself for 70 to 80 years and past 70 with some trouble. That is what Moses said in Psalm 90, with some trouble.

> **[10]The days of our years *are* threescore years and ten; and if by reason of strength *they be* fourscore years, yet *is* their strength labour and sorrow; for it is soon cut off, and we fly away.** Psalm 90:10

God established longevity over 3,000 years ago.

The average life expectancy in America is around 76 right now. We still have not exceeded God's parameters, and won't, as an average, until the coming of the Lord and the day of the Lord in the first resurrection. You can try to live to be 120, as an average, if you want to, and you'll be dead before you get there! It is appointed to a man once to die, and then the judgment.

> **[27]And as it is appointed unto men once to die, but after this the judgment:** Hebrews 9:27

We have our part in the first resurrection. Blessed are they who have part in the first resurrection because they shall not taste of the second death (Rev. 20:6).

> **[6]Blessed and holy *is* he that hath part in the first resurrection: on such the second death hath no power, but they shall be priests of God and of Christ, and shall reign with him a thousand years.** Rev. 20:6

Isn't that good news?

> **[8]We are confident, *I say,* and willing rather to be absent from the body, and to be present with the Lord.** 2 Cor. 5:8

> **[20]According to my earnest expectation and *my* hope, that in nothing I shall be ashamed, but *that* with all boldness, as always, *so* now also Christ shall be magnified in my body, whether *it be* by life, or by death. [21]For to me to live *is* Christ, and to die *is* gain. [22]But if I live in the flesh, this *is* the fruit of my labour: yet what I shall choose I wot not. [23]For I am in a strait betwixt two, having a desire to depart, and to be with Christ; which is far better:** Philip. 1:20-23

Isn't that a great hope? Takes care of anxiety and fear, doesn't it.

Eye has not seen, ear has not heard nor has it entered into the heart of man what God has prepared for them that love Him (1 Cor 2:9).

> **[4]For since the beginning of the world *men* have not heard, nor perceived by the ear, neither hath the eye seen, O God, beside thee, *what* he hath prepared for him that waiteth for him.** Isaiah 64:4

> ⁹**For we are labourers together with God: ye are God's husbandry,** *ye are* **God's building.** 1 Cor. 3:9

I want to be there, how about you? That is my hope: the redemption of my body to what God has prepared for me is the hope that I have.

> ²³**And not only** *they,* **but ourselves also, which have the firstfruits of the Spirit, even we ourselves groan within ourselves, waiting for the adoption,** *to wit,* **the redemption of our body.** Romans 8:23

I'm a happy Henry. I used to be a sad Henry, and now I'm a happy Henry, because whether I live or whether I die, I know that I am the Lord's.

Attention Deficit Disorder

There are three ranges: the lower range, the mid range, and the high range. The high range is hyperactivity. We primarily deal with ADD in children. Dealing with ADD in adults is more difficult. ADD is coming out of a **dumb and deaf spirit.** There are many classes of psychological diseases that fall under the category of dumb and deaf. Jesus cast out a dumb and deaf spirit from a person who could not speak (see Matthew 11:5; Mark 7:32, 37; Mark 9:25; Luke 7:22).

> ²⁵**When Jesus saw that the people came running together, he rebuked the foul spirit, saying unto him,** *Thou* **dumb and deaf spirit, I charge thee, come out of him, and enter no more into him.** Mark 9:25

Epilepsy

The **dumb and deaf spirit** is also found in *Epilepsy.* I have not failed to see healing in cases of epilepsy in 15 years of ministry. Every epileptic that has come to us has been healed although there is never any guarantee for healing. These healings I make reference to have been documented through EEG tests in which the Alpha, Beta and Theta brain waves were normal. These individuals have never had another seizure and are not on any medication. But in order to get that healing, we had to go back to the gospels to learn how to do it. In these cases, it wasn't a spiritual root causing the problem. I had to cast an evil spirit out. I don't make a big deal out of it, but I've cast out legions of them. That's what God wants done. I am well able, as every believer should be, to deal with it if necessary.

Psychologists have been able to document that many of our personality characteristics including rage, anger, predisposition to mental disorders and certain diseases, can be found in humans without any genetic component, but it can still be inherited. There is not a genetic or a defective gene that has been isolated, but the condition is still passed on in families. We consider those situations to be *inherited familiar spirits* that follow families to create various breakdowns in the psyche or the soul.

Dumb and deaf spirits rule over the second heavens and try to control the minds of men. Your mind is the Lord's, your spirit is the Lord's, and your body is the temple of the Holy Ghost. You are the Lord's and the enemy of your life, Satan, wants to rule you in your thoughts.

I don't believe the devil can read your mind. That would make him omniscient and he's not. His kingdom can project thoughts into your head out of the realm of the spirit, and what you do with those thoughts is up to you.

Paul said in 2 Corinthians 10:5 that we are to bring every thought into captivity, casting down every imagination and every thought that would exalt itself against the knowledge of God.

> **⁵Casting down imaginations, and every high thing that exalteth itself against the knowledge of God, and bringing into captivity every thought to the obedience of Christ; 2 Cor. 10:5**

I have to subject my thoughts to higher thoughts all the time. His ways are higher than my ways, and His thoughts are greater than my thoughts (Isaiah 55:8).

> **⁸For my thoughts *are* not your thoughts, neither *are* your ways my ways, saith the LORD. Isaiah 55:8**

The most man's wisdom could ever be just begins to approach the foolishness of God according to Scripture.

> **²⁵Because the foolishness of God is wiser than men; and the weakness of God is stronger than men. 1 Cor. 1:25**

That means we have a long way to go.

My mind has to be renewed by the washing of the water of the Word (Ephesians 4:23; 5:26) and I have to bring every thought into captivity of the knowledge of God (2 Cor. 10:5).

It says in 2 Timothy 1:7 that God has not given me the spirit of fear, but of power, love and a sound mind.

> **⁷For God hath not given us the spirit of fear; but of power, and of love, and of a sound mind. 2 Tim. 1:7**

What do you think I am holding out for? Power, love and a sound mind!

Knowing God's Word

When we get into certain difficulties we find that at some point in our family trees, or in our own lives, our minds and our spirits have been opened up to the other kingdom. We've listened to those voices, and we have followed modalities of thought, and precepts that are diametrically opposed to what God has said in His Word. *The biggest problem that I find in the Christian Church today is that Christians do not know the Word of God.*

A workman that needeth not be ashamed rightly dividing the word of truth (2 Tim 2:15).

> **¹⁵Study to shew thyself approved unto God, a workman that needeth not to be ashamed, rightly dividing the word of truth. 2 Tim. 2:15**

This comes from sitting down with the Word and letting God speak to you. Study the Scripture for yourself. Don't be swayed by new doctrines or whims that come along—study!

When I first came back to God, I would sit down every morning at 6:00 until 7:30 before I went to my business. Week after week, month after month, for 1 1/2 hours, I plowed into that Word. After months of study, the Bible exploded for me from cover to cover. That's where you begin. That's God's will and that's God's Word and if you mix it with your faith, and take it into your heart, you will never be the same. You will change your life, your families' lives, your city, your church, and your world.

In *occultism*, the real thing is hidden and something false is offering itself as if it were the real thing.

Most of the mental diseases that we have identified in mankind today are the result of separation from God's Word, which is the mind and will of God concerning all things. The revealed will of God and the living Word for mankind to follow can be found in the pages of Scripture. When we follow other ways of thinking, other gods and other spiritual leaders that are not set up by God, ordained by God, in covenant with God, anointed by God, or established by God, we have opened up our spirits to forces that are designed to steal our faith and bring us torment.

ALL FEAR COMES FROM NOT TRUSTING GOD AND HIS WORD.

The Word says:

⁶Be careful for nothing; but in every thing by prayer and supplication with thanksgiving let your requests be made known unto God. Philip. 4:6

¹⁸In every thing give thanks: for this is the will of God in Christ Jesus concerning you. 1 Thes. 5:18

³⁴Take therefore no thought for the morrow: for the morrow shall take thought for the things of itself. Sufficient unto the day *is* the evil thereof. Matthew 6:34

We are so busy dragging the past around with us, and projecting it to the future, that we forget to occupy today. If our minds, spirits, and souls are filled with fear and confusion, projection and avoidance, we are no earthly good today. We are preoccupied with dragging this junk around, and projecting it into the future. That's why we need Prozac, Valium, and sleeping pills. That's why we have ulcers.

Forget the past, forget the future.

LET GOD BE GOD TODAY IN YOUR LIFE!

The evil of today is sufficient unto itself (Matthew 6:34).

³⁴Take therefore no thought for the morrow: for the morrow shall take thought for the things of itself. Sufficient unto the day *is* the evil thereof. Matthew 6:34

Your life hangs in the balance. *Make sure you are in the right kingdom all the time.*

Paranoid Schizophrenia

Paranoid schizophrenia is a non-genetic disease of the mind or the soul, which can be inherited non-genetically. It is a classic example of what Scripture calls double mindedness.

> **⁸A double minded man *is* unstable in all his ways.** James 1:8

"Schizo" means split or divided, and paranoid means split because of fear, delusions, and projected delusions. Paranoid schizophrenia is the result of a malfunctioning of at least two of the neurotransmitters in the body. It is the result of an over-secretion of norepinephrine, and an over-secretion of dopamine. Now there is some investigation that says it is also an over-secretion of serotonin.

God created us very chemically. He created us that way in our homeostasis, and in our glandular construction. Our glands add the secretions here and there, so that in a normal situation, our homeostasis is maintained in a very perfect way. When your thinking is interrupted both on a psychological level and a spiritual level, your body responds to that breakdown in thought or feeling, or emotions, or perceptions.

As Scripture says, you are being "tossed to and fro" (Ephesians 4:14). You may be regressing in a shield of veneer, not wanting to become vulnerable or transparent, or you may overextend into assertiveness to hide. You either withdraw or you project up front to hide what's behind. You either withdraw, hold up a shield, or you take the shield away and create a new one called a *fabricated personality.* Bullies are that way. The bully is more afraid of you than you are of him; you just don't know it. The facade he projects is there to protect his inadequacies and his fears and his feelings of rejection.

How many of us find ourselves struggling between either withdrawing in a house of fear or stepping out in fabricated personalities that we hide behind? *How many of us are really who God created us to be from the beginning?* Psalm 139 says—from the beginning, from the foundation of the world, God knew you. Before your parts were in continuance fashioned from the very dust of the earth, God knew you (Psalm 139:13-16).

> **¹³For thou hast possessed my reins: thou hast covered me in my mother's womb. ¹⁴I will praise thee; for I am fearfully *and* wonderfully made: marvellous *are* thy works; and *that* my soul knoweth right well. ¹⁵My substance was not hid from thee, when I was made in secret, *and* curiously wrought in the lowest parts of the earth. ¹⁶Thine eyes did see my substance, yet being unperfect; and in thy book all *my members* were written, *which* in continuance were fashioned, when *as yet there was* none of them.** Psalm 139:13-16

You are not an accident in your generation. God said to Jeremiah—before you were ever conceived, I ordained you to become a prophet to the nations (Jeremiah 1:5).

> **⁵Before I formed thee in the belly I knew thee; and before thou camest forth out of the womb I sanctified thee, *and* I ordained thee a prophet unto the nations.** Jeremiah 1:5

Paul told us that God ordained him to be an apostle to the Gentiles.

> **[15]But when it pleased God, who separated me from my mother's womb, and called *me* by his grace, [16]To reveal his Son in me, that I might preach him among the heathen; immediately I conferred not with flesh and blood:** Galatians 1:15-16

> **[4]According as he hath chosen us in him before the foundation of the world, that we should be holy and without blame before him in love:** Ephes. 1:4

> **[1:1]Paul, a servant of Jesus Christ, called *to be* an apostle, separated unto the gospel of God,** Romans 1:1

Like Paul, it is clear that you are no accident, and that in your generation, God has called you and elected you, and selected you, to be a viable part of His corporate body in the earth.

> **[9]But ye *are* a chosen generation, a royal priesthood, an holy nation, a peculiar people; that ye should shew forth the praises of him who hath called you out of darkness into his marvellous light: [10]Which in time past *were* not a people, but *are* now the people of God: which had not obtained mercy, but now have obtained mercy.** 1 Peter 2:9-10

Would you mind getting on with it?

In 1 Corinthians 12, we see that everyone is important to the whole picture. If I could strip the facade off you today, and drag you screaming out of your prison house, and plunk you down on this planet and release you by the power of the Holy Spirit to be what God created you to be in your generation, wouldn't that be a miracle?

I would like to ask you a question. If I strip from you all the veneers of life and all the protective mechanisms, all the defensive mechanisms, fear and rejection tragedies of your life coming from victimization, fear of man, fear of rejection, fear of failure, fear of abandonment, and unloveliness, guilt, rejection, and self-hatred; if I stripped all of that away from you, *who would you be?*

If I could strip all of this away from you, there is a good chance all of your diseases would go away. All of your diseases are the result of what you carry around; I call it the plaque of life. Just like when you go to the dentist to have the plaque on your teeth removed, it's time to do some spiritual cleaning.

We'll be looking at Fear, Stress and Physiology, and you'll find just how powerful Satan is. The power of Satan is *fear*. Do you know why? I'll give you the scripture—the devil, knowing his time is short, goes about like a roaring lion seeking whom he may devour (1 Peter 5:8).

> **[8]Be sober, be vigilant; because your adversary the devil, as a roaring lion, walketh about, seeking whom he may devour:** 1 Peter 5:8

> **[12]...for the devil is come down unto you, having great wrath, because he knoweth that he hath but a short time.** Rev. 12:12

The devil knows his time is short. His days have been numbered. Remember in Daniel 5:25-28:

> **²⁵And this *is* the writing that was written, MENE, MENE, TEKEL, UPHARSIN. ²⁶This *is* the interpretation of the thing: MENE; God hath numbered thy kingdom, and finished it. ²⁷TEKEL; Thou art weighed in the balances, and art found wanting. ²⁸PERES; Thy kingdom is divided, and given to the Medes and Persians.** Daniel 5:25-28

Satan has been numbered and he has been found wanting in the balances and his very soul and spirit person is required for judgment. That's where our archenemy is headed. And because he knows he is already judged, because he knows he has lost, and because he's a sore loser, he is going about trying to convince you, like a bully, that God has lost and he has won.

Now you can listen to that lie if you want, but that's why the enemy is so powerful – he is in fear. His greatest fear is eternal banishment to the lake of fire and that's where he's headed, and all his angels with him. That's their destiny.

In dealing with mental and psychological diseases, we find that deaf and dumb spirits can attach themselves to you and control your mind. *Why do you halt between two opinions?*

> **²¹And Elijah came unto all the people, and said, How long halt ye between two opinions? if the LORD *be* God, follow him: but if Baal, *then* follow him. And the people answered him not a word.** 1 Kings 18:21

Choose! Remember, that was Israel's great challenge; do you want to follow Moloch or do you want to follow the God of Israel? What do you want to do? In the scripture above, the people did not answer. When asked this question by Moses in the sanctification of Israel in Exodus 24:3, they said, "All the words which the Lord hath said we will do." Did they? No, they lied, and went their own way. Such is the case many times today! We hear God's word and say nothing or we say we will and we don't.

How many of us say we are following God, we're "believers," but in our real life we are following the other kingdom? We come and say, "Yea, Lord," but in real life, we forget the Lord and follow the voice of the goat, the enemy.

When you are following fear, you are not following God. 2 Corinthians 10:5 says—holding every thought in captivity, casting down every vain imagination, holding every thought up against the knowledge of God.

> **⁵Casting down imaginations, and every high thing that exalteth itself against the knowledge of God, and bringing into captivity every thought to the obedience of Christ;** 2 Cor. 10:5

Everybody quotes that one. Everyone knows that one. Do you ever quote verse 6?

You know 2 Corinthians 10:5 as well as you know John 3:16 and Hebrews 4:12. But nobody quotes Hebrews 4:13 and nobody quotes 2 Corinthians 10:6. I want you to defeat the enemy. I'm looking for something to happen inside of you.

2 Corinthians 10:6 says—having a readiness to revenge all disobedience after your obedience is fulfilled.

> **⁶And having in a readiness to revenge all disobedience, when your obedience is fulfilled.** 2 Cor. 10:6

You cannot defeat your enemy in disobedience. You cannot be healed of your disease and continue to be disobedient to God and His Word when He's told you in it what's causing your disease. You cannot expect to be healed of anxiety and fear disorders if you continue to operate in fear and anxiety and stress and tension. You can quote all the scriptures about being anxious for nothing (Phil. 4:6)

> **⁶Be careful for nothing; but in every thing by prayer and supplication with thanksgiving let your requests be made known unto God.** Philip. 4:6

and God has not given us the spirit of fear (2 Tim. 1:7),

> **⁷For God hath not given us the spirit of fear; but of power, and of love, and of a sound mind.** 2 Tim. 1:7

but unless you are prepared to make fear your enemy, you are wasting your time quoting the promises.

Are you ready to do a little circumcision? Are you ready to put to death those things that didn't come from God? Are you prepared to come before God in trust and in love, not in condemnation, and to become transparent with Him?

James 5:16 talks about confessing our faults one to another that we may be healed.

> **¹⁶Confess *your* faults one to another, and pray one for another, that ye may be healed...** James 5:16

The problem today is that we have become so dysfunctional, we don't trust each other. We don't even trust our own husbands or wives. Husbands don't talk to their wives and wives don't talk to their husbands about the deep torments of their heart.

They believe that their spouse already has so many problems, their own burdens are just one more thing to add to the situation. Just one more fight on top of the six they already have had. *Have we lost our way?*

If my wife can't talk to me, who in the world do you think I should send her to? If my family can't live in peace in my home, where do you think I should send them to, to have peace in this planet? If I can't love my wife, who do you think I should send her to, to get love?

We're in prison houses. God has not called you to bondage. He's called you to freedom. If we walk in the light together as He is in the light, then we have fellowship one with another.

> **⁷But if we walk in the light, as he is in the light, we have fellowship one with another, and the blood of Jesus Christ his Son cleanseth us from all sin.** 1 John 1:7

If you confess your sin to me, I'm going to love you in it. Galatians 6:1 says—if a brother be overtaken in a fault, those of you who consider yourself spiritual, restore such a one in the spirit of meekness and consider yourself also lest you be tempted in like manner and fall away.

> **⁶·¹Brethren, if a man be overtaken in a fault, ye which are spiritual, restore such an one in the spirit of meekness; considering thyself, lest thou also be tempted. ²Bear ye one another's burdens, and so fulfil the law of Christ.** Galatians 6:1-2

Verse 2: Bear ye one another's burdens and so ye fulfil the law of Christ.

God forbid that anybody have a problem in most churches; the one way to get the left hand of fellowship is to have a problem. We hide behind our fears because we are supposed to be "so spiritual." Maybe we should go back and take a good look at Jesus' disciples to see the kind of people He had in His ministry: thieves, betrayers, unlearned, ignorant, fearful, and the list goes on.

I had a meeting with my staff two months ago, because God is adding people to our staff as our ministry is growing. I asked them, "Are you prepared to be honest with me about every facet of your life? Are you prepared to share that with your peers? I asked this because my staff was saying, "We need ministry too." I said, "Are you prepared to be ministered to by your peers with my oversight?"

They gulped, "Well, I've got something in my life that I just want to talk to <u>you</u> about, Pastor." I said, "If that member of my staff over there is going to murder you because of this information, I don't need them, let's find out real quick. If I can't trust them with you, I can't trust them with the masses that are coming. We have a sterling reputation nationally to maintain regarding our confidentiality."

I talked to a beautiful young lady yesterday who said, "Pastor, since I've heard your teaching I now have the faith to confess the rest of my problems to my husband, things about me that he doesn't know." I asked her husband, "Are you ready to handle that?" He said, "I'm ready to handle that!" Do you know what's going to happen to that marriage? God's going to come and they are not going to be hiding in fear from a skeleton in the closet. That stuff is going to come before the altar of God and the cleansing power of God is going to come to bind and to heal.

If we had done these things years ago, we wouldn't have these problems today. If we had done these things years ago, we wouldn't be as sick as we are today. Are you ready to be transparent before God and each other?

I ate at a restaurant awhile back, and got a little food poisoning. I got really sick, and the best thing that happened to me was when that stuff came up and I regurgitated. When that poison came up out of my stomach, I was better. Now, it wasn't any fun regurgitating, was it? What would have been worse would have been to let that stuff stay down there for hours and just tear me apart. When it started to come, I gave it a little help. Then I began to feel better.

You can hold every thought in captivity. You can cast all vain imaginations down. You can know the Word of God. You can know truth, and you can be an expert in the law of God *but if you don't live it, it's heresy.* You are able to defeat all evil *when your obedience is fulfilled.*

⁶And having in a readiness to revenge all disobedience, when your obedience is fulfilled. 2 Cor. 10:6

Fear is an enemy. Self-hatred is an enemy. Guilt is an enemy. Condemnation is an enemy. Denial is an enemy. Bitterness, rage, anger, and resentment are all our enemies.

Bitterness

BITTERNESS is a principality of the enemy. Ephesians 6:12 says—our battle is not against flesh and blood but against principalities, powers, spiritual wickedness in high places, and the rulers of the darkness of this world.

¹²For we wrestle not against flesh and blood, but against principalities, against powers, against the rulers of the darkness of this world, against spiritual wickedness in high *places.* Ephes. 6:12

If we are in conflict with one another, I'm not your enemy. You're not my enemy. Do you know the problem we have? *We are not able to separate the person from their sin. Their sin is our enemy – NOT THEM!*

When someone violates us, we make him or her evil along with the evil that they did, don't we? *You've got to be able to separate people from their sin.* God didn't create you from the foundation of the world as a sinner. He created you from the foundation of the world as saints before Him and as His sons and daughters forever. Because of sin, we have become separated from Him. Even after conversion, we still have many things to work out. I want to help you begin to do that today.

Bitterness is a principality; under it and answering to it are seven spirits that reinforce bitterness.

#1 Unforgiveness

When that root of bitterness in Hebrews 12:15 gets a foothold, the first thing that happens is a record of wrongs.

¹⁵Looking diligently lest any man fail of the grace of God; lest any root of bitterness springing up trouble *you,* **and thereby many be defiled;** Hebrews 12:15

How many of you are still having flashbacks about things that have been done against you? If I mention Aunt Sally's name, you'd probably be able to give me 15 reasons why you don't like her. That is unforgiveness. After unforgiveness gets a foothold, and creates a record of wrongs, there's another dimension of the spiritual dynamics and what I am talking about comes into play, and it's called resentment.

#2 Resentment

Resentment is the record of wrongs that is now being fueled by feelings of holding on to it and starting to meditate, chewing on it. It is amazing to me that when we have feelings of resentment, we think about Aunt Sally up here (in our mind), but we feel her down here (in our heart). Why is it that you think about Aunt Sally up here, but you feel her down here? Because your mind is where your soul is, but your spirit is where your heart is. You are a spirit being; you have a soul, and you live in your body.

Resentment is a spiritual problem, not a psychological problem. Bitterness, unforgiveness and resentment are spiritual problems, not psychological problems. You can take these keys and use them in any spiritual conflict you have in your life. This gets us right here in our heart. This is what separates us from others, and it is the foundation of fear that may come later. Fear of man, fear of rejection, fear of failure, fear of abandonment, we go hide.

#3 Retaliation

After resentment gets a foothold then we have retaliation. I saw a bumper sticker the other day that said, "I DON'T FORGIVE, I JUST GET EVEN." Maybe you saw it too. After resentment has started to simmer, we find ways to get back at the person who caused it. Retaliation wants to make the person pay. It's time to get even.

#4 Anger

After retaliation gets a foothold, then anger starts to set in. Unforgiveness, resentment, and retaliation have been building and now a real strong feeling of anger comes along.

Has anyone here experienced anger towards anyone in your lifetime? Did all this other stuff come with it too?

#5 Hatred

After anger sets in, comes hatred. Hatred says this: Because I'm remembering what you did to me, because I have really been meditating on it and I really resent it, I'm going to get even. I'm going to get the pressure cooker going because I'm going to add fuel to this thing and now at this stage you don't have any reason to exist any more, especially in my presence. Hatred says, "There's not even room on this planet for you and me at the same place at the same time." Hatred says, "You and I cannot stay in the same room together."

Hatred starts to develop into the elimination modality.

#6 Violence

After hatred comes violence. Violence says this: before I eliminate you, you're going to feel my pain; you're going to hear my voice; you're going to know my hatred; you're going to experience it.

#7 Murder

Once violence erupts, the final fruit of bitterness is murder.

This can be actual physical murder, or murder with the tongue, which is character assassination or verbal abuse. Whenever I find any of these in a person's life, all the stuff from here (the mind) to here (the heart) is there. I know that if we don't deal with it, its going to go to the heart and take up residence. What am I giving you right now? Discernment.

When hatred, violence and murder are in someone's life, they feel that they are justified and everybody else is going to pay the price. Have you been a victim of this? Did you feel defiled? Have you perhaps made a victim of somebody else on this basis?

Editor's Note: I have found that if any one of these seven areas that answer to bitterness exist, all of the preceding ones will be there from the one area that I noticed; and if left unchecked, all the rest will surely come. For example, if you see hatred in a person, unforgiveness, resentment, retaliation, and anger always precede. Also, each of the seven is progressively worse than the one just preceding it. For example, violence is a much more serious problem than resentment.

Jungian Psychology

Hebrews 4:12 teaches us that the soul and the spirit are distinctively separate.

> **[12]For the word of God *is* quick, and powerful, and sharper than any twoedged sword, piercing *even to the dividing asunder of soul and spirit,* and of the joints and marrow, and *is* a discerner of the thoughts and intents of the heart.** Hebrews 4:12

That is what it says, "Is able to separate the spirit from the soul." One of the great tragedies of psychology in the teaching of Jungian psychology is that it eliminates the *spirit of man* totally and inserts in its place the dualistic compartments of the soul.

In Jungian Psychology and in modern day psychology, there is no such thing as the spirit of man. There is the idealistic compartment of the soul called the "conscious" and the "collective unconscious." In the teachings of Jungian psychology, within the collective unconscious you will find the archetypes and dark shadows. Jungian psychology identifies these dark shadows as the archetypes of our historic ancestry bringing with them the darkness and the evil that we need to come in contact with and identify with so that we can cohabit with the evil of our ancestral line generationally. This is classic Jungian psychotherapy.

I don't find these concepts anywhere in Scripture. What I do find in Scripture is that the archetypes and dark shadows are in fact evil spirits, principalities, powers, and the rulers of the darkness of this world.

> **[12]For we wrestle not against flesh and blood, but against principalities, against powers, against the rulers of the darkness of this world, against spiritual wickedness in high** *places.* Ephes. 6:12

I have a book about Carl Jung written by a secular psychotherapist in Connecticut who did research on Carl Jung. Early on in Carl Jung's investigation into Spiritualism (Spiritism) and into Eastern Mysticism, Carl Jung became a channeler for invisible entities. It's in his writings; the principle entity that he channeled was *a spirit entity called Philemon.* He also channeled two lesser spirit entities called Anima and Animus, who became the foundation of the male and female principles in Jungian psychology. In fact, these principles male/female of Anima and Animus can even be found in Christian ministry/counseling circles as a therapeutic model. These were invisible spirit entities that Carl Jung channeled, by using automatic handwriting (otherwise known as journaling), and they wrote much of our modern-day Jungian psychology through him. This means that much of modern Jungian psychology was written by invisible spirit beings. If you don't believe me you can go to any public library and do your own research on the history of Carl Jung. Over the years I have done much research into his writings that substantiates what I have just said.

Carl Jung, early on in his investigation of Spiritualism (Spiritism) and Mysticism, ran into invisible evil spirits and in his early writings he called them evil spirits. As he developed his precepts, he said: "Because of the failure of Christianity in dealing with the problems of the psyche or the soul of man, and the body, or the diseases of man, *I will create an alternative to Christianity*" because He considered Christianity to be a dead religion. In fact Carl Jung was the son of a German Protestant minister and observed his minister-father preach a gospel that seemed to offer no solution for the diseases of the soul and body. He believed that mankind had to be helped while they lived on planet earth. **Modern-day psychology includes many Jungian principles and is the fruit of the failure of the Christian Church.** Psychology has become a religion and psychologists have become the "pastors" of the Christian Church in matters of the soul. Many times even Christian psychological counselors relegate everything to the dualistic concept of the soul to the exclusion of the *spirit of man.*

Jung believed that modern man would not accept basic concepts of the Bible in view of their scientific way of thinking. He deliberately took the words "evil spirit," changed the concept, and called them "archetypes" and "dark shadows" to accommodate himself to a more scientific approach, and *he duped mankind, including the Christian Church and lastly, even himself.*

I am a pastor and not a psychologist. I am a student of God and His Word. I'm a son of God by faith and I'm a shepherd of the Most High God by His permission.

Hebrews 4:12 says—the word of God is able to separate the soul from the spirit.

¹²For the word of God *is* quick, and powerful, and sharper than any twoedged sword, piercing even to the dividing asunder of soul and spirit, and of the joints and marrow, and *is* a discerner of the thoughts and intents of the heart. Hebrews 4:12

This scripture makes the dualistic compartment of the soul taught by Jungian psychology a heresy. You know what heresy is, don't you? It's a statement of truth that is not truth. It doesn't match up with the Word.

I'm not into inner healing. I'm not into inner healing that is taught by certain practitioners. I go far beyond that. *I'm into the sanctification of the human spirit.* I begin with the sanctification of the human spirit, and when we finally get it straight upstairs (soul), then our bodies start to conform to the Word and the life of the living God. It comes from obedience (2 Corinthians 10:6) where Scripture tells us to have a readiness to revenge all disobedience.

> **⁶And having in a readiness to revenge all disobedience, when your obedience is fulfilled. 2 Cor. 10:6**

The focus of discernment is found in Hebrews 4:12 where we learn that the Word of God is able to separate the soul from the spirit.

Now let's quote Hebrews 4:13 (which no one hardly ever quotes in conjunction with verse 12):

> **¹³Neither is there any creature that is not manifest in his sight: but all things *are* naked and opened unto the eyes of him with whom we have to do. Hebrews 4:13**

What things are naked before Him? Who are the creatures that are manifested in His sight? I'll tell you who the creatures are in this verse. It's Satan and his kingdom of the second heavens that try to rule mankind; Satan is called the god of this world, the ruler of men's spirits and the ruler of men's minds. It is the principalities and powers, spiritual wickedness in high places, the rulers of the darkness of this world. These creatures are the rulers of men's spirits and the rulers of men's minds. These creatures are the archetypes and dark shadows of Jungian psychology that reside not in the collective unconscious compartment of the human soul but reside in the human spirit because they are spirit, comparing like with like. For example, 2 Timothy 1:7 says:

> **⁷For God hath not given us the spirit of fear; but of power, and of love, and of a sound mind. 2 Tim. 1:7**

Fear is a spirit and can control our thoughts both in spirit and in soul.

But we've been called out of that darkness. We've been called out of that occultism. We've been called out of that and into the new birth. We have been redeemed through the shed blood of our Lord, Jesus Christ. Did we come all the way out of the darkness so that God could not reveal to us our enemies? You see, our enemies are not flesh and blood; our enemies are not the Russians or the Chinese. God loves the Russians and the Chinese. Our enemies are Satan and his fallen followers, the principalities, the powers, the spiritual wickedness in high places, and rulers of darkness of this world.

2 Timothy 1:7 says, "God has not given us the spirit of fear." There is normal fear that God has given so we don't play in traffic, or jump off a cliff thinking we can fly. There is a normal *fight or flight* pattern that God has developed in us.

There is also a kingdom out there that wants to be a part of your life. *The Church is incredibly ignorant about its enemy. Out of sight, out of mind seems to be a protective mentality in the Christian Church but I will tell you – out of sight, out of mind is not a spiritual principle.* Some spiritual warfare conferences are nothing more than shadow boxing. I'm here to tell you that we're going to defeat the devil and know him and his kingdom. Amen?

The devil is *not* omnipresent. We learned that from Job. The Sons of God came to present themselves before the LORD, and Satan came with them. The LORD said, "What have you been up to, Big Boy?" Satan said, "I've been walking up and down throughout the earth" (Job 1:7).

> [7]**And the LORD said unto Satan, Whence comest thou? Then Satan answered the LORD, and said, From going to and fro in the earth, and from walking up and down in it.** Job 1:7

If he were omnipresent, he wouldn't have to walk up and down on the earth. He's not omnipresent. He oversees a bureaucracy that is invisible called *the second heaven.* You're living in the first heaven; the third heaven is where God is.

Paul says—I was caught up into the third heaven (2 Corinthians 12:2).

> [2]**I knew a man in Christ above fourteen years ago, (whether in the body, I cannot tell; or whether out of the body, I cannot tell: God knoweth;) such an one caught up to the third heaven. [3]And I knew such a man, (whether in the body, or out of the body, I cannot tell: God knoweth;) [4]How that he was caught up into paradise, and heard unspeakable words, which it is not lawful for a man to utter.** 2 Cor. 12:2-4

If there is a first heaven and a third heaven, what comes in between? The second heaven. Satan is called the prince of the power of the air.

> [2]**Wherein in time past ye walked according to the course of this world, according to the prince of the power of the air, the spirit that now worketh in the children of disobedience:** Ephes. 2:2

> [4]**In whom the god of this world hath blinded the minds of them which believe not, lest the light of the glorious gospel of Christ, who is the image of God, should shine unto them.** 2 Cor. 4:4

He's called the god of mankind. His domain is the second heaven.

You need to wake up! No more shadow boxing. I'm going to resist the devil today. No, I'm not; I'm going to defeat fear in my life. That's my enemy. I'm going to defeat bigotry in my life because that's my enemy. I'm going to defeat self-hatred in my life because that's my enemy. I'm going to defeat anger in my life because that's my enemy. These are powers that answer to Satan and serve him.

If I'm around someone who has violence, do you know what I'm looking for? I don't tell them to stop being violent; they couldn't stop if they tried. When I am around people who are like that, I want to find out what happened. Where's that root? I'm looking for the creature. I must divide. If I can get you right spiritually, then your mind will catch up.

I'm a student of the psychology of man, not from a Jungian perspective but from a biblical perspective. I do a lot of ministry with people once we get them changed spiritually, and get the critters and creatures removed. Then we have to come back and help them get their minds renewed.

Teaching on Memory

We think on two levels. Did you know that you are a spirit? Your spirit man thinks and your intellect thinks independently of your spirit man. That's why Hebrews 4:12 says—the Word of God comes to separate the soul from the spirit. Why? To get God's Word to enter into your human spirit so your mind is renewed by the washing of the water of the Word as you continually apply it. When your mind and your spirit were one in a way of thinking that lined up with Satan's mind, you followed Satan.

As a work of the Holy Spirit, Who shall lead you into all truth, your spirit and your soul now become one in God's way of thinking, following God. But in the process of becoming one in God's way of thinking, there's a great gap that has to be worked out. This is the stuff that tears at you. This is the stuff that doesn't want to let you change your way of thinking. Changing your thinking is really scary because your mind will pitch a fit.

Now, let me help you understand how this works.

When I have ministered to somebody who has been subjected to some kind of tragedy, or victimization, and the result was wounding of their human spirit, they still remember the tragedy. I can't take your memory away from you, because it is your soul. The Bible says your soul will be saved. How is your soul saved? Your soul is part of your brain cells. When you die, your brain cells die with your body but the mirror image of the soul thoughts remain with your spirit which returns to God to await the resurrection. In fact, the Bible says in that day (resurrection) you will be known as you were known.

> [12]**For now we see through a glass, darkly; but then face to face: now I know in part; but then shall I know even as also I am known.** 1 Cor. 13:12

> [14]**I am the good shepherd, and know my** *sheep,* **and am known of mine.** John 10:14

> [39]**But we are not of them who draw back unto perdition; but of them that believe to the saving of the soul.** Hebrews 10:39

> [20]**Let him know, that he which converteth the sinner from the error of his way shall save a soul from death, and shall hide a multitude of sins.** James 5:20

This is how it works. We have short-term and long-term memory. Short-term memory and long-term memory are made up of units of memory called "memes." You have individual memes, you have mass memes, and you have cultural memes (inherited or learned).

There is a Christian leader in the world right now named George Otis, Jr. I don't know if you know who he is. He is doing sociological and spiritual mapping of the planet with respect to spiritual bondage involving mass memes and cultural memes.

There are principalities that rule nations. We know that from Daniel. You know that the prince of Persia and the prince of Grecia were invisible principalities ruling from the heavenlies on behalf of Satan over nations (Daniel 10). Another invisible principality that rules over nations is Gog, as found in Ezekiel 38-39. In my opinion, this invisible principality that serves Satan is the invisible ruler over Islam today.

How is Satan the god of this world? He controls the minds of men with a gospel that is not the gospel of our Lord, through the modalities of religiosity, ethnicity, sociology, and the gods of this world. He controls minds yet he and his kingdom are an invisible spirit form.

How many of you have ever changed your theology in your life?

How many of you have discovered in your life that you had something called "stinkin' thinkin' "? Were you proud of it? How many of you have ever changed your mind? It's a woman's prerogative, but it's a little more difficult for the men to do. It's just a way of life for the women! Just kidding.

How many of you remember the erroneous thinking of your past? I'm not asking you to meditate on it. How many of you would remember the error of your ways? When you became born again and your heart opened up to God and you had a new life and the Word of God came to bring the mind and will of God to your life, were you still able to remember your atheistic ways? We don't lose the memory of that. No, we don't, because it's part of your soul.

When people have a broken heart and their spirit has been injured, through ministry we remove the pain in the heart. They still have the memory here in the mind, but the pain down here in the heart no longer exists. How is it one day they have the memory and the pain, and then after the Lord comes to heal, they still have the memory but no pain? What has been removed? The creature inside spiritually that was reinforcing the damage and the thought (Hebrews 12:13).

A meme is a unit of memory. Mass memes can include mass hysteria. Another mass meme is gossip. I want to help you think here because some of you have been programmed in your long-term memory by your enemy, and he wants you to follow his thinking all the way to the grave. That way, he can continue to keep these diseases on you that are the result of "stinkin' thinkin'." Behind spiritually rooted diseases are always feelings, emotions, and thoughts. Your enemy is banking on the fact that he's got you right here in your mind, and here in your heart. He's got to have you because, without you, his kingdom cannot exist on this planet (Genesis 3).

Do you know the enemy wants to use you as a medium of expression? Does that scare you? Do you know many people are channelers for the devil and don't even know it? When you hate your brother, you are a channeler for the devil. When you slander your brother you are an oracle for Satan. We're not always taught that, are we? This is why your mind needs to be renewed by the washing of the water of the Word.

²³And be renewed in the spirit of your mind; Ephes. 4:23

²⁶That he might sanctify and cleanse it with the washing of water by the word, Ephes. 5:26

In short-term memory you "take a picture"—that's a meme. A unit of memory is an electrical, chemical occurrence that happens in the brain. In short-term memory, it doesn't become fixed. However, in long-term memory we have something that happens that's now being reinforced by meditation, being reinforced by repetition, being reinforced by a locking in of consciousness, so that something happens in the electrochemical occurrence.

There is a factor of genetics that kicks in involving RNA. Something called "protein synthesis" occurs and that memory becomes biologically a part of your brain cells, not just as a flash point or a picture in short-term memory. It has now become part of you biologically. That's how your soul is preserved. The mirror image is taken like a negative, and the human spirit picks up on it and you become one with it spiritually and psychologically.

Proverbs 23:7 says—so as a man thinketh in his heart so is he. Well, I changed my heart recently and my poor head is catching up slowly. I follow God not just because my mind agrees; I follow God because my heart mixed with faith agrees based on the Word of God. The areas of your thinking that don't match God's knowledge need to become subjected to a superior way of thinking, God's thinking. Will you always remember your "stinkin' thinkin'," or your error, or your ignorance? Yes, but as a work of the Holy Spirit this old way of thinking, even though you remember it, is not inferior. This is how truth is established and error is dispelled.

Your enemy wants to control you through long-term memory. Do you know who else wants to control you through long-term memory? Don't be offended; God does! Would you rather be possessed by God or possessed of the devil? Would you rather have the mind of Satan or the mind of Christ?

I Corinthians 2:16 says that we are to put on the mind of Christ.

¹⁶For who hath known the mind of the Lord, that he may instruct him? But we have the mind of Christ. 1 Cor. 2:16

What do you think that is? We go up and take His brain cells and stick them in our head? No, it means that we are to know the will of the Father and the Word of God. Then we are able to conform to His nature, and to His image, so that when we think, it's like Him thinking; when we speak it's like Him speaking and when we act, it's like Him acting so that it is the totality of the restoration of a man and a woman of God.

In the total restoration of a man and woman of God, this is how I see it in the Word of God; total expression of renewal and restoration from the works of darkness into the works of life. That's the way God sees me in my generation; that my will should match the Father's will, and my word should match the Word of God, and my actions should be as if it were the Holy Spirit so that the will and the Word and the action of God can be performed through me as a way of life. I'm to be a total extension of the Word, the will and the action.

Isn't it amazing that we have been created in God's image? I want to break some past memes here, OK? Some of you have been conforming to the mind of Satan, the mind of death, the mind of antichrist, to things that are diametrically opposed to what God says. You've not been given the spirit of fear (2 Tim. 1:7). You are not to let a root of bitterness spring up and trouble you. (Heb. 12:15) We must guard what becomes a part of our long-term memory.

What is meant by—holding every thought in captivity in 2 Corinthians 10? In your creation, the way you are, isn't it amazing we usually do things by thinking about them first? If you were to create something called a Styrofoam cup, an object that would hold water, the first part of the concept would come from where? Your mind. Then you would find a friend and say, "I've just invented a cup." You would express what? The concept originating in your mind, and then after you articulated it in writing or speech, the final stages should be what? Do it, create it, make it.

That's God's very essence: He thought it, He spoke what He thought, and He did it. The three members of the eternal Godhead were in perfect agreement. *The Father willed it—the Word said it—and the Holy Spirit did it.* If you're in fellowship with the Godhead, and you're in fellowship with God by His Word, you should be an extension of the will, the Word and the power as a way of life. When the world sees you, they ought to see an extension of the Godhead at every point they turn. Would that be something idealistic to think about or do you think that is Scriptural?

We have got a ways to go before we can unravel diseases. We need to be weighing and considering. I want you to be holding every thought in captivity. I want you to be doing some X-raying of your thoughts, emotions, parts and pieces of your existence. If you are afraid to go there, don't be. *You're already tormented into it anyway.* God wants to get inside you, so don't shut Him out. He wants you well, in your right mind, in health, sanity, and to be the fulfillment of 1 Thessalonians 5:23.

> **[23]And the very God of peace sanctify you wholly; and *I pray God* your whole spirit and soul and body be preserved blameless unto the coming of our Lord Jesus Christ. 1 Thes. 5:23**

There's that word sanctify, there's that circumcision word, that burning fire of the Holy Spirit word, that conviction word, there's that thing that makes you whole. *God wants to sanctify you <u>wholly</u> in spirit, soul, and body.* God just doesn't want you fixed in one dimension; He wants you fixed in every dimension of your creation. It begins deep on the inside, as a man thinketh in his heart so is he (Proverbs 23:7).

> **[7]For as he thinketh in his heart, so *is* he... Proverbs 23:7**

Summary

I want to bring you into a place of focus. We have established the Biblical standard, I hope, for healing. It is God's will to get involved in your life. The second thing we established is that the church has been a miserable failure in dealing with it. Number three, in reading Ezekiel 34, we established that God the Father, by the Spirit of God speaking through the prophet Ezekiel, established the fact that He was ticked off about it and He had a few things to say against the spiritual leaders. They were not healing the sick. They were not taking care of the diseased. They were not searching for the ones who were lost over the cliff.

We also found in both the Old Testament and the New Testament that it's God's will that we prosper in spirit, soul and body. We've given you an insight into the reality of spiritual roots. We've established a foundation for our thinking about spirit and soul and how it affects our physiological existence. We are moving into a place of looking into various diseases.

I want to say that I represent the gap between allopathic medicine and no help at all. I deal with disease; with disease that has a spiritual root with various psychological and physiological manifestations. I deal with the etiology of over 70 to 80 different so-called incurable diseases in America and the world.

God and I have taken that word incurable, and done this to it: *When you say incurable, you have made the devil greater than God.* As a minister, I cannot bring myself to say that. I believe all things are possible. *I believe mankind has disease because we have become separated from God and His Word and fallen into disobedience to Him.*

I consider all healing of spiritually rooted disease to be a factor of sanctification. I believe that all disease that has a spiritual root is a result of lack of sanctification in our lives as men and women of God. I believe all healing of disease and/or prevention is the process of being re-sanctified.

Remember what we read from 1 Thessalonians 5:23: "May the God of peace sanctify you wholly in spirit, in soul and in body." I also believe that God cannot heal, He will not heal, unless we measure up to His standard of holiness. I don't think He has to. I don't think God is going to bless us and let us keep our sin. I'm not into legalism. I'm not into the works of righteousness. I'm into a heart change—the circumcision of the human heart, the submission to the living God because we *want* to submit, not because we have to.

I believe that there is a connection between sin and disease. I believe that because Deuteronomy 28 says so. Disobedience to God and His Word, and not staying in covenant with Him, will open the door to the curse. In Deuteronomy 28, in the section on curses, we found all manner of disease. When men came to obedience to God and His Word, in covenant with Him as His children, we found blessings, and I found not one disease listed. *I consider all disease to be a curse, and not a blessing. I consider all absence of disease to be a blessing.* Choose this day what you shall have, blessings or curses, life or death (Deut. 30:19-20).

> [19]**I call heaven and earth to record this day against you,** *that* **I have set before you life and death, blessing and cursing: therefore choose life, that both thou and thy seed may live:** [20]**That thou mayest love the LORD thy God,** *and* **that thou mayest obey his voice, and that thou mayest cleave unto him: for he** *is* **thy life, and the length of thy days: that thou mayest dwell in the land which the LORD sware unto thy fathers, to Abraham, to Isaac, and to Jacob, to give them.** Deut. 30:19-20

With respect to forgiveness of sin and healing of disease, Psalm 103:3 says, "The Lord who forgiveth us of all our iniquities and healeth us of all of our diseases."

> [3]**Who forgiveth all thine iniquities; who healeth all thy diseases;** Psalm 103:3

In one verse, we have forgiveness of sin and healing of disease right together. In the New Testament, James 5:14-15, we're told concerning sick people in the Church:

> [14]**Is any sick among you? let him call for the elders of the church; and let them pray over him, anointing him with oil in the name of the Lord:** [15]**And the prayer of faith shall save the sick, and the Lord shall raise him up; and if he have committed sins, they shall be forgiven him.** James 5:14-15

Right here we have the connection between sin and healing. Jesus had just healed someone and He said this:

> [14]**Afterward Jesus findeth him in the temple, and said unto him, Behold, thou art made whole: sin no more, lest a worse thing come unto thee.** John 5:14

Right here, in the harmony of just three scriptures, I see a direct relationship between lack of sanctification, disease, and sin.

I was reading the other day in 2 Chronicles 29 and 30. It was really interesting because in the days of King Hezekiah, He brought the Word of God back to God's people. The Levites had not been doing the sacrifices; there had been no shedding of blood for the remission of sins by the priests. The people had been serving the gods of pagan nations and Hezekiah the King came to re-establish the righteousness of God in God's people. It was interesting because they brought the Levites together. They brought the singers together, the priests together, and as they sacrificed for sin, a worship went up to God. It was a spontaneous worship and thanksgiving, in conjunction with establishing a fellowship and relationship with God and the sacrifice, which provided the shed blood for sin.

The LORD looked down and He heard and in 2 Chronicles 30:20:

> [20]**And the LORD hearkened to Hezekiah, and healed the people.** 2 Chron. 30:20

The LORD heard and He healed, but sanctification had to occur first. In order for you to be able to come to a place of receiving healing from God, you have got to be in fellowship with Him. In fellowship, you are in contact with all three members of the Godhead. You're in fellowship with the Father, the Lord, and the Holy Spirit through the communion of the Holy Spirit (2 Corinthians 13:14).

¹⁴The grace of the Lord Jesus Christ, and the love of God, and the communion of the Holy Ghost, *be* with you all. Amen. 2 Cor. 13:14

Much of the Church body today is trying to receive from God through prayers and petitions, but they are not in fellowship and they are not in obedience.

Jesus said that loving Him involved obeying Him (John 14:15).

¹⁵If ye love me, keep my commandments. John 14:15

Fellowship with God involves being obedient to Him, not out of Phariseeism or legalism, but out of a heart that wants to know and be in fellowship with God by faith. Fellowship with the Father, fellowship with the Word, Who is the Son, and fellowship with the Holy Spirit is what God desires.

Out of the fellowship comes worship; we only worship two members of the Godhead. We don't worship the Holy Spirit; he doesn't speak of himself. He only honors the Will and the Word. In worship, we worship the Father, and the Son who is Jesus. The work of the Holy Spirit is separate.

We're only to contact one member of the Godhead in petition. Jesus said—in that day you shall ask me nothing but you shall ask the Father in My Name and He shall give you what you ask (John 16:23).

²³And in that day ye shall ask me nothing. Verily, verily, I say unto you, Whatsoever ye shall ask the Father in my name, he will give *it* you. John 16:23

The disciples said, "Teach us to pray." Jesus said—Boys, say it like this (Matthew 6).

⁹...Our Father which art in heaven... Matthew 6:9

Petition is made to the Father in the Name of the Lord Jesus Christ.

However, the Church doesn't seem to be getting many answers. This is a statement of the problem. I don't see a well Church trying to save a sick world. I see a sick Church trying to save itself. It should be a well Church trying to save a sick world. This is what I see in Scripture.

Re-establish your relationship with God and you'll be in worship. When fellowship and worship are in place, then when you come before God in the name of the Lord, you're going to have His attention. It won't cost you anything.

There will be people who hear this that will never be the same. There are some of you who are dealing with things in your life and, when you apply the principles that I have given you, and you go before God and the Word, you'll walk away from certain diseases just like you never had them. This does not happen to everyone, because some of us are still working out our problems. We are still working them out, thinking about it, doing that circumcision, doing that repentance, getting before God, getting back in fellowship, getting to a place where we are going to be honest with God about our problem and getting to a place where we are ready to come before Him to deal with it.

The Bible tells me in John 8:36: "Who the Son sets free is free indeed." Support groups are not the answer. *Support groups magnify what the enemy is doing in our lives and* often *make no provision for freedom.* I don't mind bearing your burden, but I don't want to carry you forever in it. It is not God's will that you be sick forever.

The 5 R's of Freedom

1. Recognize
2. Responsibility
3. Repent
4. Renounce
5. Resist

#1 Recognize

Recognize the problem—have discernment. Isaiah 5:13 says—(God said) my people have gone into captivity because they have no knowledge. Could we say they had no discernment? Hosea 4:6 says—(God said) my people perish for lack of knowledge. Could you say lack of discernment? Hebrews 5:14 tells us—but strong meat belongs to those that are full aged, even those that by reason of use have their senses exercised to <u>discern</u> both good and evil. Not just good, you must be able to discern evil also.

> [13]**Therefore my people are gone into captivity, because** *they have* **no knowledge: and their honourable men** *are* **famished, and their multitude dried up with thirst.** Isaiah 5:13

> [6]**My people are destroyed for lack of knowledge: because thou hast rejected knowledge, I will also reject thee, that thou shalt be no priest to me: seeing thou hast forgotten the law of thy God, I will also forget thy children.** Hosea 4:6

> [14]**But strong meat belongeth to them that are of full age,** *even* **those who by reason of use have their senses exercised to discern both good and evil.** Hebrews 5:14

You say, "Pastor, I'm afraid of evil." Shame on you. Where did you get that from? Watching too much of the Exorcist? Why would you be afraid of evil? Are you telling me Satan is greater than God? "Well, Pastor, something bad might happen to me." Yea, it might. So what? Why are we afraid of evil?

If I told you that you had a particular disease because you had a root of bitterness against someone and had not resolved it, what would I have given you? *Discernment.*

If I told you that you had Lupus because you hated yourself and felt guilty about it, what would I have given you? *Discernment.*

If I told you that you had Breast Cancer because you hated your Mama, what would I have given you? *Discernment.*

If I told you that you had Ulcerative Colitis because you were in fear and anxiety, what would I have given you? *Discernment.*

If I told you that you had Malabsorption because of anxiety and fear also, what would I have given you? *Discernment.*

All right, so you hate Aunt Sally. What's going on if you have hatred toward Aunt Sally? What did we teach you earlier? What was the principal that brought the hatred into play? Bitterness. What was one of the fruits of bitterness? Hatred.

If you found someone who was violent in your family, what could you immediately go to them and say that would be absolutely true? You could tell them, "You have a root of bitterness."

If you have somebody who is angry and hostile, what can you tell them? "You have a root of bitterness." If you find someone who has resentment, what could you tell them? "You have a root of bitterness."

When you see hatred, anger, resentment, unforgiveness, and retaliation, you can also tell them this: *"that if you don't get this under control in your life, the chances of you getting a disease as a bad fruit of this is very likely in your lifetime."*

Now what have you given them? **Wisdom**. Knowledge to put into action.

There are two gifts of the Holy Spirit taught in 1 Corinthians 12 that you need to understand. One is the gift of Wisdom, and the other is the gift of Knowledge. What am I giving you now? You may not be realizing it, but I'm operating in the gift of Knowledge and the gift of Wisdom in your life right now. If you had ears to hear, you could hear. In fact, I'm also operating in the gift of Faith, Discerning of Spirits, Knowledge, Wisdom and if needs be I can operate in the gift of Healing and the gift of Miracles. I operate in all of these gifts as the Holy Spirit wills, because He's working with people through our ministry.

Do you know that every believer should be participating at some level in this area? 1 Corinthians 12 teaches that *the Church is designed to heal the Church.* Ephesians 4 says that, as a pastor, I'm supposed to equip you and bring you to the place where you can do that (regarding the body of Christ healing itself). I first have to be able to demonstrate it. **Knowledge ties the past to the present but Wisdom takes the present and moves it to the future.**

If you can really figure out what I am saying, I'm taking your past, helping you to understand your past and where it fits in today, so that you can move ahead with God into the future according to Wisdom. Do you understand?

We're taking your past, and bringing it to the present so you can see what in the world is going on in your present state. Then God, through Wisdom, can take you into the future to change your circumstances. Now it's going to take Faith and the work of the Holy Spirit to do the rest of it, but we have to be able to teach first, because…faith *cometh* by hearing, and hearing by the word of God (Romans 10:17).

> [17]**So then faith *cometh* by hearing, and hearing by the word of God.** Romans 10:17

Remember that in Jeremiah 3, God said He would give you pastors according to His heart that would teach you, lead you, and give you understanding.

> [15]**And I will give you pastors according to mine heart, which shall feed you with knowledge and understanding.** Jeremiah 3:15

What am I? I am a pastor; you are the sheep of His pasture and I'm an under-shepherd that cares for you just as much as He does. I'm not here to fill your head with a bunch of knowledge. I came here to break the power of the devil over your lives and release you. Your freedom was paid for 2,000 years ago on the cross, and the power of God was released into your life so you can get on with it. I want you to be free. He wants you to be free.

Do you want to be free? Do you really? I've found many people like being sick because it is the first attention they have received in their life. Get them on the phone, "How are you doing today." They say, "Ohhhhhh, I'm sure glad you asked that." The phone call goes on for thirty minutes.

Do you want to be well? Do you want to be sane? GOOD! If I come along and put my finger on that stuff, those creatures from Hebrews 4:13, if I come along and put my finger on some of that stuff that's making you sick, what are you going to do with it? You say, "Pastor, that was a nice time, I'll see you" and you walk out the door and take all those crispy critters with you. It's a lot of work keeping up with a zoo like that!

> [13]**Neither is there any creature that is not manifest in his sight: but all things *are* naked and opened unto the eyes of him with whom we have to do.** Hebrews 4:13

#2 Responsibility

After you *recognize*, the Holy Spirit comes to convict you from discernment and then the second "R" is take *Responsibility.* I deal with a lot of people from coast to coast, and not everybody wants to take responsibility after discernment. Do you know what really bugs me? This gets my sanctification really close to being lost. When somebody looks at me and says to me after discernment, "Well, Pastor, bless God, that's just the way I am." What happened to the scripture that says, "From glory to glory we're being changed?" (2 Corinthians 3:18).

> [18]**But we all, with open face beholding as in a glass the glory of the Lord, are changed into the same image from glory to glory, *even* as by the Spirit of the Lord.** 2 Cor. 3:18

"Well that's for somebody else, Pastor. If God wants to change me He's just going to have to do it." Let me tell you, brother, God couldn't do it if He tried. You won't let Him.

Are you interested in change? Are you locked into those memes that I taught you about earlier? Is long-term protein synthesis locked in; are you rigidly set in your ways not only spiritually but intellectually?

"Bless God I'm angry, I always have been angry, and I always am going to be angry, and if you don't like it, I'll eat you for lunch." Are you going to lock yourself into, "Well, I'll forgive them if they forgive me first." What are you going to do?

I like to say it this way: "I don't care what somebody else did to you, *somebody has to get spiritual here*—who is it going to be?"

Somebody's going to have to get spiritual. Do you think the other person needs to get spiritual first, or do you need to get spiritual first? "Well, if my husband would just go to church with me, I'd go too." Take *responsibility.*

#3 Repent

What is the third "R" that you need to be free? *Repent.* Acts 3:19 says, "Repent therefore, be converted that your sins may be blotted out when the times of refreshing shall come from the presence of the Lord."

> [19]**Repent ye therefore, and be converted, that your sins may be blotted out, when the times of refreshing shall come from the presence of the Lord;** Acts 3:19

Do you want the times of refreshing to come from the Lord in your life? Are you tired of the blistering heat of disease? Are you ready for that oasis? You won't get there unless you go here first—*repent.*

#4 Renounce

After you have *repented,* which means taking *responsibility* after recognition and discernment, the next step is to *Renounce.* A lot of people repent but they don't mean it. A lot of people have remorse but they don't change on the inside. To renounce literally means to "turn away from." There are many scriptures in the Bible where God said—get away from idols, get away from heathen practices because they will be your ruin.

> [2]**Ye know that ye were Gentiles, carried away unto these dumb idols, even as ye were led.** 1 Cor. 12:2

> [20]**But *I say,* that the things which the Gentiles sacrifice, they sacrifice to devils, and not to God: and I would not that ye should have fellowship with devils.** [21]**Ye cannot drink the cup of the Lord, and the cup of devils: ye cannot be partakers of the Lord's table, and of the table of devils.** [22]**Do we provoke the Lord to jealousy? are we stronger than he?** 1 Cor. 10:20-22

Get away from evil, *renounce* it as fast as you can. Develop a perfect hatred for evil in your life. Separate yourself from the evil. Love yourself, but hate the evil. Love your neighbor, but hate the evil he does. Learn to separate yourself and others from their sin.

#5 Resist

Number 5 of the 5 "R's" to freedom is to *Resist*. James 4:7 says, "Submit yourself, therefore to God. *Resist* the devil and he will flee from you."

> [7]**Submit yourselves therefore to God. Resist the devil, and he will flee from you.** James 4:7

What comes first? *Resist* the devil and he will flee or submit to God. Is that what we are doing here? *Submission to God first; then you have power over your enemies, not before.*

Remember, earlier I quoted from 2 Corinthians 10:6: "Having a readiness to avenge all disobedience after your obedience is fulfilled." Do you remember what Samuel told Uncle Saul? I Samuel 15:23 "Obedience is better than sacrifice, for rebellion is as the sin of witchcraft, and stubbornness is as idolatry."(Self-will, self-exhortation, witchcraft, and idolatry.) That's a tough scripture isn't it? "Obedience is better than sacrifice."

> [22]**And Samuel said, Hath the LORD *as great* delight in burnt offerings and sacrifices, as in obeying the voice of the LORD? Behold, to obey *is* better than sacrifice, *and* to hearken than the fat of rams. [23]For rebellion *is as* the sin of witchcraft, and stubbornness *is as* iniquity and idolatry. Because thou hast rejected the word of the LORD, he hath also rejected thee from *being* king.** 1 Samuel 15:22-23

Discussion of Specific Diseases

As we move on to discussing specific diseases, I want you to prayerfully allow God to deal with you. If you need to repent, repent. If you need to acknowledge in discernment, acknowledge in discernment. This is a private thing. God knows your heart. He already knows what's in there; you don't have to tell Him. He knows the thoughts of your heart. He knows the stuff that is causing you trouble. It is no surprise to Him.

Scoliosis

I have done a lot of research with Scoliosis, and we have seen many healings of curvature of the spine. I didn't see all the implications until recently when I was digging into some medical information and research. I bumped into something called proprioception. Proprioception is tied to the emotional cortex of your brain, down through the thalamus gland, and keeps you balanced. It also is tied to the centers of feel, touch, and the five physical senses. It allows you to be coordinated. In Scoliosis, it has been discovered that in 50% to 60% of all cases proprioception malfunction is involved.

There is a neurological misfiring; one muscle stiffens, one remains normal; the normal one is now considered weak. If this happens in an adult, there is no cure. In children, if they are treated while they are young enough, they can be put in special body braces and it slows down or stops the process. Scoliosis progresses from childhood at the rate of one degree of spine curvature per year. Because the normal side is now considered weak in one side of the back muscles, the stiffened one is now considered strong and pulls. The weak side is unable to maintain the balance and the spine starts to bend.

Most Scoliosis cases are an "S" curve. I dealt with a case of inverted Scoliosis years ago. When I was first starting in ministry a young man was brought to me with an inverted spine. His spine was actually out here with his stomach. You could take a basketball and put it on his back and it would fit right into the curvature of his spine.

I'll tell you, and I pray you can receive it, that Scoliosis, like Epilepsy, is the presence and the fruit of an *evil spirit. You will not get Epilepsy healed, and you will not get Scoliosis healed unless you cast out an evil spirit.* I had to cast the evil spirit of Scoliosis out of this young man in the name of Jesus.

Sciatica

There is another disease where an evil spirit has to be cast out; it's called *Sciatica,* an inflammation of the sciatic nerve that accounts for 50% of lower back pain in most people. Medical observation indicates the left side is most usually affected; occasionally the right side.

If so many people had not received healing over the years, you probably would think I just got off a spaceship. Casting out evil spirits is found in Matthew, Mark,

Luke and John and the book of Acts. I figured one day that I would just trust God and give it a shot. I thought I would just speak to one and cast it out. It obeyed me and left. That was interesting and exciting.

Matthew 10:1 explains how Jesus empowered the disciples in this matter:

> **10:1And when he had called unto *him* his twelve disciples, he gave them power *against* unclean spirits, to cast them out, and to heal all manner of sickness and all manner of disease.** Matthew 10:1

In Luke 10:17-20, we see that the seventy were given the same power, and they weren't even disciples:

> **17And the seventy returned again with joy, saying, Lord, even the devils are subject unto us through thy name. 18And he said unto them, I beheld Satan as lightning fall from heaven. 19Behold, I give unto you power to tread on serpents and scorpions, and over all the power of the enemy: and nothing shall by any means hurt you. 20Notwithstanding in this rejoice not, that the spirits are subject unto you; but rather rejoice, because your names are written in heaven.** Luke 10:17-20

I believe that's for today, and I've seen the results of that belief. *If you do not believe it's for today, then for you, it's not.* Matthew 9:27-38 is another scriptural teaching about healing that we must examine.

> **27And when Jesus departed thence, two blind men followed him, crying, and saying, *Thou* Son of David, have mercy on us. 28And when he was come into the house, the blind men came to him: and Jesus saith unto them, Believe ye that I am able to do this? They said unto him, Yea, Lord. 29Then touched he their eyes, saying, According to your faith be it unto you. 30And their eyes were opened; and Jesus straitly charged them, saying, See *that* no man know *it.* 31But they, when they were departed, spread abroad his fame in all that country. 32As they went out, behold, they brought to him a dumb man possessed with a devil. 33And when the devil was cast out, the dumb spake: and the multitudes marvelled, saying, It was never so seen in Israel. 34But the Pharisees said, He casteth out devils through the prince of the devils. 35And Jesus went about all the cities and villages, teaching in their synagogues, and preaching the gospel of the kingdom, and healing every sickness and every disease among the people. 36But when he saw the multitudes, he was moved with compassion on them, because they fainted, and were scattered abroad, as sheep having no shepherd. 37Then saith he unto his disciples, The harvest truly *is* plenteous, but the labourers *are* few; 38Pray ye therefore the Lord of the harvest, that he will send forth labourers into his harvest.** Matthew 9:27-38

If we are to pattern who we are after Christ, then these scriptures include some very important elements that are relevant for today:

1. Belief that the Lord is able to do it.

2. According to your faith be it unto you.

3. A person had a devil that would not allow him to speak.

4. Jesus cast the devil out, then he could speak.

5. The religious leaders of the day accused him of casting a devil out by the power of the devil (this is what blasphemy of the Holy Spirit is).

6. Jesus set the pattern of ministry which was to teach and preach, heal every sickness and disease, and cast out evil spirits.

7. Jesus was moved with compassion for others.

8. God's people are scattered as sheep with no shepherd.

9. The fields are ready for harvest and the laborers are few.

10. Will you help?

Mark 6:7-13 teaches us that Jesus gave the power necessary for dealing with unclean spirits and healing to His disciples.

> [7]And he called *unto him* the twelve, and began to send them forth by two and two; and gave them power over unclean spirits; [8]And commanded them that they should take nothing for *their* journey, save a staff only; no scrip, no bread, no money in *their* purse: [9]But *be* shod with sandals; and not put on two coats. [10]And he said unto them, In what place soever ye enter into an house, there abide till ye depart from that place. [11]And whosoever shall not receive you, nor hear you, when ye depart thence, shake off the dust under your feet for a testimony against them. Verily I say unto you, It shall be more tolerable for Sodom and Gomorrha in the day of judgment, than for that city. [12]And they went out, and preached that men should repent. [13]And they cast out many devils, and anointed with oil many that were sick, and healed *them.* Mark 6:7-13

There are many, many people literally running around these days who no longer have *Epilepsy, Scoliosis,* or *Sciatica* problems because this ministry dared to believe that Matthew 10:1 and Luke 10:17-20 are true for today.

I'm not exactly sure what the spiritual root for *Scoliosis* is. But I have known for 14 years that you have to minister deliverance in order for *Scoliosis* to be healed. In the case of the young man with the inverted spine, I knew it was an evil spirit. I didn't deal with spiritual roots; I just said, "In the name of Jesus, you spirit of *Scoliosis* come out of him. I break your power." After that I laid hands on him and commanded that spine to straighten.

I will never forget as long as I live, the tears of rejoicing in his mother and father's eyes, and the looks on their faces, as he snapped and his spine became straight as an arrow. They all left rejoicing. He was 14 years old. I will never forget that day. In that day, I knew of a certainty that God was still on the throne and that He still answers prayer.

Epilepsy

They brought a young lady to me in 1985. She was about 21 years of age and had been experiencing grand mal epileptic seizures for many years. They heard that God was using this ministry, honoring our work, and people were being healed.

I had a member of my staff that day who said, "Pastor, this situation is like the one that the disciples couldn't cast out. They went back to Jesus and He said that this one cometh out but by prayer and fasting" (Matthew 17:14-21). The young lady was supposed to be there by 7:00 that night, and it was 10:00 in the morning when my staff member asked me, "Don't you need at least 3 days of prayer and fasting before you can defeat this?"

I said, "What!!???" They replied, "Well, that's what the Bible says." I staggered for a moment and I said, "You know what? I live a prayed and fasted life with Christ. That woman could die in 24 hours, let alone 3 days." Today is the day of salvation, now is the appointed time, she's coming, let's go for the gold. In Matthew 17, Jesus taught that my faith concerning this type of ministry was all that was necessary, and so I did as Jesus had taught us to do.

> [14]**And when they were come to the multitude, there came to him a** *certain* **man, kneeling down to him, and saying,** [15]**Lord, have mercy on my son: for he is lunatick, and sore vexed: for ofttimes he falleth into the fire, and oft into the water.** [16]**And I brought him to thy disciples, and they could not cure him.** [17]**Then Jesus answered and said, O faithless and perverse generation, how long shall I be with you? how long shall I suffer you? bring him hither to me.** [18]**And Jesus rebuked the devil; and he departed out of him: and the child was cured from that very hour.** [19]**Then came the disciples to Jesus apart, and said, Why could not we cast him out?** [20]**And Jesus said unto them, Because of your unbelief: for verily I say unto you, If ye have faith as a grain of mustard seed, ye shall say unto this mountain, Remove hence to yonder place; and it shall remove; and nothing shall be impossible unto you.** [21]**Howbeit this kind goeth not out but by prayer and fasting.** Matthew 17:14-21

They brought her to me; she was unsaved and she was living with her boyfriend in sin. She had had two abortions, and I had to talk to her about these issues. She decided to accept the Lord because I told her if she accepted the Lord, the chances of Him healing her would be pretty good. "You have come all this distance. I think He really wants to do this." I broke the power of the *dumb and deaf spirit* and cast it out of her and commanded the *spirit of epilepsy* to be gone. I didn't know if it had gone or not; I didn't see any visible evidence.

I said, "Goodbye." One week later she went to her doctor in Asheville, North Carolina. He ran an EEG on her and her alpha, beta and theta brain wave tests were all normal. The last time I heard about her, she was serving God internationally with Youth With A Mission (YWAM). Saved, healed, and now serving God. She never had another epileptic seizure, ever again. That was the first of several encounters with people who had epilepsy. So far, we've never lost a healing of epilepsy in the history of our ministry, although there is never a guarantee. Everything is in God's hands by faith.

Everybody that is ministered to doesn't get well. There are reasons for that. The reasons why they didn't get well is what this ministry is all about in America today. We're picking up in situations where people don't get well after prayer.

My ministry began where prayer, and standing on the Word, and jumping on it did not work. That's when God began to teach me about the spiritual roots of disease, and the spiritual blocks to healing.

It's not that God does not want to heal; it's that He would have to deny Himself, and His holiness, to do so in our lives when those spiritual roots and/or spiritual blocks exist. He's not going to compromise our heart change in the name of blessing. He would be an unfaithful Father if He let us keep our sins and blessed us anyway. However, there is evidence in Scripture that God healed and delivered people who did not qualify. That is His sovereignty and must be recognized.

> **[15]For he saith to Moses, I will have mercy on whom I will have mercy, and I will have compassion on whom I will have compassion.** Romans 9:15

Sometimes God heals and delivers people first and straightens them out later. However, it is my observation that God is first interested in our sanctification as a prelude to healing and deliverance.

We would not honor Him, and we would not serve Him, because He would have condoned evil in our lives. Do you really respect anyone who condones evil in their own life? You think about it; when your kids were growing up and Mommy and Daddy said, "Don't do this and don't do that," did they really appreciate it?

No, but when they became older, did they appreciate it?

Do we have respect for people who try to get us in trouble? Do we have respect for people who uphold evil in our lives and jeopardize our very existence? We would not respect God if He did that, would we? We wouldn't serve Him. *We do expect God to be holy.*

Attention Deficit Disorder

We're still learning about ADD, involving the spectrums from the lows to the mediums and the highs. We have more experience in the hyperactive range than the lower range, though we have had a couple of cases in the lower and medium ranges.

We understand ADD to be a neurological interruption. We also understand that ADD is or can be familial or inherited. It seems to run in family trees. We have a very strong feeling that it is tied to a dumb and deaf spirit that is putting a person into bondage.

ADD, dyslexia and homosexuality have something in common. Don't think that because I've merged dyslexia and ADD with homosexuality, that anybody's at risk of becoming a homosexual because they have ADD. They do, however, have a common thread. There is a *double mindedness* that comes and this is an inherited family curse. "A double minded man is unstable in all his ways" (James 1:8).

> **[8]A double minded man *is* unstable in all his ways.** James 1:8

When you find ADD, you'll also find it in the parents and grandparents. You won't find it in just one place. You'll find it right down the line. It's the same with dyslexia. It involves a type of double mindedness, and confusion, and the prime root of the confusion is gender disorientation because of an inversion of Godly order in the home. The home is ruled by matriarchal control rather than patriarchal authority as God intended.

The home is ruled by the female, not the male, and the confusion that comes out of it is producing ADD, dyslexia, and homosexuality. When the male does not rule the home in love, the female has no choice but to take the reins.

The minute she does, Satan's entire kingdom comes to help her. She was never designed to rule the home; she was designed to follow a patriarch, a Godly one I might add. I'm not a chauvinist, and I do not send females back into the oppressive rulership of ungodly males in the name of the LORD. When the female is being oppressed, I call for immediate separation and resolution.

I will protect the children and the female first before I'll protect the male. My position, as a pastor, is that the male should be protecting the female and the children to begin with so I hold him to a higher level of responsibility.

You see, the female and the children should follow the male as he follows Christ. The head of the woman is to be the man, and the head of the man is Christ. But the head of Christ is the Father, and nobody quotes the rest of that scripture. It doesn't stop with Christ; it stops with the Father.

> **³But I would have you know, that the head of every man is Christ; and the head of the woman *is* the man; and the head of Christ *is* God.** 1 Cor. 11:3

That brings the male back into the rulership, not just as the husband, in a similar relationship that Christ has with the Church as our Husband. The husband is called to represent God as the father to his family just as if it were God Himself. It's a tough job, but it is the job God has called a man to do.

I also have observed various standpoints of rebellion as part of this profile. Historic family rebellion exists in families that have been involved in occultism and false religions. Historically, it's an interrupter of the thoughts. It interferes with self-esteem. *It involves much self-rejection, self-hatred and guilt.* It often involves dyslexia and other various breakdowns of perception. Many times you'll find color blindness, which is also inherited, tied to it. You can also have other peripheral problems that come with this family profile.

I'll give you one testimony of success in the healing of ADD. I've been asked about ADD in adults versus ADD in children. I have no experience in the healing of ADD in adults. I have not had the first adult ever come to me with ADD. I do have experience at the children's level. One case in particular is astounding.

A child was brought to me. The child's school had said they needed a meeting with the parents because this child was so disruptive that he had to be placed in the back of the school room in a chair with his face against the wall. He was totally isolated in a classroom and they still could not contain him.

When the parents got the letter and came to me, it was very obvious that the next step the school counselors would recommend would be to put the child on the drug *Ritalin*.

Ritalin is a very dangerous drug. This drug is the shame of our school systems in America because it's a lazy way out of a problem. The information that I have on children who are on Ritalin is that a national organization's research concerning children on *Ritalin* showed that 50% of them, at some time in their lifetime, end up afoul of the law and in jails. This has been directly related and attributed to the drug, not to ADD. There is a psychotic value that comes with this drug that's horrific. It's a Pandora's Box, and yet it is currently the "drug of choice" for ADD.

I had been doing some pastoral studying, been involved in certain levels, and I was aware of an alternative methodology that would satisfy the school system. They don't like it, and they don't want to be involved in it because it takes work on their part. It takes an effort and cooperation with the parents and teachers. It's a technique called *focusing*.

In the hyper range of ADD, the child is fine as long as he or she is concentrating on an object of interest. The nerve synapses and the flow of focusing are normal, but when the child is not motivated, the neurological flow is interrupted, and there is what's called *ranging*, free-floating thoughts and impulsive realities. The child just does whatever comes to mind.

This particular child had straight "Fs"; antisocial, disruptive, mouthy, rebellious, you-name-it behavior. I went with the parent to the school counselor to propose an alternative. The parent did not want the child on *Ritalin* because of its psychotic side effects and potentially dangerous implications. With *focusing*, and with "counseling" (actually, we were talking about ministry—I'm not into counseling, I'm into ministry), we explained that we felt this child's ADD could be resolved.

Focusing is a treatment, at the secular level, but you will hardly ever hear about it because it is so much easier to give your children the drug *Ritalin*. That's the quick way, but *Ritalin* doesn't solve the problem. The Bible says, in Proverbs 22:6—train up a child in the way he should go: and when he is old, he will not depart from it.

> **⁶Train up a child in the way he should go: and when he is old, he will not depart from it.** Proverbs 22:6

That is what focusing does.

We took this particular child and made up a chart. It had a row for every day of the week and every week of the month. We charted the next nine-week period of the school semester. The chart had three columns. The first column had a smiling face. The next column had a face with a straight line for the mouth, and the next column had a frowning face.

I brought the child in and said, "This is the deal, if we can't help you through ministry and focusing, they are going to put you on *Ritalin*, which is a drug." I explained to the child the ramifications of the drug and the consequences. *This is part of focusing...education,* but this is not threatening to the child. Children understand when you take the time to talk to them. You may not think they do, but they really are listening and you can reason with children if you take the time to meet them on a level they can understand.

We asked the child, "If you could have anything today, what would you like?" He said, "A SEGA/video game player." "Of course, you want a SEGA!" We told the child, "For every day that you turn your homework in and you behave well in the classroom, the teacher is going to evaluate you and if you have succeeded she's going to put a smiling face in that column for that day. If you come home with a smiling face, your parent is going to give you $2.00 toward your goal to purchase the SEGA. The day that you just barely make it is a straight line and you don't get any dollars. The day that you blow it, and you really blow it, and get a frowning face, you will lose one dollar from one of the days you got a smiling face.

"At the end of the nine-week period, if you have more smiling faces than you have straight lines and frowning faces, then you will receive your prize. The alternative if you don't is *Ritalin,* because the school will require it. *This is your choice."*

That's where we began. For the first two weeks, it was kind of rough. Remember that we are establishing new memes—new focusing, new concepts— and that takes time. But things started to shift. I'm here to tell you that, with ministry and focusing, in conjunction with the teacher's cooperation as well as the child's and the parents', this works. In the second nine-week period, the child went from "Fs" to the AB honor roll. The third nine-week period, the child maintained a position on the AB honor roll, and by the fourth grade period the child was still on the AB honor roll. He became student of the year, and for the last nine weeks was the teacher's assistant. He went from the back of the room to the front of the room, all through focusing, prayer, and ministry and we didn't have to go to drugs. That's significant **and this is a more excellent way.**

That's not the rest of the story. He felt so good about himself, was so proud when he walked up in front of that assembly at the end of the school year and got the certificate for Student of the Year, that something wonderful happened on the inside of him and he never let go of his achievements.

Part of the profile for ADD is *self-rejection.* This young man started to be a winner and he liked being a winner. He did not want to be a rebel anymore. He liked being the teacher's pet. Suddenly a new life had begun, and he knew he wasn't on drugs and didn't need to be on drugs and that was very important to him.

The second year came up and they brought him to me again and I said, "OK, you know how we won this battle last year. This year, there'll be no reward. You only get one SEGA in a lifetime. You know how God met you, and you know how you came through with flying colors last year. This year do you think you can make it through just by focusing and observing how you feel about yourself? He said, "Pastor, I think I can do it. I might blow it every now and then." I said, "Well, I blew it yesterday myself."

We've got the mentality that white collar is better than blue collar. That is hogwash. We are so success oriented, and driven to success, that we've forgotten the bigger picture. Our children are paying the price of our drivenness to perform and to demand perfectionism. It's time to stop it. One of the things I do in ministry is to ask parents to "lay off" your children.

Teach them the ways of the Lord and to be what God wants them to be from the foundation of the world. Pray for your children, instruct them in the ways of the Lord, and then release them. Leave them alone. They'll hear God in due season. You did.

It's amazing to some of your parents to see you serving God today. They're shocked. You know what? The greatest sinners sometimes make the best pastors, too. It's amazing whom God will save. Those saintly ones that you were once compared to—some of them are still stuck in the mud!

There is an important distinction that needs to be made here. I am not a counselor, and the members of my staff are not counselors—we are ministers.

> ⁶**Who also hath made us able ministers of the new testament; not of the letter, but of the spirit: for the letter killeth, but the spirit giveth life.** 2 Cor. 3:6

Now you can be a minister and not be an ordained pastor or evangelist. The Bible makes a provision for ordinary saints to minister the gospel of reconciliation.

> ¹⁴**For the love of Christ constraineth us; because we thus judge, that if one died for all, then were all dead:** ¹⁵**And *that* he died for all, that they which live should not henceforth live unto themselves, but unto him which died for them, and rose again.** ¹⁶**Wherefore henceforth know we no man after the flesh: yea, though we have known Christ after the flesh, yet now henceforth know we *him* no more.** ¹⁷**Therefore if any man *be* in Christ, *he is* a new creature: old things are passed away; behold, all things are become new.** ¹⁸**And all things *are* of God, who hath reconciled us to himself by Jesus Christ, and hath given to us the ministry of reconciliation;** ¹⁹**To wit, that God was in Christ, reconciling the world unto himself, not imputing their trespasses unto them; and hath committed unto us the word of reconciliation.** 2 Cor. 5:14-19

Every saint has been given authority to be ministers of the kingdom of God. The word *counselor* is secular. The word *minister* is scriptural and we make the distinction very clearly. However, this does not exclude proper leadership made up of the members of the five-fold ministry to oversee the ministry of the saints and instruct it.

Do you know that if I'm a counselor, I immediately come under the authority of the state? If I'm a minister, I have freedom. As a counselor, I'm considered a professional, but as a minister I'm considered a non-professional? *I like my non-professional status.*

I'm from Georgia and I'm very active in my community. In the state of Georgia, if you are a counselor and are aware of even a suggestion of molestation in a family you have to report it to the law immediately. It's a felony not to do so. As a pastor, I don't have to report even a suspicion of molestation, which gives me the ability to get involved with the family and find out what's really going on.

A psychologist or a teacher has to report to the law, but in the state of Georgia, I don't have to because I'm not considered to be a professional. This is a provision for spiritual involvement by the state. I'm also given the ability to get involved without government scrutiny. I think that's wonderful, don't you? In the state of Florida, pastors are required by law to call the authorities at even the suggestion or implication of molestation. This is a tragic situation because no provision for God's wisdom and restoration is possible without intervention of government. Many lives are destroyed including false accusation.

I'm going to tell you why it's tragic. I'm certainly not against preventing molestation, but without proper investigation many innocent people's lives are damaged forever. This is where a grand jury is very important, so that you can have scrutiny of legal problems without the press and the rest of the world being dragged into it to destroy people's lives. So I think we've got a glitch in the system when it comes to this area.

I know the intent of the state is to protect the children at all costs. But there isn't a week or a month that goes by that some father, pastor, teacher, or counselor is falsely accused by some individual who has a grudge and knows that's "the way to get even."

The Immune System

God created your immune system to maintain your body. God created your bodies to be able to fight invaders. The average person develops a mutant cancer cell or two at least 200 times in a lifetime. Because you have a healthy immune system and the killer cells are active and in full volume, they recognize that mutant cell or the viruses or the bacterium and they attack it and destroy it. God created your immune system to protect you, not to destroy you. In all autoimmune diseases, the white corpuscles decide that a part of your body is the invading enemy and needs to be destroyed.

Crohn's Disease

Crohn's and *Ulcerative Colitis* mirror each other but they are two different classes of diseases. Does anybody know any one with *Crohn's Disease?* Does anybody know anyone who has *Ulcerative Colitis?*

Ulcerative Colitis and *Crohn's* mirror each other in that they both involve ulceration of the colon and extreme bleeding. *Ulcerative Colitis* is confined to the colon, but *Crohn's Disease,* although it's primarily in the colon, can appear in the ileum, the esophagus, and at any point of the gastrointestinal tract in advanced cases of spreading.

Crohn's is a disease in which the white corpuscles decide it's not virus, bacterium, or mothers-in-law, but it is the lining of the colon that is the enemy of the person. In all autoimmune diseases, the white corpuscles are involved.

In our literature, if you'll remember, we discuss something we call *"white corpuscle deviant behavior."* It's a term that I coined to let you know that something God created, that is supposed to take care of invading enemies, has now decided that we are the enemy and is attacking various parts of our body. *The spiritual implications are incredible in that as we attack ourselves spiritually, the body eventually agrees and starts attacking itself in destruction.*

In the case of *Crohn's*, it can be diagnosed by the excessive presence of white corpuscles. In the case of *Ulcerative Colitis*, you won't find the proliferation of white corpuscles at all. It's easy to distinguish in diagnosing from a medical standpoint the difference between *Crohn's* and *Ulcerative Colitis*. In *Crohn's Disease*, the white corpuscles start attacking the lining of the colon, initially, causing ulceration. It is a very serious disease. The root behind *Crohn's* is *extreme self-rejection coupled with guilt. Crohn's* also has a component of hopelessness, because the individual doesn't know how to solve the problem they are tribulating over. There's a lot of conflict built into it. *Crohn's Disease* is a disease coming out of massive rejection, abandonment, lack of self-esteem, *and/or drivenness to meet the expectation of another. In fact*, Crohn's Disease *involves a great degree of codependency and false burden bearing.*

Ulcerative Colitis

In *Ulcerative Colitis* the dendrites are flaring in the lining of the colon. Do you know what dendrites are? Envision my arm as a nerve and at the end of each nerve is something called a dendrite. It looks like five fingers. Here are my muscles and here's a nerve and I want to clap my hands. Clap! Clap! Clap! I want to clap my hands, and raise my hands. I want to do something, but I've got to make this arm move. Now in conscious thought, I can do whatever I want, such as dance, talk, or whatever.

At the end of the dendrite is something called a nerve synapse. I like to say it crudely; it's like you're submerging the dendrite in battery acid. There's an aqueous material that acts as an electrical conductor, and on the other side is a receptor cell that causes your muscles to move. It carries the message that I'm going to clap my hands, or do whatever I want to do. There is a receptor cell, and the nerve transmission goes down like an electrical current. Your nervous system is like a bunch of electrical cords. It is the electrical part of your creation. There's an electrical impulse which travels down your nerve into the dendrite, arcs across the nerve synapse, connects to the receptor cell and my hands go clap, clap, clap!

However, stress and anxiety, things that are bugging you long-term, lack of trust, even feeling like you don't belong, can cause the dendrites to pulsate. Pulsation involves irritation, inflammation and ulceration. That's what produces *Ulcerative Colitis*. It is an *anxiety disorder*; the fruit of it is hemorrhaging of the lining of the colon.

You go to the doctor and he may give you chemotherapy, prednisone, or other steroids or drugs, all of which have incredible side effects.

Ulcerative Colitis is an anxiety disorder, rooted in extreme fear and anxiety and dread, causing a flaring of dendrites in the lining of the colon which irritates it in a manner similar to an ulcer. It causes an ulceration of the lining of the colon, producing severe bleeding. That's what *Ulcerative Colitis* is. The only way to get *Ulcerative Colitis* healed is to *deal with the anxiety disorder and the fear behind it.*

Diabetes (autoimmune disease)

I'll tell you what the spiritual root is behind *diabetes: extreme rejection and self-hatred coupled with guilt.* In many cases that we have ministered to in the past 10 years, we've found that there was *direct rejection by a father and sometimes, a husband, or a man in general.* We're not just talking about a little bit of rejection but stuff like "you ain't no good", "you ain't never going to amount to a hill o' beans" and then some choice language to go along with that.

We've had tremendous success in seeing *diabetes* healed. There has to be an absolute change in that person, allowing them to receive the love of God, in order for that to happen. *Diabetes* can be inherited because an unloving spirit can be inherited. A broken spirit (heart) is implicated also.

Fear can be inherited, allergies can be inherited; many of the things that we deal with can either develop in our lifetime, or we can inherit it from our family tree. Now when I see that happening in a child, I can go back to the father and mother, grandfather and grandmother, on both sides, and I'll find some abuse. I'll find some victimization, I'll find rejection, I'll find somebody not being nurtured somewhere. That can be inherited, not only from a genetic standpoint but also from a spiritually inherited standpoint. That is what I would be looking at in that case.

The Bible says in Ezekiel 18:17 that the children do not have to die for the sins of the father but in Exodus 20:5 it says the curse which is the result of that sin shall be passed on to the third and fourth generation.

> [17]**...he shall not die for the iniquity of his father, he shall surely live.** Ezekiel 18:17

> [5]**Thou shalt not bow down thyself to them, nor serve them: for I the LORD thy God *am* a jealous God, visiting the iniquity of the fathers upon the children unto the third and fourth *generation* of them that hate me;** Exodus 20:5

Lupus

Lupus is an autoimmune disease in which the white corpuscles attack the connective tissue of the organs. I ministered to a beautiful lady in California who has been healed of *lupus.* She was medically diagnosed, documented through her physician's case history and testing, and is now healed of *lupus.* Today, I can still remember how her voice sounded when calling me on the phone about 4 years ago, she said, "Pastor, I just got back from the doctor, and he can find no evidence of *lupus* in my body; it's gone." *Lupus is rooted in extreme self-hatred, self-conflict, and includes guilt. Performance also may be implicated.*

Multiple Sclerosis

Multiple Sclerosis occurs when the white corpuscles decide that the myelin sheath of the nerve is the enemy. Recent investigation has shown it's not just the myelin sheath that's affected by the attack of the white corpuscles, but that the nerve itself is damaged. This is recent information I did not know previously. I thought it was just the myelin sheath. The myelin sheath is like the insulation around the nerve, just as rubber insulates the outside of an electrical cord.

Multiple Sclerosis occurs when the white corpuscles come like a modern day Pac-Man, and take a bite out of the coating around the nerve, effectively short-circuiting it. It isn't that there is a problem with the muscles; it's that the nerve that causes the muscles to work has been short-circuited during the nerve transmission process. That's called sclerosis and in *Multiple Sclerosis* there are many of these holes created. The recent medical information is that the nerve itself has also been severely damaged in advanced cases of MS.

In a small percentage of cases the person eventually dies because even the muscles that are necessary for respiration are no longer functioning. However, 85% of these people live a normal lifespan. Generally nerve tissue does not regenerate; that's why certain parts of your body do not heal. That's why it would take a creative miracle by God and ministry to restore this type of damage.

MS is rooted in deep, deep self-hatred, and guilt, and spiritually it is very close to *diabetes* in that it involves a father's rejection. I want to say something to you. **The father is responsible for the spiritual welfare of the family. The father, not the mother, is responsible for his daughter's value system and her self-esteem.**

I don't give men many breaks, because I know the tragedy of my own life. I've had to learn this thing the way the Word teaches it; not the way my generation has lived it. I've had to have some paradigm shifts in my thinking as a human being and a man of God. I have to represent God the Father to my children. I have to be to my wife as Christ is to the Church. I don't have a choice.

Rheumatoid Arthritis

This is an autoimmune disease, and affects the joints of the skeleton, the tissues, the cartilage, and the connective tissue of the skeleton. It acts on the body like this: your white corpuscles decide that the bacteria and the viruses are not the enemy and they attack your joints and cartilage instead.

In *Rheumatoid Arthritis,* basically there is a proliferation of white corpuscles that congregate in the connective tissue of the skeleton and, like a Pac-Man, start to eat away and destroy the material. It is degenerative, and this is so classic that I end up saying it just the way I'm going to say it: *as the person attacks themselves in self-hatred, so the body conforms to that spiritual dynamic and attacks itself in return.*

Most people, lots of people, wish they were dead, and will say so if you talk to them long enough. They don't believe they belong on this planet. They don't believe God loves them. They don't believe their mother-in-law loves them. They don't believe their father and mother love them. They don't even love themselves and when you get into it, they are attacking themselves spiritually. There is a spirit of infirmity that comes, that agrees with them, and mutates the biogenetic character of the white corpuscles so that they take an assignment from the devil, not from God who created them, and they are on a mission of destruction.

The only way to be healed from Rheumatoid Arthritis, and other autoimmune diseases, is to accept yourself once and for all and to get the self-hatred and the guilt and the lack of self-esteem and the junk out of your life. When you don't accept yourself, you hate yourself, and you have called the living God who loved you from the foundation of the world, a liar. You have declared that He made a mistake in saving you. When you say that, you have called God a liar and the devil agrees. He's right there to bless you with the opposite of your Father in heaven's blessing and that's where the *"spirit of death"* comes in.

Can you say this? I want to hear you say it. "I shall live and not die to declare the glories of my God in my generation." What glory is there? Say it, "What glory is there if the grave takes me prematurely?"

> [17]**I shall not die, but live, and declare the works of the LORD.** Psalm 118:17

> [18]**For the grave cannot praise thee, death can *not* celebrate thee: they that go down into the pit cannot hope for thy truth.** Isaiah 38:18

Does God get any glory out of losing you prematurely off this planet? I want to give you some shocking theology. God doesn't need you in heaven right now. You are of no earthly good to Him up there and He doesn't need your help. He has birthed you by His will in the generations of your ancestry and He's called you by His Spirit. He's redeemed you to Himself for His glory in the earth to establish His kingdom, His love, His grace and His mercy through you until you just book it into heaven when you've finished all of that in your generation. I consider it error to even suggest that God needs disease as a vehicle to get you to heaven. There is much evidence to the contrary in Scripture.

Rheumatoid arthritis is another disease when the body attacks the body. As the person is spiritually attacking himself or herself, the body conforms to that spiritually and you've got it. It will be very difficult to be healed of *Rheumatoid arthritis,* or any other autoimmune disease, as long as you are buying that lie and allowing guilt and self-hatred to rule your thoughts and lives. It's not possible because God is not going to honor it, because He says—you are fearfully and wonderfully made (Psalm 139:14-18).

> [14]I will praise thee; for I am fearfully *and* wonderfully made: marvellous *are* thy works; and *that* my soul knoweth right well. [15]My substance was not hid from thee, when I was made in secret, *and* curiously wrought in the lowest parts of the earth. [16]Thine eyes did see my substance, yet being unperfect; and in thy book all *my members* were written, *which* in continuance were fashioned, when *as yet there was* none of them. [17]How precious also are thy thoughts unto me, O God! how great is the sum of them! [18]*If* I should count them, they are more in number than the sand: when I awake, I am still with thee. Psalm 139:14-18

Psalm 139 also says—His hand is upon you from the foundation of the world. Before your parts in continuance were fashioned from the dust of the earth, He knew you and He ordained that you be here in your generation. So accept it and get on with it.

Out of darkness, out of bondage, out of the fall of Adam and Eve, He has gathered you to Himself. The Father gathers His children to Himself. **You are going to have to accept His love and yourself in it.**

I don't care what your poor head tells you. Let God be true and every man a liar.

> 'God forbid: yea, let God be true, but every man a liar... Romans 3:4

"Yeah, but Pastor, you don't know what they did to me in 1948." No, but I know what God is doing for you this year! He's going to heal you. Get all your theology straightened out so you can get on the right side of faith, not fear.

Autism

Autism is a disease that I have been asked to get involved in, and I am studying four case histories now. We are about ready to get involved with autistic children in ministry. I'm looking forward to it. Our initial investigation has to do with a neurological breakdown coming out of rejection and rebellion. The entrance points, considering some of the younger ages of autistic children, are something we're not sure about. I have information coming to me all the time from research but I'm not really in a position to give you a definitive answer today.

Autism is an interesting one. I got a call from Pennsylvania recently, from a gal we've been working with. Her autistic son is now cutting himself. That's self-hatred, and brings a new component into this disease. I believe *autism* is a result of rejection, and the other components of *autism* involve rebellion and anger. They are almost the same principles that eventually produce *schizophrenia*. However, *autism* is not *schizophrenia*. Recent medical research indicates that an imbalance in a particular neurotransmitter secretion is implicated.

Parkinson's Disease

We have enough insight on this disease initially and spiritually to give me the faith to move ahead in actual ministry now. The only way we know that we're going to get this one is to get involved and start applying the principles that we see and see if God will honor that insight and give us the healing.

In New York State, there is a family of three generations with *Parkinson's disease.* Two brothers have already died, and in the three generations they all have Parkinson's.

I'm a member of the Parkinson's Foundation of America because I'm tapping into what they're doing. Current research is pointing at a deficiency of dopamine as the cause. When we have either under- or over-secretion of various neurotransmitters, I have always found either a genetic or spiritual component that's behind it. Either way, it has a spiritual root. I consider *Alzheimer's, Parkinson's* and *autism* to be spiritually rooted diseases.

In the case of *Parkinson's,* my initial investigation indicates unresolved rejection, massive amounts of abandonment and rejection, and hope deferred. As a point to ponder, personal and family involvement and spiritual error may be implicated.

Addictions

We've had some success with healing dopamine reductions in addictions. In dealing with addictions, dopamine is very important to pay attention to because dopamine is the pleasure neurotransmitter of the human body. The body produces it very slowly, while serotonin can be replaced very quickly. In fact cocaine is a very unusual drug because cocaine is not chemically additive. *Cocaine is psychologically and spiritually addictive.* I'll tell you why.

The mechanisms of cocaine are that when a person takes a hit of cocaine it releases dopamine in mass. It is equivalent to a massive orgasm. There is a huge release of dopamine that can never be duplicated a second time. That is why once they've had their first hit they will never have the same rush ever again. They try and try, but what they don't understand is that they'll never have it because the high is coming from the release of dopamine. It's not the drug that gives them the fix; it's dopamine being released that gives them the biological fix. That's why people on cocaine are very tormented.

All addictions are rooted in the need to be loved.

Masturbation

Masturbation is a big issue. Masturbation usually begins in childhood, not necessarily because of lust, but coming out of families that are full of strife. You see, a child learns that when a house is filled with argument and strife, and the tension is building, that an orgasm will give him or her a type of physical release from that tension. There's also a release of dopamine because when you have an orgasm, dopamine is the neurotransmitter that, when it is released, gives you that fulfilled feeling. It's a neurotransmitter and it gives you a neurological-biological "fix."

A child growing up in an atmosphere full of tension and strife will get temporary relief from masturbating, but what comes in behind it are the feelings of uncleanness and guilt. It's the same thing with cocaine. Right after it come feelings of uncleanness and guilt. We have a vicious cycle of release and condemnation. Masturbation and cocaine are very similar in their spiritual implications. A release, and fulfillment, and guilt. A release, fulfillment, guilt, and condemnation. Your enemy certainly knows how to work you over!

Those are some of the mechanisms of dopamine and cocaine, but what does that have to do with *Parkinson's Disease?* I'm not sure, but we're going to find out.

I just don't like losing. I've had so many victories in fighting disease that I just figure we'll just win them all one of these days. I think if we get an army here in the body of Christ, we might defeat the devil at some level. But if we don't start, it ain't gonna happen.

Those of you hearing this are experiencing a new frontier. This is a new frontier, where God is moving in mankind. I'm learning more every day. I don't have all the answers, but what I do know, and what has been proven to be true, I'll share with you.

Alzheimer's Disease

Alzheimer's disease, on the other hand, according to recent research in the medical community, seems to involve a proliferation of white corpuscles that are congregating at critical nerve junctions in the brain.

Wherever I find white corpuscles congregating and causing trouble, either eating at linings of flesh, eating the myelin nerve sheath as in *MS*, eating at the connective tissue of the organs as in *lupus*, eating at the cartilage connective tissue of the skeleton as in *rheumatoid arthritis*, destroying pancreatic function as in *diabetes*, eating at the lining of the colon and ulcerating it as in *Crohn's disease*, or congregating in a nonbacterial inflammation, as in *prostatitis*, or congregating in the brain and producing nonbacterial inflammation and interruption of nerve transmissions in *Alzheimer's*, I know the spiritual root. Whenever I find white corpuscles that are attacking the body, and not doing what God created them to do, I have—without exception—found various degrees of *self-hatred and guilt*.

If we could stop the white corpuscles from collecting at critical nerve junctions of the brain, *Alzheimer's* might not continue to exist. If we can get dopamine levels back up to where they need to be, then *Parkinson's disease* might not continue to exist. That's elementary, and God will give us the understanding as to the spiritual roots so that healing can happen. I know God wants to heal *Alzheimer's*.

The medical prognosis for many of the "incurable diseases" is very bleak. During a weekend seminar I did in New York City a year ago a doctor attended. We were discussing the "best" the medical community can expect to offer is ***disease management*** because in my teaching I had made a statement that the best allopathic medicine could offer was various forms of disease management. He came up to me and said, "Pastor, you're being very generous with my profession. The medical profession can only hope to achieve *disease management*, and we're a long way from even doing that." So, if we're not even getting disease management from the medical profession, how will we see cures?

A national magazine discussing the frontiers of medicine for the next millennium included the following observation that in the areas of cancer, disease, aging, strokes, AIDS, fertility, alternative therapies, gene therapies, organ transplants, mental illness and more – the best that we can look forward to, nationally and internationally, from the medical community is either miracle drugs or genetic engineering.

In their mind, there is no other alternative left except for gene therapy or miracle drugs. That's all you have left to look forward to. The rest of it has been exhausted. There is no hope. There are no solutions. That's what the medical community is telling us. I am reminded of the Scripture that says—physician, heal thyself (Luke 4:23). They can't even do it.

> **23And he said unto them, Ye will surely say unto me this proverb, Physician, heal thyself: whatsoever we have heard done in Capernaum, do also here in thy country.** Luke 4:23

Do you know what is really amazing, in terms of the longevity of life? The profession that has the lowest life expectancy in America is our physicians. Their average longevity is only 56 years. The people that you are looking to for healing are the ones that die first. That is a national statistic. Is that not sobering?

Cholesterol

America has been on a yo-yo. You need some cholesterol to grease your veins. The worst thing you can do is remove all of your cholesterol. Because you have high triglyceride levels and/or high cholesterol levels, does not mean it's caused by what you eat. If you're avoiding fatty foods to keep cholesterol down, that's not the issue. Why is it that some people eat whatever they want and never develop a problem with high cholesterol? Why do others have a problem?

It's because certain people have a predisposition to high cholesterol, and others don't. *There is a spiritual component to high cholesterol.*

I ministered to a lady a few years ago that had a triglyceride level of 378 and within 48 hours of ministry it had dropped to 178. What changed? Let me give you an example of how this works. Here are the veins; the inside is hollow and blood runs up and down inside, like a drinking straw. In people who have a predisposition to high cholesterol, something is on the inside that's reaching out and grabbing the cholesterol and binding it to the cell wall. That plaque finally thickens and thickens and thickens until you have the potential closure of the vein or the artery. The mechanisms that caused that plaque to form and to collect have a spiritual root.

This is my spiritual diagnosis: *Cholesterol is directly related to people who are very, very angry with themselves.* There is a high degree of self-deprecation; they're against themselves, they're always putting themselves down. It is more than merely putting themselves down; they are very hostile with themselves. They are very angry with themselves.

I dealt with a woman one time and she is totally well today. In fact, she is a member of my staff now; however, she was sick for 55 years. She had 17 different major "incurable" diseases and she has been healed of all 17. She had so much self-hatred and self-anger at one point that she burnt her flesh and carved it with knives. Her flesh was literally mutilated with fire, knives, razor blades, and glass.

I've got some good news for you; she's a wonderful lady. She is gloriously saved, gloriously healed, and she loves herself today. She serves God working 12-16 hours a day in our ministry. She's been marvelously healed and delivered by God. That *was* a high level of self-hatred wasn't it? Self-mutilation and self-hatred. Self-mutilation is a national epidemic today, especially among the youth.

It all begins with rejection. ***The beginning of all disease is the separation from God, separation from your own self and separation from others.***

Shingles and Hives

Behind all skin eruptions, which would include many rashes, humps and bumps, hives, and *shingles,* you are going to find the over-secretion of histamine, and in conjunction with it, a congregating and a proliferating of white corpuscles. Shingles is an *anxiety and fear* disease, coupled with an autoimmune component involving *self-rejection.*

Hives are a direct manifestation of fear and anxiety. Your skin is very responsive. Right behind the epidermal layer of your skin is your immune system, blood vessels, nerves, and every facet of your existence, just beneath the layers of your skin. You have white corpuscles that can congregate, and histamine. Systemic histamine can be created anywhere in the body: in localized sinuses, skin, internal connective tissue, etc. Histamine can be over-secreted and when you have an over-secretion of histamine, you have swelling, edema, and pain. Hives and *shingles,* in conjunction with dendrite flaring, give you a double problem. You've got your nervous system, you've got the secretion of histamine, the chemical part of you, the electrical part of you connecting, expressing itself as an extension of your anxiety and stress.

Definition of *shingles:* an acute central nervous system infection involving, primarily, the dorsal root ganglia and characterized by the vesicular eruption and neuralgic pain in the cutaneous areas supplied by peripheral sensory nerves arising in the effected root ganglia.

Etiology incidents in pathology: herpes zoster is caused by the varicella zoster virus, the same virus that causes *Chicken Pox,* and may be activated as local lesions involving the posterior root ganglia by systemic disease. Many latent viruses are often released in conjunction with fear, anxiety and stress. So thus, *shingles* and hives, for example, are considered to be anxiety disorders even though there may be viruses implicated in the profile.

That is very interesting to me because we are looking at some autoimmune characteristics right off the top. It may occur at any age, but is most common after age 50. Inflammatory changes occur in the central root ganglia and in the skin of the associated dermatome. In some instances, the inflammation may involve the posterior and anterior horns of gray matter meninges and the dorsal and ventral roots. There is no specific therapy.

We've had some success with it. I told you it had an autoimmune component attached to it before we got into this discussion, didn't I? I said this one was straight anxiety, but coupled with anxiety, self-rejection, and self-hatred. What does a virus do with that? What triggers these things to come up? What allows a virus to work?

When you look at classes of viruses, then you see they are almost like a phylum that has a particular object of its attention. I don't have all the answers to viruses, but I certainly am following their persnickety ways around mankind. They are interesting, because they seem to be on a mission and their mission is highly destructive and very calculated and has become a real pain to mankind. Also there seems to be an intelligence behind viruses that defies imagination.

In conjunction with other factors such as fear, anxiety, stress, lack of self-esteem, there are other problems that are of a non-viral order. What does a virus do? Why does it attach itself to other spiritual problems? I don't have an answer to that. I would certainly like to know. In the meantime, in ministry, I would say that with all viruses, we have had to come and do deliverance.

Rosacea

Rosacea has more of an autoimmune component to it, rather than anxiety which involves self-hatred. Rosacea is a chronic disease of the skin of the face.

Acne

Recent information on acne is really interesting. They have just come out with a statement this past year in the medical community that adolescent acne is the result of peer pressure. It's not just that the child is in puberty and the oil glands are exploding and presto! We have acne. What they have discovered, for the most part, is that adolescent acne is rooted in *anxiety and fear coming out of peer pressure. Simple acne is coming out of fear of man. Fear of rejection, and fear of man. In puberty and adolescence, it's peer pressure and peer pressure is fear.*

You know I've got six kids and four are teenagers. I'll tell you, they are overly concerned about what their buddies think. I mean, do you know what designer labels are? Kids are vicious with each other. Children are vicious, and children are more afraid of their peers than they are of you as parents.

That's why in church, as a pastor, I try to get the children in my church to get to know adults. I don't ship them off to a children's church, but get them involved in the congregation of the saints in worship. I get them into fellowship, so that they can have alternative peer pressure. They are not just stuck with the tunnel vision of kids that maliciously shame them, but with adults who will love them.

There can be an antidote to this problem. That's my position. I want my children to grow up knowing adults, not just other children, if I can find some spiritual adults I can trust my children with, that is.

Ovarian Cysts

Breast Cysts

Systolic Acne

Systolic acne is a different ball game. You will find this occurring mainly on the back, mostly in females; it is like cysts that erupt. *Systolic acne, ovarian cysts,* and *breast cysts* have something in common as a spiritual root. We've seen great success with *breast cysts, ovarian cysts, and systolic cysts,* nationally in our ministry. *Ovarian cysts, breast cysts* and *systolic acne* are taught together because of a common root.

I have found it true, without exception, that these conditions are coming out of the breakup of the relationship between the girl and her mother. Unresolved issues involve a great breach, and there is no fellowship. It carries right down into the reproductive area. It involves a full issue of femininity. It is involved even to the degree that the girl may question her own femininity, or the female part of her creation. The mother has breached it at that level.

Many times there is great bitterness, anger and great resentment toward the mother. I have found it true, coast to coast, that the people who have been healed of *ovarian cysts, breast cysts,* and *systolic acne* have had to get things right before God concerning their mothers.

Endometriosis

You know I've had some success in the area of *endometriosis* and yet, for the life of me, I haven't figured out the root yet. I don't have any idea. I wish I had more to say about it because it shows up all the time in conferences. To this date I still don't know. I have ministered and I have taken a position just because I really didn't know anything else to do. *I have found self-rejection and self-hatred.* I've had some success. I had a tremendous feeling about it several years ago and this was the leading; that it has to do with self-hatred and self-rejection. I don't have enough evidence yet to document what I'm saying, so let's let that one slide into the investigative mode for the moment.

(Audience comment on endometriosis: I've done a lot of studying on this because I've been very concerned about abortion. Apparently one of the factors, or

*results, of abortion is endometriosis because it has to do with the hormonal
interruption. Abortion is not a normal miscarriage and so there are a lot of factors
that come into play. It seems that a lot of women who have had an abortion,
whether chemical or otherwise, wind up with endometriosis.)*

Herpes

When we get into *Herpes,* we've got more than one kind. We've got Simplex:
whether it be genital herpes or fever blisters, and they are viral. Now are you saying
that *shingles* is viral? That's what the doctors say. When I get into *herpes,* which are
viral, I still get into a spiritual problem. There are several cases of *herpes* that I've
dealt with. It's amazing that *herpes* seem to go into remission, but under stress they
erupt. Bacteria can be destroyed easily but viruses are difficult to destroy because they
mutate, change, hide, and even go dormant for years. Again, there seems to be an
intelligence behind them that defies imagination.

Viruses

I want to tell you what viruses are. A virus does not have as its origin its own life.
It is a mutation of what is already genetically in another life form and then mutates
after its aberration. Viruses are an aberration of genetic materials producing various
kinds of interference with human flesh. That's what a virus is. It is a mutant genetic life
form that seems to have a mind of its own. It is difficult to destroy and, in the case of
HIV, it can remanufacture itself in a different form by taking the genetic code of a
living organism, and using the genetic material of a living organism, to produce its
own genetic form.

I have finally come to this conclusion, and I couldn't document this even if I tried,
but in ministry I have been attacking viruses from this basis and have been getting
healing in incurable diseases that are virally related.

I consider viruses to be *spirits of infirmity* and consider them to be a
physiological expression of the work of evil spirits, working in conjunction with man's
flesh and genetics. That's the only thing I have been able to figure out. *A virus has an
intelligence behind it that defies imagination.* A bacterium, just floating around, will
duplicate itself and it's still a bacterium and it kind of has a "life form." However,
viruses seem to be very intelligent; behind a virus there is some type of intelligence,
and it's not God.

I have been attacking viruses as spirits of infirmity, and I got that from the Bible.

> [11]**And, behold, there was a woman which had a spirit of infirmity eighteen
> years, and was bowed together, and could in no wise lift up** *herself.* [12]**And when
> Jesus saw her, he called** *her to him,* **and said unto her, Woman, thou art loosed
> from thine infirmity.** Luke 13:11-12

Jesus cast out spirits of infirmity with His words. Jesus knew something then that
I don't know, but I'm here 2000 years down the road with some advanced technology

to help me try to figure it out, and I'm coming to the same conclusions that He did. There's something alien that is an intelligent, invisible being that afflicts man's flesh and tissue. You can't kill it, you can't destroy it, but you can divert it. And so I have tried casting it out, and it has worked. Why is it that we have a virus sitting around, hanging out, doing no physical harm and then it's released because of another spiritual problem called fear, anxiety and stress and it does damage to the body? Do you think there's a connection?

Is it possible to make a virus go dormant forever if we deal with other spiritual problems? That's an interesting question, and I certainly will be pursuing it to see how much success we have long-term.

Our Statement Concerning Diagnosis and Success of Diagnosis

The only thing we can do here, in any investigation of disease, is first of all to acknowledge that we are dealing with hypotheses. Even from the secular standpoint of ministry, we have to see how many cases in the long-term are healed, and stay healed, based on the information that we have. The more case studies we get into, the more we will know. I will tell you that this ministry is on the cutting frontier of disease, yet we have a long way to go in getting enough case histories under our belts that we can see established, complete patterns. From the standpoint of investigation, I hope without making this a big issue, that you can hear where I'm coming from and where I'm going on this issue.

Cancer

I will tell you up front that I don't have all the answers to cancer. It's one of the most feared diseases of this generation. And yet, there are some cancers that we have had some insight into.

Editor's Note: Cancer that is the result of metastisizing of cells to other parts of the body is an unfortunate by-product of the disease and may have nothing to do with the root of the original source.

Colon Cancer

I'm coming to the conclusion that it is deeply rooted in bitterness and slander with the tongue. The Bible says that—life or death is in the power of the tongue. Every word that we've spoken that is evil will be held in judgment against us.

> [21]**Death and life *are* in the power of the tongue: and they that love it shall eat the fruit thereof.** Proverbs 18:21

> [36]**But I say unto you, That every idle word that men shall speak, they shall give account thereof in the day of judgment.** Matthew 12:36

There are a lot of strange things happening between the lips and the anus, and in between all kinds of things can go wrong for many spiritual reasons. If you poop on enough people, it comes back to you. I'm rapidly looking at colon cancer cases and looking back to past generations, because it is clear that it can be inherited. I believe colon cancer is an inherited disease. I'm looking back to see if we can trace the history of conflict in families. Family conflict similar to the Hatfield's and the McCoy's, where unresolved bitterness, unresolved antagonism, and words of frustration and anger have occurred causes damage throughout the successive generations.

Do you know that when you speak evil against someone that is a curse and what you speak against another returns? Can I give you a scripture? Jesus said—those sins that you retain are retained and those sins that you remit are remitted (John 20:23).

> [23]Whose soever sins ye remit, they are remitted unto them; *and* whose soever *sins* ye retain, they are retained. John 20:23

Do you know that when you retain another person's sins, and you don't forgive them, that you in fact have retained that curse on yourself? You read that scripture— whatever is bound on earth shall be bound in heaven and whatever is bound in heaven shall be bound on earth (Matthew 16:19).

> [19]And I will give unto thee the keys of the kingdom of heaven: and whatsoever thou shalt bind on earth shall be bound in heaven: and whatsoever thou shalt loose on earth shall be loosed in heaven. Matthew 16:19

The Lord's prayer says—if you do not forgive your debtors the Father in heaven will not forgive you yours (Matthew 6:9-15).

> [9]After this manner therefore pray ye: Our Father which art in heaven, Hallowed be thy name. [10]Thy kingdom come. Thy will be done in earth, as *it is* in heaven. [11]Give us this day our daily bread. [12]And forgive us our debts, as we forgive our debtors. [13]And lead us not into temptation, but deliver us from evil: For thine is the kingdom, and the power, and the glory, for ever. Amen. [14]For if ye forgive men their trespasses, your heavenly Father will also forgive you: [15]But if ye forgive not men their trespasses, neither will your Father forgive your trespasses. Matthew 6:9-15

So the sins that you retain are retained. You are holding the other person under the bondage of your judgment. But by the same judgment that you judged others, you yourself are judged. That's what the Bible says.

> [7:1]Judge not, that ye be not judged. [2]For with what judgment ye judge, ye shall be judged: and with what measure ye mete, it shall be measured to you again. Matthew 7:1-2

> [2:1]Therefore thou art inexcusable, O man, whosoever thou art that judgest: for wherein thou judgest another, thou condemnest thyself; for thou that judgest doest the same things. Romans 2:1

When we get into the area of gossip and slander, tale bearing, sedition, anarchy, division making, causing trouble, not promoting peace, being an instrument of division and anarchy, I wonder if these sins may be the cause of colon cancer?

The cancers that I am most familiar with are breast, ovarian, Hodgkin's, leukemia, and prostate. I have one case of pancreatic cancer in my portfolio, and I never got to minister in that situation. The person went off into alternative realities and didn't stay in touch with me.

Skin Cancer

I don't know if there is a spiritual root or not; the evidence seems to involve care of the temple (our body) and keeping the skin covered properly to protect it from ultraviolet rays.

Liver Cancer

I haven't yet had the opportunity to minister to someone with liver cancer.

Editor's Note: Additional information has come to me concerning liver cancer. Since this seminar was taught, an individual e-mailed me the following scripture.

> [21]**With her much fair speech she caused him to yield, with the flattering of her lips she forced him.** [22]**He goeth after her straightway, as an ox goeth to the slaughter, or as a fool to the correction of the stocks;** [23]**Till a dart strike through his liver; as a bird hasteth to the snare, and knoweth not that it *is* for his life.**
> Proverbs 7:21-23

There seems to be some indication that these scriptures have to do with an individual, in this case a man, who was lusting after a female, either in his mind or actual fornication of adultery, or following seduction. The individual who e-mailed me indicated a close family member died from liver cancer and even though it was not known if actual fornication or adultery had occurred, it was known that this individual was heavily into pornography. The question I'm asking myself in this note is: is this a warning from the Word of God concerning the fruit of being addicted to pornographic material?

Breast Cancer

Let me say something that will really shock you. I don't mean to scare you, and every time I say this certain ladies end up being scared, so please—don't be scared. I'll tell you, 10% of all breast cancer in America is caused by mammograms.

A big uproar happened about a year ago when the AMA said you don't have to have mammograms until at least age 50. The feminist radicals immediately objected and said that women must have them throughout adulthood. However, the medical community had come to the startling conclusion that 10% of all breast cancer was caused by mammograms. That's why the feminists backed off. Startling isn't it?

Why 10%? Most of the women who fell into that category had what is called a "predisposition to breast cancer." A healthy cell has two enzymes called anti-oncogenes. They are tied directly to the immune system. There are three classes of cells in the human body: healthy, which have two anti-oncogenes present; predisposed, which have one anti-oncogene present; and compromised, with no anti-oncogenes.

A healthy cell will never become cancerous. You cannot develop cancer with both of the anti-oncogenes present. Something has to come and destroy them. In the case of someone who is genetically predisposed, there is only one anti-oncogene present. A compromised cell is where one or two of the anti-oncogenes have been destroyed by some intrusion into the cell, either by toxic chemicals from outside the body or toxic chemicals manufactured by the body internally for some reason, such as a result of bitterness.

The ladies that develop breast cancer from mammograms had an inherited predisposition for cancer with only one anti-oncogene. The X-rays from the mammogram destroyed the one remaining anti-oncogene, the cell became compromised, and breast cancer began. As a pastor I would tell any lady, "if you're going to get a mammogram, it might cost you a little money, but go to an oncologist first and get tested."

I know they are saying that they have reduced the radiation dosage and they've changed radiation mechanisms so that now the mammograms are safe and won't destroy the anti-oncogenes that are present because of an overdose of radiation. That's what they tell you when you ask the questions. My recommendation is that you check it out first, especially if there is any history of breast cancer in your family tree.

When I talk about healings that have taken place with breast cancer, I'm talking about an individual who had gone to an oncologist in conjunction with a geneticist, and had their breast tissue tested. If the oncologist finds that the breast tissue is compromised (no anti-oncogenes are present) then it would be necessary that you be re-tested after ministry to see if there be any changes. In ministry, we deal with the spiritual roots, and come before God, and meet the spiritual conditions for healing to take place. In re-testing in this particular case, it was found that both anti-oncogenes were present in the cell after ministry, where before they were medically proven to be missing. That's a miracle!

One of the first cases of breast cancer I got involved with was in 1984. A lady came to me a couple of days before her scheduled surgery for a radical mastectomy. I got involved in her life, and it took awhile to figure out what the spiritual roots of her cancer were. There had been competition between the females in her family, I mean sibling rivalry, and the girls were competing with their own mother for supremacy. It was a mess. There was a tremendous amount of bitterness and bickering. I got with her before God and helped her to forgive her sisters and her mother. She had a strong root of bitterness.

Concerning a root of bitterness, there is an old saying: *"It eats at them like a cancer."* If you have this type of festering resentment and bitterness on a long-term basis, then your body will produce toxins that will eventually accumulate to the level and volume that they will destroy the anti-oncogenes of the immune system at the cellular level in the breast tissue.

The target cells in females are in the breast tissue, because it's the breasts that are the nurturing aspect of a female. When the female is no longer nurturing, or she is being nurtured yet is turning into a spiritual alley cat, there is a problem. It's a tragedy. When the resulting toxins develop, they destroy the anti-oncogenes.

In this lady's case, after I began ministering to her, we came before God, looked at all the things she was doing, and she repented before God for this long-term historical feud. Her mother had a history of the same type of behavior with her own sisters. These females had hated one another for generations. It was a cat fight all the way.

She had the mastectomy surgery, and coming out of the surgery we were still doing ministry, dealing with spiritual roots and blocks and coming before God. Her doctor said to her, "I'm going to put you on chemotherapy for 5 years." She came and told me her doctor wanted to put her on chemo for 5 years.

I said, "Well, if your anti-oncogenes are present, and if God has healed you, you are wasting your time." I suggested that she get re-tested. She went back to her doctor and said, "I think I want my cells tested to see if both anti-oncogenes are present now." He said, "Where did you hear that?" He said, "This is new."

She said, "My pastor told me." She asked him, "Doctor, if both my anti-oncogenes are present in genetic testing, can I get cancer?" He said, "NO." She said, "Then why do I need chemotherapy?" He said, "For our protection." She said, "What if I don't want it?" He said, "You'll have to sign a disclaimer relieving us from all responsibility." She said, "I'll do it." So they tested her and both anti-oncogenes were present, where before they had not been. **That's a miracle!** I tell you, we are now 10-12 years down the road and she's still alive today. Praise God! There are many other cases.

Breast Cancer is coming out of the sins of conflict and bitterness between the female and either her mother and/or her sisters or mother-in-law. *Systolic breast cysts* are very similar. Many women get *breast cysts* and think it's cancer.

DISCLAIMER: This profile represents a large percentage of breast cancer cases but there are many other causes for breast cancer also.

Ovarian Cancer

Ovarian Cancer is coming out of a woman's hatred for herself and her sexuality. Unclean and unloving spirits that accuse her in the cleanness of her sexuality can lead her into self-bitterness and self-loathing concerning her own sexuality.

Uterine Cancer

Uterine cancer possibly may be caused by promiscuity and uncleanness. However, behind the promiscuity and the uncleanness is the need to be loved and that's another issue.

Hodgkin's Disease and Leukemia

Hodgkin's Disease and *Leukemia* are very similar. They are similar because in *Hodgkin's* (Lymphatic) and *Leukemia* (Blood), the root cause is the same. The factors are the same. I have found that *Hodgkin's Disease* and *Leukemia* many times are caused by deep-rooted bitterness coming from unresolved rejection by a father. I have always found a breach between the person who has that disease and their father. I've never found a mother involved in the breach. Abandonment by a father, literally or emotionally, is also implicated.

Prostate Cancer

Prostate cancer is coming out of anger, guilt, self-hatred and self-bitterness. All cancer that has a spiritual root involves some type of bitterness against someone for some reason. It involves long-term, lingering, festering and damage leading towards death. Hate is the 5th part of bitterness. You wish that someone didn't exist. God says, "If they don't exist neither do you."

> [14]**We know that we have passed from death unto life, because we love the brethren. He that loveth not** *his* **brother abideth in death.** [15]**Whosoever hateth his brother is a murderer: and ye know that no murderer hath eternal life abiding in him.** 1 John 3:14-15

Your enemy has as much of a right on this planet as you do. God loves you and your enemy and He might save both of you! You might be an enemy to somebody else. What's good for the goose is good for the gander. In conclusion, though, the bitterness is more directed towards one's self although others may be indicated in the profile.

Remember 2 Timothy 2:24-26:

> [24]**And the servant of the Lord must not strive; but be gentle unto all** *men,* **apt to teach, patient,** [25]**In meekness instructing those that oppose themselves; if God peradventure will give them repentance to the acknowledging of the truth;** [26]**And** *that* **they may recover themselves out of the snare of the devil, who are taken captive by him at his [the devil's] will.** 2 Tim. 2:24-26

There are a lot of people blaming God for their problems, and He's not guilty. Let's get this straight: the Word of God says, in James 1:13—God does not tempt man with evil, neither can He be tempted with it.

> [13]**Let no man say when he is tempted, I am tempted of God: for God cannot be tempted with evil, neither tempteth he any man:** James 1:13

I'm going to get Daddy off the hook if you don't mind, and put the deceiver back in the frying pan. I want to make sure that I sow seed into your lives that the Holy Spirit can use, that the Father can use, and that the Lord Jesus, Who is the Word, can use, that They might bring you into a place of defeating your enemy and bearing fruit in your generation and your lifetime, not to mention extending your life expectancy without disease.

I've said many times in teaching and seminars that since Adam and Eve mankind has been on probation for almost 6000 years.

God has been trying the reins of men's hearts to see if there would be any that would seek after Him so that He may show Himself strong on their behalf. Your hearts are being tried.

> **⁹For the eyes of the LORD run to and fro throughout the whole earth, to shew himself strong in the behalf of *them* whose heart *is* perfect toward him. Herein thou hast done foolishly: therefore from henceforth thou shalt have wars.** 2 Chron. 16:9

> **²Examine me, O LORD, and prove me; try my reins and my heart.** Psalm 26:2

Will you choose the good, or will you choose evil? Will you repent? Will you take responsibility or will you go into rebellion? The bottom line, whether we like it or not, is submission to the living God: out of our free will, because we want to, and because we're in love with Him. He is in love with us. He tells us so over and over in His Word.

When we step outside the parameters of the covenant, outside the holiness of God, then God gives us over to our enemies.

Read the history of the Jews. When they didn't like God, they went out and followed the gods of the Amorites, Moabites, Syrians, Egyptians and all the rest. God would say, "OK, if you don't want Me as Father, let them be your Father. Let them bless you."

What was the blessing? The Curse. When God's people had enough of it and they were sick and dying and in captivity they would come running back to Daddy and say, "Daddy, we're sorry, we repent, we repent, we repent." And God would say, " I forgive you."

When we step outside the commandments of God, we open ourselves up to the "blessing" of the devil. It's as simple as that. When you start to hate your brother, you receive the recompense of the reward. Through one man sin entered into the world and death by sin. (Romans 5:12) Through one man's disobedience sin came, and through another man, Christ Jesus' obedience, we are free. We are either obedient sons and daughters of God or we are disobedient sons and daughters of God.

Does the devil have a legal right to you after conversion? I'm not sure about that, but I'll tell you what; I sure see evidence of it. Many people struggle with the reality and the question, "Can a Christian have an evil spirit?" I'm not sure I have the answer to that but I'd raise this question, "Can an evil spirit have a Christian?"

Proverbs 26:2 says—as a bird by wandering and the swallow by flying so the curse without a cause does not come.

> **²As the bird by wandering, as the swallow by flying, so the curse causeless shall not come.** Proverbs 26:2

Your enemy does not have the right to oppress you just because he's out there. Somebody has to open the door and invite him in. Go back to Genesis 3: Satan used the serpent as a medium of expression. He did not have access to this planet until Eve invited him in, and Adam agreed. In your life, the evil one does not have the right to oppress you; he only takes that right because you give it to him, many times through ignorance, or lack of knowledge. Proverbs 26:2 says—the curse without cause does not come.

God has set parameters of protection around mankind against the devil. The only way the devil can get at you through his kingdom is if you invite him in at some level. **These are called the doorpoints of entrance.** If this were not the case, then the Christian wouldn't have a chance. Satan could have killed us all and it would have been over with. However, Satan does not have that ability. God forbade him to bring death in the discourse with Job. But in Job's life there was a spiritual root problem. Job had a hedge of protection, and Satan challenged that protection. God had no choice but to let Job be sifted so that he could be purified at the level of that testing. When you read Job, especially in chapter 3, Job said—the thing that I have feared greatly has come upon me.

> **²⁵For the thing which I greatly feared is come upon me, and that which I was afraid of is come unto me.** Job 3:25

Faith and fear are equal in this dimension: both demand to be fulfilled.

Hebrews 11:1 teaches us about faith:

> **¹¹:¹Now faith is the substance of things hoped for, the evidence of things not seen.** Hebrews 11:1

Fear is the substance of things *not* hoped for and the evidence of things not yet seen. Faith is God's future for you. Fear is Satan's destruction of your faith and ultimately your future.

> **⁶But without faith *it is* impossible to please *him:* for he that cometh to God must believe that he is, and *that* he is a rewarder of them that diligently seek him.** Hebrews 11:6

That's what the Word says. Job had a root problem. Chapter 3, he was full of fear. In chapters 40-41, in the discourse concerning Behemoth and Leviathan, the great parable of his spiritual condition, we find he had pride and he had spiritual arrogance. You know that, because he took God on for size and discourse. God came back with, "Where were you, big boy, when I did this, this and this?" God turned the captivity of Job around when Job finally was humbled and he prayed for his friends. He received twice as much as he had when he began, and his captivity was turned around. Could God turn around your captivity? Yes, He can.

Editor's Note: It must be understood and distinguished that not all growths are cancerous. There are two types of growths: one is fibroid tumor (benign) and the other would be considered cancerous (malignant). *It is my observation that when a tumor does not become malignant, it involves bitterness against one's self. But, when it becomes malignant, it involves bitterness against others.*

Osteoporosis

The root for *osteoporosis* is envy and jealousy, which matches the Word. (Remember the testimony in the early part of this teaching about the lady from New Jersey who was healed of osteoporosis?) The Word says that envy and jealousy is the rottenness of the bone (Proverbs 14:30).

> [30]**A sound heart *is* the life of the flesh: but envy the rottenness of the bones.**
> Proverbs 14:30

The fruit of the root of envy and jealousy is rottenness of the bones and that is not only a physical problem but a spiritual problem. The healing and prevention of *osteoporosis* begins in eliminating envy and jealousy from your life. Envy and jealousy are sins.

Spondylolysis

Spondylolysis is progressive degeneration of the vertebra of the spine. That entire scenario is rooted in self-hatred. *Spondylolysis* is the degeneration of the vertebra caused by *self-hatred.*

Arthritis

Arthritis (Involving Inflammation of the Joints)

Basic simple *arthritis* is inflammation of a joint usually accompanied by pain, swelling and frequently changes in structure. It might be noted that this differs from *osteoarthritis* and other forms of *arthritis* by the type of manifestation and that there is a different spiritual root behind each of the types.

The spiritual root for simple *arthritis* involves bitterness against others.

Editor's Note: To help you understand, it seems to be that when you have bitterness against yourself, it involves degeneration but when you have bitterness against others, it involves swelling and inflammation. It is the swelling and inflammation that produces the deformity.

Osteoarthritis

Osteoarthritis is progressive cartilage degeneration in joints and vertebra and usually does not involve inflammation. The cartilage is the other material between the vertebra. *Osteoarthritis* is the result of *self-bitterness* and *not forgiving one's self.* It's holding a record of wrongs against yourself, and also can involve an element of guilt.

Degenerative Disc Disease

Degenerative disc disease is usually caused by anything dealing with the disc, apart from accidents and injury that is degenerative in nature. Inherited or degenerative disc disease is *usually tied to an addictive personality* involving drugs, both legal and illegal, and may be included in the inherited profile. Somewhere in your past, there may be someone who was a drug runner or put drugs or alcohol to someone else's lips to make them drunk, or your own usage of such.

> **15Woe unto him that giveth his neighbour drink, that puttest thy bottle to *him*, and makest *him* drunken also, that thou mayest look on their nakedness! 16Thou art filled with shame for glory: drink thou also, and let thy foreskin be uncovered: the cup of the LORD's right hand shall be turned unto thee, and shameful spewing *shall be* on thy glory.** Habakkuk 2:15-16

These scriptures are not just about getting someone else drunk, contributing to their demise, but it is very clear that there is a "woe" (curse) that comes upon someone because we have not contributed to a person's welfare. I wouldn't want to be a bar owner for too long.

I've dealt with many cultures and nationalities in ministry and I've observed another characteristic. Have you ever noticed people coming out of the "Hippie" days? Many of them have back problems. I have observed degenerative disc disease and back problems coming out of drug addiction and in profiles of families who were addicted to various drugs. It's an observation. I've dealt with some of these people regarding their addictions and have had some success; with others I haven't. The first place that I look when ministering to someone with degenerative disc disease, apart from injury, is into the drug profile. There's where I've had more success.

Alcoholism

Have you ever wondered why some people can drink and are not alcoholics and others drink and are alcoholics? First of all, alcoholism is not a genetically inherited disease. However, there is a genetic component that has to be paid attention to that is born out of an alcoholic family. Did you know alcoholism runs in families because *there is a curse in that family that produces it?* Molestation runs in families. Victimization runs in families. *There are familiar spirits that travel in families.*

A national statistic reports that 35% of all females in America have been molested at some time or another, and that 25% of all males have been molested at some time in their life. That is a national statistic in America. It brings a rollover. The possibility that a person who has been molested will molest someone else in their lifetime is very, very good, unless they are saved by the blood of Jesus Christ and delivered.

When a child is born into an alcoholic family, he has what is called a *deficient chemical* in the basal (nerve) ganglia. The basal ganglia is at the top part of your spinal cord, where your brain sits. In here are various neurotransmitters that are connected directly to your central nervous system via the cerebral processes.

There are four major classes in neurotransmitters that can be found in that area.

One has to do with painkillers. When a person is born with an inherited predisposition for alcoholism there is a defective chemical coming out of the birth. It's not normal. It's like it needs something to give it completeness as a chemical. Alcohol is a chemical; it's a drug. When this defective chemical comes in contact with alcohol, there is a chemical reaction and a brand new chemical is formed. This new chemical stays permanently in the basal ganglia; it's called THIQ. This new neurotransmitter produces a permanent craving for alcohol.

A person who is an alcoholic is actually allergic to alcohol. Alcoholism is an allergy. That is the reason it only takes one drink to start this thing moving.

I've had some success with alcoholism and some failures. The success with alcoholism comes first of all from the Lord delivering the person, in conjunction with them just having had enough. There has to come a time in the person's life where they make a quality decision to just say "NO." I know God meets us and honors us in that decision.

I've seen unsaved people get free of alcohol. I'm not necessarily in agreement with the 12-Step Program and I'll tell you why. They teach, "Once an alcoholic, always an alcoholic" and I disagree. The people who have been delivered and healed through our ministry concerning alcoholism need no support groups, and they are not drawn to alcohol ever again. I think when you say, "Once an alcoholic, always an alcoholic," you have just said to God that He cannot deliver you and that He cannot save you to the uttermost. I cannot go that route. Although 12-Step Programs have done some good, there has to **be a more excellent way,** a greater grace, and that is to be free.

Psoriasis

Psoriasis is an autoimmune disorder in which the white corpuscles are congregating on the skin, creating the scaling, the flaking, the redness, and the hardness. Psoriasis is rooted in *self-hatred, lack of self-esteem and conflict with identity*.

Nonbacterial Inflammation

About three years ago, in ministering with people, we bumped into a new disease that's just now being recognized by the medical community. It's a combination of two diseases that have merged into one. Its root is a combination *of anxiety, fear, guilt and self-hatred* producing something called *nonbacterial inflammation*. Inflammation comes from bacterial intrusion. When you have bacterial intrusion, you go to the doctor and he puts you on antibiotics. What if you have inflammation and he puts you on antibiotics and there is no bacterial material intrusion? If you continue taking the antibiotics you're not going to have any relief and after awhile you're going to end up with *Candida*. Continuous usage of antibiotics destroys the body flora and you need some body flora to maintain your balance. You don't want to destroy all the bugs! Some are helpful!

Interstitial Cystitis

Interstitial cystitis is a swelling and inflammation of the bladder tissue of females. It is very painful, nonbacterial, and the current treatment for it is to give an antibiotic. The antibiotic is prescribed, not because there are bacteria present, but because a certain antibiotic has been developed that has anti-inflammatory properties. The purpose of the anti-inflammatory is to bring down the swelling. In *interstitial cystitis*, what you have is the over-secretion of histamine, producing swelling, and the proliferation of white corpuscles producing inflammation and swelling. In males it is called *Prostatitis*.

Prostatitis

Prostatitis also is a disease that involves nonbacterial inflammation in males. Prostatitis is pretty serious because it can lead, at some point, to prostate cancer. Again, *prostatitis* involves two dimensions as does *interstitial cystitis* and those are excessive secretion of histamine and a proliferation of white corpuscles on location.

In these nonbacterial inflammation diseases the spiritual root, as mentioned, is fear and anxiety, which causes excessive histamine secretion and self-rejection and self-hatred coupled with some guilt produces the proliferation of white corpuscles.

We ran across an individual in New York City 2 or 3 years ago who was light sensitive, was in a highly exhaustive state, had swelling and edema, and the doctors couldn't figure what it was. We diagnosed him spiritually with this new disease so that the spiritual roots caused a combination of an over-secretion of histamine and a proliferation of white corpuscles in various parts of his body; and there were spiritual roots behind it.

He talked to a member of my staff earlier last year, and related that he had been to a doctor at New York City Hospital who had said, "This is a brand new disease that we have been studying and we are diagnosing you with it. We don't understand much about it, but it has to do with autoimmune and histamine problems."

He said, "I sat in that office for over 30 minutes and every word they said you had already told me a year before, almost word for word."

Skin

Skin rashes, itching, hives, blotching, swelling. How many of you have had a rash appear on your arm—you scratched, it itched, and you went to the doctor? He prescribed a topical salve for you. Did you ever look at the ingredients of the topical salve? When you look at the small fine print on the tube that you squeeze, it's an antihistamine. When you have an over-secretion of histamine in your body, whether it involves your skin, sinus, or an internal organ or tissues, you have swelling. When you have swelling, you have pressure on your nervous system and you have pain, discomfort, and irritation. The spiritual root behind this is fear, anxiety and stress over some issue in your life.

Sinus Infections

Sinusitis involves the over-secretion of histamine. We deal with histamine disorders from a standpoint of sinus, skin and systemic. Systemic would be internal. When histamine is over-secreted, it produces swelling, edema, and runny noses. When you get sinus problems and you go to the doctor, you are given an antihistamine, which is a drug. The side effects of antihistamine can include a personality change for a minimum of 24 hours. Secondly, it can also include feelings of rage and anger. Antihistamines are extremely addictive. I've had to help many people stop using antihistamines before I could get to the root problems of their *sinusitis.*

What happens in *sinusitis,* and the result of taking antihistamines, is that you become chemically addicted to the drug. When the drug which was initially prescribed to combat the over-secretion of histamine wears off, the initial problem no longer exists, but your body is now craving the drug. Your body mirrors the sinusitis symptoms: runny nose, watering eyes, etc., just to get the drug. Now you've got a double problem. The exception is if you have a nasal obstruction from a birth defect that prevents proper drainage.

The root behind sinus infection and *sinusitis* is *fear and anxiety.* All histamine, whether involving skin, sinus or systemic, is over-secreted in conjunction with *stress, anxiety, and tension.* That whole area of *insecurity* produces an excessive histamine secretion in the human body.

PMS

PMS and menopause are not the same. Menopause is part of life. I do believe God can make a provision for you in menopause so that you don't have a hormonal tragedy. There is much debate about estrogen therapies and I have mixed emotions about it. I would say that it is probably best if you could go the more natural route. You'd be better off because of the cancer risk.

PMS is another story. PMS basically comes from a tightening of the muscles of the uterus and uterine walls producing pressure, pain, distress, and discomfort. Part of it is tied to fear. *Fear of pain.* The first area of ministry in PMS we do is start to pray peace and ask God to take away the *fear* of pain and discomfort. We ask God to bring the person to full relaxation of the muscles in that area. It's nothing more than muscular tension. Complicating the syndrome also can be feelings of uncleanness around a person's sexuality because of a stigma attached to the monthly cycle.

You can get pills to "treat" PMS. What are they going to do for you? They are a neurological blocker, designed to give you muscle relaxation. Personally, I believe that the root behind PMS is part of the curse on females. Not all females have PMS, just as some do not have pain in childbirth. They have pressure but not the pain. Most people that have PMS that we've run into are pretty introspective females. They are females that are really bound with *introspection, phobic realities* in their minds, and *stress.*

I also found another ingredient in PMS: sometimes females don't like being females. I find that some females really get hostile at "that time of the month" because they just don't like going through it. Although I recognize hormonal shifting can be a factor, this can be overamplified by a spiritual and emotional conflict. As a result of the mind-body connection, the hormonal shift is now magnified and complicated by thoughts, thus increasing the problem. On the other hand, when I deal with people who have MCS/EI, many of them have not had a menstrual cycle for years. One of the first signs of healing in females with MCS/EI is they get regular cycles back. One gal called me after 8 years of no female cycle. "Pastor, I had my period!" I said, "Glory to God." I had another one say, "Oh no, it's here." I got one response of rejoicing and one saying, "Oh no." I'll tell you what's worse than PMS—not having your cycle—if that's any consolation!

Fibromyalgia

It goes with the MCS/EI profile. When you find MCS/EI you'll find *primary fibromyalgia syndrome* (PFS) almost without exception. PFS is often a misunderstood disease. The first time I ran across someone with PFS, I thought they had the worst thing in the world. It can be very painful. It can be localized, generalized, or all over your body. Somebody said that PFS is what causes MCS/EI. I still hear that, or I hear that *candida* causes MCS/EI. But that is not true. They are by-products of a whole different root problem.

I have a Merck Manual, which is a physician's desk reference on disease. I also have a Physician's Desk Reference (PDR) on disease and drugs, and a good college textbook on pathophysiology, and many books on anatomy and physiology. We don't have to be in the dark about the enemy. When somebody comes to me about disease, I want to be able to help them in addition to what their doctor's doing. I have discovered, through this ministry, that in some cases I know more about the etiology (cause) of certain diseases than some people's doctors do.

The doctor can tell you where it is, and what it's doing, and how to drug it or cut it out but he still does not know why you have it. If you go to the doctor's desk reference many times it will say: "etiology unknown." The cause of the disease is unknown.

I believe God knows what causes our diseases and in the case of 70 to 80 different "incurable" diseases, God has revealed why people have those diseases. Doctors consult with us concerning their patients from coast to coast. There are doctors who consult with us for their own health and healing. Some doctors send their patients to us by phone for insight and ministry. The reason I'm sharing this with you is because I want to bring you into focus. You don't have to be ignorant about what you don't know. You just need to know where to look it up!

The term *myalgia* indicates muscular pain, in contrast to *myositis*, which is pain due to inflammation of muscle tissues, ligaments, tendons and white connective tissue.

Fibromyalgia is an appropriate term for pain where inflammation is absent. What does that tell me? PFS is pain that does not have inflammation or swelling as its cause. There is no pressure on the nerve from edema or swelling. Most of the pain that we have comes by pressure of swelling or edema on an adjacent nerve. Pressure on the nerve produces pain. Right off the bat, I know that the pain in PFS is not due to inflammation or swelling, or an infection, and not from bacteria. It is true pain in which no inflammation is present.

PFS is a term used to describe pain in fibrous tissues, muscles, tendons, ligaments, and other "white" connective tissues. This is a quotation from pp. 1369-1370 of the Merck Manual (16ᵗʰ edition as published by Merck & Co. in Rahway, NJ, 1992):

> **Etiology:** Primary Fibromyalgia Syndrome (PFS). The condition occurs mainly in females...is particularly likely to occur in healthy young women who tend to be stressed, tense, depressed, anxious, and striving...

What's the difference in male and female in body parts? There are few differences, as far as bone, muscles and tissue and structure. We have the same nervous system. We have the same muscles and ligaments, don't we? Sexually we're different, but basically from a nerve standpoint we are the same. Then why do you think this condition is basically a female condition?

In MCS/EI, 85-90% of the individuals who suffer this disease are female and only 10-15% are male. Why is that? It's the same reason why nearly 100% of all PFS patients are female.

The Bible says in 1 Corinthians 11:8—man was not made for woman but woman was made for the man.

> ³**But I would have you know, that the head of every man is Christ; and the head of the woman *is* the man; and the head of Christ *is* God...⁸For the man is not of the woman; but the woman of the man. ⁹Neither was the man created for the woman; but the woman for the man. 1 Cor. 11:3, 8-9**

Now that doesn't mean that the man has the right to be chauvinistic or oppressive; this has to do with God's order in creation.

I want to tell you something: I have not found one woman during my ministry who does not want to follow a spiritual man unless she has a hatred of men or a distrust. God created her to follow an example of nurturing. When the woman is not nurtured, when she has no one to follow, and she is made the spiritual head of the home by default, she goes down in stress and anxiety and never surfaces again.

Somebody's got to take care of the family. Somebody's got to represent God. Somebody's got to do nurturing. Somebody's got to communicate. Somebody's got to spout off somewhere. Somebody's going to be emotional. Most female disorders are the result of a lack of nurturing and protection (covering) by a male in which the female is saddled with the problems of life without any help, emotionally or spiritually. Occasionally, drivenness and perfectionism may be implicated. If it is, it's an attempt to receive love and feel complete through works.

The reason why is because anxiety and stress and fear come upon a woman under those circumstances because she was not made to be the stronger vessel. The Bible says—she has been created to be the weaker vessel (1 Peter 3:7).

> [7]**Likewise, ye husbands, dwell with *them* according to knowledge, giving honour unto the wife, as unto the weaker vessel, and as being heirs together of the grace of life; that your prayers be not hindered.** 1 Peter 3:7

It doesn't mean that she's weak upstairs. It doesn't mean that she's weak before God; it means that, in the God-ordained order of things, she is designed to respond and be a helpmeet to her husband. The husband was designed to lead in all things, and to establish the kingdom of God in righteousness, in justice, and in love in their home. The Proverbs 31 woman was no slouch but her husband was known and did sit in the gates with the elders of the city. Also, "the heart of her husband doth safely trust in her...she will do him good and not evil all the days of her life." This reality is only possible **if** the man takes his rightful place in the home in love.

> [11]**The heart of her husband doth safely trust in her, so that he shall have no need of spoil.** [12]**She will do him good and not evil all the days of her life.** Proverbs 31:11-12

When a man molests his daughter, when he beats his wife, when he won't listen to his children, he violates the protection mechanism and his family does not know where to turn. Fear and anxiety comes, and disease results.

Men, we need to take the time to get our priorities re-established. If you want your wife to love you, you'd better get hot toward God first. *Let God teach you how to represent the Godhead in your family.*

Also according to the Merck manual definition of PFS it is "likely to occur in healthy young women who tend to be stressed, tense, depressed, anxious...striving," driven, perfectionists, and who are moving all the pieces around. "Symptoms can be exacerbated by environmental or emotional stress, or by a physician who does not give proper credence to the patient's concerns and discharges the matter as 'all in the head.'" You want to get a flurry of PFS? Let somebody be insensitive to your problem. What comes in? More hopelessness, despair, anxiety, and stress. The root behind *fibromyalgia* is fear, anxiety, stress, drivenness, and perfectionism, for the most part, unless there is a specific organic reason.

Fibromyalgia works like this: Let's pretend that my arm is a nerve and around my arm is tissue but there is no inflammation so there's no contact. At the end of your nerve are something called dendrites. They are called dendrites because the word dendrite translated means digit or finger-like. When I want my hand to move, my thought process causes a nerve impulse to be sent. The impulse runs down the nerve to the dendrites, arcs over a nerve synapse to a receptor cell on the corresponding muscle that hooks up with the nerve, and the whole process causes my hand to move. The short version is that I think about it, and it happens.

In *fibromyalgia*, the nerve impulse is initiated without conscious thought. There is no intended corresponding muscular reaction required. What triggers it is *the spirit of fear in the realm beyond consciousness*. Even if you know it's there, you try to ignore it. It's there, and it initiates nerve impulses through the hypothalamus, which is sensing the problem upstream in the soul and the spirit, and all of a sudden you've got something happening. What happens in PFS beyond conscious thought is that the nerve impulse runs down the nerve into the dendrites and pulsates. And it dead-ends. That is what causes the pain. You can't do anything with it.

The only way you can get rid of it is to allow God to deliver you from the anxiety, fear and stress. The Bible says—be anxious for nothing (Phil. 4:6).

> **⁶Be careful for nothing; but in every thing by prayer and supplication with thanksgiving let your requests be made known unto God. Philip. 4:6**

God has not given you the spirit of fear, but of power, love, and a sound mind (2 Tim 1:7).

> **⁷For God hath not given us the spirit of fear; but of power, and of love, and of a sound mind. 2 Tim. 1:7**

That's the mechanism of PFS. The spiritual root can be found in females who do not feel covered, protected, nurtured, don't feel safe, are always looking over their shoulder, are driven, anxious, moving the pieces of their life around, and are insecure.

Sleep Disorders

Proverbs 3:24(b) says—your sleep shall be sweet.

> **⁸I will both lay me down in peace, and sleep: for thou, Lᴏʀᴅ, only makest me dwell in safety. Psalm 4:8**

> **²⁴...yea, thou shalt lie down, and thy sleep shall be sweet. Proverbs 3:24**

> **⁵Thou shalt not be afraid for the terror by night... Psalm 91:5**

I claim that. I claim sweet peaceable sleep without fear at night. If you're not able to sleep there might be a physical reason, but many times there is a spiritual reason.

The hypothalamus gland is the brain of the endocrine system. The hypothalamus gland is very important because it will make or break you in all areas of disease. The hypothalamus gland controls many things in your body.

> **It is one of the centers that maintain the waking state and sleep patterns.** (Principles of Anatomy & Physiology, by Gerard J. Tortora and Nicholas P. Anagnostakos, Second Edition, Harper & Row, 1978)

Right here in this book on anatomy and physiology, you find where the problem begins. When you have problems in your mind, the hypothalamus is going to respond to what you are thinking about.

Sleep disorders can be caused by the hypothalamus responding to your spiritual and emotional state. Torment can interrupt and perplex you, and can stimulate your hypothalamus to keep you awake. I'll tell you why. The hypothalamus is the main gland that is involved in *fight or flight*, the first stage of the General Adaptation Syndrome in the fear profile.

We will be teaching later on fear and anxiety disorders (fear, stress, anxiety, and physiology). There are three stages of an anxiety disorder in the General Adaptation Syndrome: (1) the *fight or flight* stage; (2) the *resistance stage;* and (3) the *exhaustion stage*.

You will find that when you are tormented inside, deep in the spiritual or in the emotional part of your soul, it can be beyond your conscious thought in *fight or flight*. Life's circumstances, which include tragedy, torment, victimization, fears, phobias, unrest, uncertainty, and all the other vicissitudes of life, come to project themselves into the future, and that threatens your existence. That's enough to keep you awake all night.

The Bible tells you—take no thought for tomorrow (Matthew 6:34).

> **³⁴Take therefore no thought for the morrow: for the morrow shall take thought for the things of itself. Sufficient unto the day *is* the evil thereof.** Matthew 6:34

If you're not worried about tomorrow, you will sleep tonight.

If you're worried about tomorrow, you will not sleep tonight. What is the worst thing that can happen to you? You can die and go to heaven—to be absent from the body is to be present with the Lord (2 Corinthians 5:6-8).

> **⁶Therefore *we are* always confident, knowing that, whilst we are at home in the body, we are absent from the Lord: ⁷(For we walk by faith, not by sight:) ⁸We are confident, *I say,* and willing rather to be absent from the body, and to be present with the Lord.** 2 Cor. 5:6-8

So what if you lose everything tomorrow? The same God that got you this far can start over again and probably do better. The Bible says—He that would try to save his life shall lose it and he that would lose his life will save it (Matthew 16:25).

> **²⁵For whosoever will save his life shall lose it: and whosoever will lose his life for my sake shall find it.** Matthew 16:25

I think that we have been majoring in minors and minoring in majors. I think it's time to get rid of the rudiments of the world's way of thinking and get back into line with the thinking of God.

> **⁶Be careful for nothing; but in every thing by prayer and supplication with thanksgiving let your requests be made known unto God. ⁷And the peace of God, which passeth all understanding, shall keep your hearts and minds through Christ Jesus.** Philip. 4:6-7

You say, "Well. I don't like what's happening to my life." Maybe you're under the chastening of the Lord, and if you don't go through it, you're never going to get through it!

I want to tell you something about problems. How many of you like problems? How many of you like stress in your life? I have learned something about problems. They are always going to be there. The second thing I've learned about problems is that when I've got a problem, if I lose my cool and lose my peace, *I still have that same problem to deal with.* If I still have to solve the problem, then I might as well just be cool. It is much easier to solve the problem when you haven't lost it and you have your peace. You're going to have to solve it anyway. You can run from it, but it will follow you.

What I'm saying to you is this: if you have a problem, it may not just be the enemy trying to oppress you. It may be God trying to lead you into the next stage of His will for your life.

You may never get there if you don't face the issue. You might as well get a good night's sleep before you do. That problem will still exist tomorrow, just as well as tonight. If it's going to be there tomorrow, why don't you have your peace tonight and get your rest?

It's that stuff that's upstream that destroys your peace and your sleep, and your hypothalamus is agreeing with you. The Bible says—many are the afflictions of the righteous, but the Lord delivers us out of them all (Psalm 34:19).

> [19]**Many** *are* **the afflictions of the righteous: but the Lord delivereth him out of them all.** Psalm 34:19

Certain sleep disorders can be from two sources: fear and anxiety, or torment from victimization. Of course, it could be from fear because you watched "The Exorcist." You've been down to that place that rents movies for $3.00, and you've been watching horror films. You've opened your spirit up to the spirits of fear, anxiety, torment, tragedy, and horror and you wonder why that stuff is coursing through your spiritual dynamics. You have a responsibility to guard your heart in order to receive protection from God in regard to torment.

Isaiah 33:13-16 says,

> [13]**Hear, ye** *that are* **far off, what I have done; and, ye** *that are* **near, acknowledge my might.** [14]**The sinners in Zion are afraid; fearfulness hath surprised the hypocrites. Who among us shall dwell with the devouring fire? who among us shall dwell with everlasting burnings?** [15]**He that walketh righteously, and speaketh uprightly; he that despiseth the gain of oppressions, that shaketh his hands from holding of bribes,** *that stoppeth his ears from hearing of blood, and shutteth his eyes from seeing evil;* [16]**He shall dwell on high: his place of defence** *shall be* **the munitions of rocks: bread shall be given him; his waters** *shall be* **sure.** Isaiah 33:13-16 [italics for emphasis]

Scripture is telling us that there is no protection for you from God if you don't hide your eyes from seeing the shedding of blood and hold your ears from what's happening in evil. When you watch that junk on your video machine and your TV, movies about mutilation, horror and murder, there is no protection from God for you from the sleeplessness and the projection of tragedy. You have brought it upon yourself. So if you watch "As the World Squirms," then be prepared to squirm.

I guard my heart as to what I look at. I won't watch anything that would make me condone evil. I don't watch rapes on TV. I don't watch violence on TV. I will get away from it, turn it off and I've taught my children to do their own censorship also. When you open your eyes and your heart to that evil garbage, you are desensitizing yourself to the Spirit of God and condoning evil in your heart. You say, "Well, I'm not doing it. I'm just watching it." God says that you are wrong! You are an accessory to evil. What you condone is what you establish.

Isaiah 33:13-16 tells us very specifically what God thinks; God doesn't pull any punches.

The TV button goes off just like that! We're very careful. I won't watch anything that has to do with murder or evil and that includes sexual issues, also including pornography. I won't do it. I'm supposed to be saving lives, not destroying them. I'm supposed to be establishing righteousness in the earth not enthroning evil.

If you have a fear of evil you are a sitting duck for everything invisible traveling in the second heaven. Remember what Job said in Job 3:25—what he feared the most came upon him.

> **25For the thing which I greatly feared is come upon me, and that which I was afraid of is come unto me.** Job 3:25

You need to take an assessment of your fears, because fear demands to be fulfilled. *Fear and faith are equal in this dimension: both demand to be fulfilled.*

Sometimes in ministry, I have had people sitting in observing, especially in the areas of dealing with evil spiritual powers. If I sense that people are afraid of the devil, or afraid of principalities and powers, I ask them to leave the room. Why? They are on the wrong side of this battle.

Remember when Jesus went back to His hometown? He did very few miracles. He only healed a few sick folks. Do you know why? Great was their unbelief and doubt. If you are receiving this teaching in unbelief, I'm wasting my time. In fact, you could douse the Spirit of God by unbelief and doubt. That is why I ask some to leave the room. Do you understand what I'm saying? I can't help you any more than Jesus could when He went back to His hometown, if you do not believe.

Multiple Personality Disorder

I have with me a testimony of MPD from a woman who had 14 multiples documented by a clinical psychologist in a major city in America a few years ago. She had been in therapy for 14 years to accomplish what is called integration and fusion. Integration and fusion is where the therapist tries to get all the personalities to agree to hang out with each other and agree with each other, and in Christian therapy, to get them saved. That's what it is.

When I read the Bible, it tells me that type of therapy would make a person more double minded.

[8]A double minded man *is* unstable in all his ways. James 1:8

I want what God wants – for the person to be single-minded. I think what God intended in creation was for us to be an extension of who He created us to be from the foundation of the world, not a unified combination of personalities from life circumstances.

[4]According as he hath chosen us in him before the foundation of the world, that we should be holy and without blame before him in love: Ephes. 1:4

This individual after 14 years of integration and fusion therapy with the clinical psychologist was still a mess. The amount of time it took to get her free through our ministry was one sentence long. It was over.

I had 14 personalities all talking to me. I listened to these characters talking to me out of this woman and I said to myself at 8:45 that night, "Let's see, there are 14 of them, maybe I can get one out every hour. That's 14 hours. That's not going to fly too well. Maybe I can do one every 30 minutes. That would make it 5:00 AM in the morning by the time we're done."

The Spirit of God dropped down in my heart and prompted me to say this, "Listen guys, if you think I'm going to mess with you all night long, you've got another thought coming. Here's the deal, you're gonna join your little demon hands together inside this woman and go 'boogie, boogie.' Book it in the name of Jesus!" One of them spoke out of her. A voice came out of her and said, "We know we have to obey you." They were gone and it was over just like that.

Remember Jesus cast out 7 devils from Mary Magdalene? Do you believe that really happened? Do you believe that really happened or that's just there to make us have a story to tell?

[2]And certain women, which had been healed of evil spirits and infirmities, Mary called Magdalene, out of whom went seven devils, Luke 8:2

Could you accept the fact that I cast 14 devils out of this woman?

I'll tell you what the Lord said; He said that the things He did, we shall do, and greater things than He did, we would do because He went to the Father and He sent the Holy Spirit to come and allow us to get this job done. Are you listening to me?

[12]Verily, verily, I say unto you, He that believeth on me, the works that I do shall he do also; and greater *works* than these shall he do; because I go unto my Father. [13]And whatsoever ye shall ask in my name, that will I do, that the Father may be glorified in the Son. [14]If ye shall ask any thing in my name, I will do *it.* John 14:12-14

Migraines

We have known for quite some time the spiritual root for *migraines*. But we didn't know the whole picture until recently when I started to do some research on the drug of choice given to America today for migraines: *Imitrex*. In my study about *Imitrex* and its mechanisms in the human body, I have found "the rest of the story." *Imitrex* is prescribed 70 to 80% of the time for migraines.

A migraine is a type of headache pain known as psychogenic pain. Psychogenic means that it is not caused by any known organic reason. It's not pain because of injury. It's not pain because of any organic reason. It comes and it goes and it's incredibly painful. It brings with it nausea, flashing lights, and a complete shutting down of one's ability to cope with life.

Our success with migraines without drugs, I think, is second to none in America. Let me explain to you its mechanisms and let me give you the root. In order to show you how that works, I'll give you the mechanism of the drug *Imitrex*.

There are two parts to migraines. First, there is a reduction in the secretion of serotonin, and second, there is an increase in histamine secretion. This is triggered by *guilt resulting from conflict in your life in conjunction with fear.*

It's not the conflict itself that you're having that triggers the migraine. It's the conflict that you have with yourself over the conflict that triggers the migraine, either real or imagined.

You may have guilt because you think you spent too much money, and you got in a little argument with your husband over how much you spent. That argument, about that little infringement in finances, is not what causes the migraine. It's the guilt that you have with yourself that produces the migraine.

Migraines are triggered in people that have conflict with themselves about conflict in life or conflict with others. It's rooted in guilt. *All migraines are rooted in guilt.* Out of guilt comes fear, and it is always in that order. *It's guilt first and then fear.*

Here's the mechanism. As you enter into guilt over some issue, the hypothalamus gland senses that you are in conflict with yourself. A mechanism of *self-hatred* sets in causing the pineal gland to slow down the secretion level of serotonin. This causes a lowered serotonin level. The conflict develops in the realm of the soul and the spirit and fear now starts to move. Anxiety concerning the issue starts and histamine begins to be over-secreted in the cranial region.

Serotonin is a *vasoconstrictor*. When your serotonin levels are normal, they maintain the diameter of your blood vessels just the way God intended and they carry your blood supply into each region of your body.

Histamine is a *vasodilator*. As the serotonin levels are decreased and histamine is increased, you have a resulting dilation of the blood vessels. A swelling of the blood vessels puts pressure on sensitive nerves and that's what produces the migraine.

Imitrex is a compound drug that is designed to be an antihistamine and a serotonin enhancer. Serotonin and histamine are antagonistic to each other in that they are in opposition to each other in body functions. They repel each other. They don't coexist together. When serotonin levels are reduced because of the guilt, then histamine levels are allowed to increase because of the fear. Histamine and serotonin are incompatible with each other in the human body. What happens when the drug *Imitrex* is given is this: first, histamine is reduced and then serotonin is enhanced. Vasodilation reduces, vasoconstriction is broken, the blood vessels return to normal and the migraine is over. That's the mechanism behind migraines and this is the mechanism of *Imitrex* drug therapy.

In ministry, our desire is that you don't have to take *Imitrex*. First of all, it costs a lot of money and secondly, it's a form of *pharmakeia*/sorcery. Thirdly, it does not solve the root problem. There has to be **a more excellent way.**

Let's look at scriptures that define drugs in the Word. These scriptures have to do with works of the flesh that are considered to be sin by God.

> [19]**Now the works of the flesh are manifest, which are** *these;* **Adultery, fornication, uncleanness, lasciviousness,** [20]**Idolatry,** witchcraft, hatred, variance, **emulations, wrath, strife, seditions, heresies,** Galatians 5:19-20

> **pharmakeia, Greek 5331, Strong's,** *far-mak-i'-ah;* **from Greek 5332 (pharmakeus);** *medication* **("pharmacy"), i.e. (by extension)** *magic* **(literal or figurative) :- sorcery, witchcraft.**

> **pharmakeus, Greek 5332, Strong's,** *far-mak-yoos';* **from pharmakon (a** *drug,* **i.e. spell-giving** *potion***); a** *druggist* **("pharmacist") or** *poisoner,* **i.e. (by extension) a** *magician* **:- sorcerer.**

In Strong's, the word witchcraft is #5331 in the Greek, the word *pharmakeia*. It is from the root numbered word 5332. 5332 is the Greek word *pharmakeus* which means a drug, i.e., spell-giving potion that: a druggist ("pharmacist") or poisoner, i.e., a magician :- sorcerer. Going back to the main word 5331, it literally means as defined in the Strong's – medication (pharmacy).

If you were God, would you want to maintain your child on the earth through a drug, or deal with the spiritual problem so your child wouldn't have a migraine to begin with? If you were God what would you do? You'd solve the root problem, wouldn't you? This is **a more excellent way.**

In ministry, we come alongside people and start dealing with the guilt and the self-conflict. We address the spiritual dynamics that are tormenting them. We want to get the situation before the Lord, get them delivered, and get them fixed, so that when they are faced with conflict and failure, they can have God's peace. They are no longer bound by guilt and conflict. They have been delivered; they have been healed. They no longer have lowered serotonin levels. Fear is not there because anxiety is gone. Histamine is not secreted and a migraine does not develop. Our ministry helps people recognize these dynamics to the degree that in the "walk-out" stage of ministry on their journey to total freedom, many of them are able to quickly stop a migraine before it gets a foothold. This is **a more excellent way.** This is true discernment and spiritual warfare that produces long-term freedom.

Learning to deal with migraines, as with allergies, can take time. However, now that you know the cause and the process you have the knowledge and the power of God to help you.

Cell Wall Rigidity vs. Cell Wall Permeability

We minister to folks with a class of diseases *involving cell wall rigidity versus cell wall permeability.* Classic angina, asthma, and retention of toxins in the bloodstream fall into this same category. When you have cell wall permeability, it means that in the process of osmosis or diffusion (that material in the bloodstream that is necessary in the cell enters through the semi-permeable walls of the cell and the waste by-product is exchanged on the same basis; it leaves the cell through semi-permeable walls), in normal tissue, free flow goes unhindered. When you have cell wall rigidity, you have stiffening of the cell walls and osmosis is hindered. Behind this is a very definite spiritual root. In the case of toxic retention at the cellular level, toxins build up in concentration and are retained as the cells lose their ability to dispose of waste products.

Asthma

In the case of *asthma,* there is stiffening of the cell walls of the alveoli. This causes an entrapment of carbon dioxide and an exclusion of oxygen. Thus you have breathing problems and find yourself gasping for air.

The inhalant medication given by a physician is a neurological blocker, which basically short-circuits the process and allows a relaxation of those cell walls. The carbon dioxide is then released and oxygen starts to be absorbed. You begin to breathe normally. Those are the mechanisms of what happens when drug therapy is applied to the problem. The process of osmosis or diffusion is normalized.

We have known for many years that *asthma is a fear-anxiety manifestation.* It can be inherited. There can be a genetic component. We have observed from medical journals that the hypothalamus gland, when it senses fear and anxiety, causes a hormone called ACTH to be secreted. This hormone goes into the bloodstream and docks at a receptor cell in the alveoli. This produces the stiffening.

Asthma is one of the fastest growing childhood diseases in America. I've known the root problem of *asthma* for over a decade. When I taught it, people would look at me and laugh. "Well, that's not what the medical community says. You are out to lunch." I might be out to lunch but many people are well. Now the medical community is agreeing with me.

The findings from research of the John Hopkins University Research Team, in the fall of 1996, confirmed our spiritual diagnosis of asthma and that changed the conventional wisdom concerning asthma for the past 50 years. You've been taught that many asthmatic attacks are a response to an exposure to allergens, irritants, pollen, dust, and danders— things that you take into your respiratory system through breathing.

John Hopkins University research has conclusively proven that nothing that you breathe causes an asthmatic attack. Something is happening in the lungs, in the alveoli, that is causing stiffening, an entrapment of carbon dioxide, and an exclusion of oxygen. Thus we see the respiratory difficulty, the gasping for air, and all that goes with the drama of the situation.

Usually the type of fear and anxiety that produces *asthma* has to do with *great fear concerning relationships*. We have ministered to many people who no longer have *asthma*. John Hopkins University is still trying to figure out what this invisible reality is that triggers the stiffening. I'll tell you what it is—*a spirit of fear* and it is able to control your physiology through the hypothalamus.

Editor's Note: Since this seminar was taught, evidence has led me to observe the depth of this spirit of fear. In fact, my conclusion is that fear of abandonment and the resulting insecurities is the key issue behind asthma.

Angina Pectoris

The word *angina* comes from the Greek word meaning strangling. *Angina* is a cell wall rigidity disease but does not involve osmosis or diffusion. *Angina* involves the hardening and stiffening and narrowing of blood vessels and produces faulty circulation. *Angina pectoris* occurs when coronary circulation is reduced for some reason. Stress and anxiety (spiritually speaking, fear) produces a constriction of vessel walls and is a common cause. Also implicated is strenuous exercise or a heavy meal. Apprehension and dread increases the problem. The bottom line is that fear, anxiety and stress is a common culprit. Remember what the Word says in Luke 21:26:

> **²⁶Men's hearts failing them for fear, and for looking after those things which are coming on the earth: for the powers of heaven shall be shaken. Luke 21:26**

Hypertension (High Blood Pressure)

Again we a have cell wall rigidity which produces a vasoconstriction of blood vessels, coupled with an increase of cardiac output, which increases the blood pressure. It is again caused by *fear and anxiety*. On page 305 of chapter 9 in the Pathophysiology textbook on the subject called "Stress and Disease" – One of the physiologic effects of the catacholamines is a peripheral vasoconstriction of blood vessels in the cardiovascular system. Also on page 309 in the section entitled "Examples of Stress-Related Diseases and Conditions," under the target organ or system, the cardiovascular system is listed and one of the corresponding diseases listed that is a result of stress is *hypertension* (high blood pressure).

Our position is still the same—God has not given us the spirit of fear but of power, love and a sound mind"(2 Tim 1:7).

⁷For God hath not given us the spirit of fear; but of power, and of love, and of a sound mind. 2 Tim. 1:7

We have to go back into a person's life and find out where the open doors are, either inherited or personal. It is these open doors that allow the spirit of fear to come in, and to take over that person's life, and control them at this level.

Toxic Retention

When you have cell wall rigidity, the body will retain various toxins at the cellular level and will not cleanse itself properly because the process of osmosis or diffusion is hindered. We ran into this by accident. When we started to review the case histories of people healed of MCS/EI, we came up with a startling observation. When the doctor re-checked their blood, the toxin levels were normal. They had not used any drug therapies or modalities of cleansing to cause the cells to be cleansed of toxins. As these individuals walked out of their disease spiritually, the toxins went away.

As I started to get into it, I realized that when the mechanisms that produce cell wall rigidity were gone, full cell wall permeability now existed. *God designed the body to cleanse itself as part of its creation.* When the spiritual roots are dealt with, that is exactly what happens.

Have you not read the scripture—if you drink any deadly thing, it shall not harm you?

¹⁸...and if they drink any deadly thing, it shall not hurt them... Mark 16:18

Do you know why? It is because when you are in a right relationship with God your body cleanses itself of toxins. I'm not talking about going out here and doing something presumptuous like drinking something poisonous. I'm talking about a normal lifestyle and things that you are exposed to. God created your body to cleanse itself of impurities. The spiritual root of the toxic retention is fear and anxiety.

Editor's Note: I am for a clean environment and do take a stand that government and industry should be responsible in protecting us from excesses of chemical intrusion. And I am fully aware of the possibility of chemical injury. However, the majority of toxic blood cases that I have reviewed do not include exposure at this level. In fact the many cases of MCS/EI that involved diagnosable toxic levels, after ministry and walk-out, the toxic reality was gone and tissue was normal. This has been an astounding fruit in our investigation of cell wall rigidity vs. cell wall permeability.

NOTE: *Even though many people are well today from MCS/EI and toxic retention including the corresponding allergies and all that goes with it, it does not mean that everyone who started to apply our principles has gotten well. The reasons are many because people's life circumstances can be complicated and not everyone has continued with our program to its conclusion. I am not responsible, nor is any other person trying to help someone responsible, for the failure of insight to work when that person withdraws from the insight. That doesn't make the insight invalid, it just indicates that there is breakdown at a different level.*

Allergies

An *allergy* is a hypersensitive reaction to any antigen (any substance that produces a reaction). This is a strong area where our ministry sees victory, much victory over *allergies*. I'll tell you how it works.

DEFINITIONS:

- Antigen – any substance that, when introduced into the body, stimulates the production of an antibody.

- Allergen – a substance that causes an allergy.

- Allergy – hypersensitive reaction to environmental factors or substances such as pollens, foods, dust or micro-organisms in amounts that do not affect most people.

So an *allergy* is an acquired, abnormal immune response to a substance [allergen] that does not normally cause a reaction.

- Antibody – any of the complex proteins produced by B lymphocytes in response to the presence of an antigen.

Thus an antigen [allergen] is a substance that induces a state of sensitivity when it comes in contact with body tissues. A reaction called an allergy is produced.

This stage of this teaching concerns allergies that are the result of a compromised immune system. The body produces cortisol to suppress the inflammatory response to the attack. Cortisol (a steroid hormone secreted by the adrenal cortex) is over-secreted long-term and you have destruction of white corpuscles and macrophage and killer cells. Too much cortisol long-term produces cell death at this level.

Many times you have antibodies to antigens occurring in your body in relationship to a compromised immune system. Fear, anxiety and stress compromise your immune system. This is exactly what we are learning from the medical textbooks; that long-term fear, anxiety and stress can destroy your immune system and when that happens you have antigen to antibody and that's exactly what an allergy is, a hypersensitive reaction.

I'm here to give you some startling information. **Your body is not allergic to anything.** You've been had. You've been had with the biggest lie of the devil you've ever been had with. In creation, God created you to be compatible with everything that you are exposed to.

What the devil did to you through his kingdom was that he destroyed, or compromised, your immune system and set up this sequence of events because of fear, anxiety and stress. Why don't you take your life back before the LORD once and for all, and tell your friends and your neighbors and your family you've been had?

How often have you heard your friends say, "Well, I'm allergic to peanut butter, I'm allergic to chocolate, I'm allergic to dairy products, I'm allergic to this, I'm allergic to that?"

Tell them they've been had! Get involved in their life. Ask them what's bugging them. What are they afraid of? What is their stressor? Where is their conflict? What is unresolved? This is the work of the enemy in the human spirit and the human soul. Are you with me? Oh my, it's powerful, isn't it?

Look here. Here's something else that happens when you experience long-term fear, anxiety and stress. This is incredible also. This is how it affects you. I know this is kind of technical but I just wanted to show you because this is coming directly out of the medical community and their research. These are some physiological effects of long-term over-secretion of cortisol as a result of fear, anxiety and stress and as a result, the destruction of the immune system. Look what's affected. Functions affected by cortisol: *carbohydrate and lipid metabolism, protein metabolism, inflammatory effects, lipid metabolism, the immune reserve, digestive function, urinary function, connective tissue function, muscle function, bone function, vascular system and myocardial function, central nervous system function.*

Every bit of this is affected long-term by fear, anxiety and stress and we wonder why we have so many diseases that are coming out of fear, anxiety and stress.

Now you understand why the LORD needs to deliver you of all your fears. Let me show you something else here. Let's talk about the mind-body connection. I know this is not overly spiritual but you need to know what your doctor is *not* telling you. You need to know what the medical community is *not* telling you.

I'll tell you why the medical community is not telling you this; because they wouldn't know what to do with it if they did tell you about it. They don't know what to tell you, so they don't tell you anything.

Your homeostasis (equilibrium in the body with respect to various functions and chemical composition of fluids and tissues) is controlled by the release of various hormones. You are very chemical in your creation. You are very nuclear, you are very sexual, you are very spiritual, but you are also very chemical. You have a number of organs and glands, particularly in the endocrine system, which secrete a particular chemical. It kind of goes like this: a squirt here, a squirt there, here a squirt, there a squirt, squirt, squirt, everywhere a squirt, squirt.

And your enemy knows that he can control the rate of your squirts by your thoughts, and by your soul, and by your spirit. Your enemy knows that things like bitterness and guilt and fear, if allowed to remain within your consciousness, can be used of him to control you. When your spiritual dynamics are compromised by the enemy in a manner that he can control your body, and he can control your chemistry; then he can put depression or any other psychological or biological malfunction on you when he feels like it.

He can do this because depression, by definition, is no more and no less than a chemical imbalance in the body caused by a chemical imbalance induced externally or internally.

Your enemy knows that if he can get you "unspiritual" and he can manipulate you in areas of lack of sanctification, then he can control your very thought process.

When Satan can control your thought process, he can also control your chemistry. When you have *serotonin* deficiencies, you don't feel good about yourself because there is a deficiency of the chemical that God created in you to make you feel good chemically. For every thought that you have, conscious or unconscious, there is a nerve transmission, a secretion of a hormone or neurotransmitter somewhere in your body to react to it.

And when you start listening to that fear, you start listening to that self-hatred, you start listening to that guilt, and you start listening to that rejection, your body is secreting chemicals in response to those spiritual attacks that are counterproductive to your peace.

Your enemy knows this very well. *It's about time you know what your enemy knows about you so that you can defeat him at the pass.* You don't have to be a victim, nor do you have to be ignorant, nor do you have to die of a disease and go to heaven to find out why you died.

Mitral Valve Prolapse

Reflux

Mitral Valve Prolapse and *Reflux* are identical in their spiritual root cause and manifestation.

In the case of *reflux*, there is a sphincter muscle at the top of your stomach (lower end of your esophagus) and when it does not stay closed, you reflux stomach acid up into the esophagus and this action creates heartburn and even esophageal ulcers.

In the case of *mitral valve prolapse*, the mitral valve in the heart does not open and shut correctly. This allows blood to flow backward into the atrium, causing the heart to work harder. That's why it's called mitral valve prolapse. The root problem behind *reflux* and *mitral valve prolapse* is *anxiety*.

When you have anxiety, the hypothalamus sets into motion not only an imbalance of the endocrine system, but anxiety and fear immediately affect the sympathetic nervous system, the involuntary nervous system and the central nervous system.

Behind a valve is a nerve, and behind a sphincter muscle is a nerve, and if the nerve malfunctions both the valve and the sphincter muscle will not do what they were designed to do. It's caused by a neurological misfiring. The root behind it is *fear and anxiety*. Many people have been healed *of mitral valve prolapse* and *reflux* through our ministry.

CFS (Chronic Fatigue Syndrome)

a.k.a. CFIDS (Chronic Fatigue Immune Dysfunction Syndrome)

Chronic fatigue syndrome is not Epstein-Barr Virus. Epstein-Barr Virus is mononucleosis, the old college disease. Epstein-Barr Virus is just a new name for it. It used to be called "Mono." Now it is called EBV. Epstein-Barr Virus is not CFS, or CFIDS.

CFS, almost without exception (and this has also been verified by the CFS National Organization in Charlotte, and others who have become "specialists" in CFS) involves a diagnosis *of hypoglycemia/low blood sugar.* You will find that CFS and *hypoglycemia* are often linked together in the diagnosis. Hypoglycemia has an autoimmune component. It is not considered an autoimmune disease proper, however, it has an autoimmune component. This indicates that it would have a similar spiritual root to other autoimmune disease that we need to address.

Whenever we minister to someone with an autoimmune disease, we find without exception, degrees of *lack of self-esteem and/or guilt.* A person has conflict with himself over his identity, drivenness, performance, conflict and guilt that, at some level, causes an autoimmune disease. *CFIDS (or CFS) is an anxiety disorder coupled with an autoimmune override,* which triggers *hypoglycemia.* The problem with CFS is that the *hypoglycemia* is also a disease all by itself.

Some people are going to have *hypoglycemia* and not be diagnosed with CFS. It makes it tough, because with *hypoglycemia* you have a neurological triggering in the bloodstream that keeps the manufactured glucose from getting to the brain. Glucose provides the energy for the firing of the brain cells, which creates in you the ability to process thought; it makes your brain work. Complicating the diagnosis is that there is evidence of people that have been diagnosed with CFS who do not have *hypoglycemia.* It is my position in ministry that if fatigue and exhaustion show up in a person without the corresponding diagnosis of *hypoglycemia,* then the person does not have CFS but is in the third and final stage of the General Adaptation Syndrome of the anxiety profile – which is *exhaustion.*

Now in the case of *environmental illness,* we have "brain fog," but it may not include *hypoglycemia.* The reasons for brain fog with *environmental illness* are different than the reasons for brain fog in CFS. In the case of MCS/EI, we have a combination of less oxygen or too much carbon dioxide coming out of *anxiety.* Specifically, hyperventilation, because in MCS/EI when we have stress our heart starts to race, we have repetitive breathing, and the respiratory rate increases. We also have potassium levels that have been depleted and the 3rd stage of an anxiety disorder called the *exhaustion stage* sets in. The long-term effect of a decrease in potassium ions is *fatigue.*

In CFS, we don't have a lower potassium level; we have a lowered level of glucose. You don't have the glucose necessary to fuel the firing of the brain cells. That's part of it. *Chronic fatigue* is the first part of the name of the disease. The symptoms are exhaustion, lethargy, lack of motivation, and lack of energy flow. The word "syndrome" basically means they don't know what causes it. *When you hear the word incurable, etiology unknown, or syndrome, you usually have a spiritually rooted disease.*

I have had to take a look at the many CFS cases that I've dealt with, and up until a couple of years ago, it looked like one member of the family tree was primarily responsible for them. I've run across people in the past few years, as we have had more

CFS cases that have surfaced, and it has not held true. I've had to modify a black and white statement to what I consider to be a majority statement. I'll give you my insight into CFS.

When we minister to people with CFS, we do ministry in what's called blood sugar profile. We minister against hypoglycemia first because the *hypoglycemia* comes to hide the real problem.

Many others doing diagnosis of CFS do not include the insight of *hypoglycemia* as the primary problem. I am shocked! It's like a form of disease occultism. Do you know what occultism is? It's when the real thing is hidden. Something comes before it that hides it. It's like the real root problem for CFS is here, and as the profile of the syndrome develops, then *hypoglycemia* comes and gets a foothold. There are such a myriad of physiological problems that the real enemy is hidden. We've learned this slowly and surely in ministry.

The first thing that we do in ministering to CFS these days is to get rid of the impostor hiding the real root problem. Behind the *hypoglycemia* is the real problem. CFS is an anxiety disorder coupled with hypoglycemia override (which would be the autoimmune rider) clouding a *very major fear anxiety disorder and is the result of drivenness to meet the expectation of a parent in order to receive love. The love is usually sought from a mother,* but not always.

CFS is a result of drivenness to meet the expectation of a parent in order to receive love and acceptance. In most cases the man or woman who comes down with CFS is not doing in life what they wanted to do but is trying instead to meet the expectations of a parent. Many times you will find behind the scenes a parent who is very controlling regarding what the child is going to be in life. It is easy to better understand CFS if you first eliminate the MCS/EI diagnosis.

I consider CFS to be a *performance disorder*. It is called "yuppie disease" or a white-collar disease. It usually hits professionals at the heighth of their careers. After they have achieved what they were supposed to achieve to meet the expectations of others, they crash. As they crash, the guilt, the self-hatred comes, the autoimmune components set in, and then we have hypoglycemia which clouds the whole issue. Now we are chasing this imaginary problem.

I have many medical books on this subject in my library. I've read them all, and no one knows the "cause" of CFS. *It's not the result of chemical exposure. The only way that I can tell you that our etiology and our diagnosis of the spiritual roots are correct is because so many people are now well!* **This is a more excellent way.** So it's kind of a reversed thing; rather than trying to get a diagnosis, let's go over here and get involved in somebody's life and see what's going on and come back through the mess and see what we have. In doing this reverse process, we've seen healing. From that standpoint, we've unraveled this mystery by getting involved with people at their spiritual and emotional levels, helping them come to grips with their innermost thoughts and innermost fears.

I consider CFS to be a fear and anxiety disorder producing drivenness to meet the expectation of someone in order to "measure up" and receive love.

There are people in the secular world that consider MCS/EI and CFS as one and the same disease. I don't agree, because they have two different components. The person who has CFS has not usually been victimized at the level we see in those with MCS/EI because in most MCS/EI cases, we have seen a breakup in human relationships, usually concerning a close family member, and usually going back to childhood. One or more of four life circumstances usually is involved:

- emotional and verbal abuse

- physical abuse

- sexual abuse including molestation

- drivenness to meet the expectation of the parent, in order to receive love in a sterile, loveless environment.

This is heavy stuff for a child to deal with while they are in the process of growing up.

Parasites

You don't usually see parasites unless somebody has a compromised immune system. When people come to me, especially with MCS/EI and they say, "Pastor, I've got parasites," I say, "Oh well, no big deal." I don't even bother ministering to the parasite issues. I'm wasting my time. If you want to get rid of parasites, let's go ahead and get the fear and anxiety dealt with because that may cause a weakened immune system.

When your immune system is healed, parasites don't stand a chance. I have had call after call after call in this ministry where people have called and said, "Pastor, I just went to the doctor, and there are no more parasites." Parasites usually get a foothold long-term because of a compromised immune system. You can have a compromised immune system because of *fear, anxiety and stress.*

Irritable Bowel Syndrome

Irritable Bowel Syndrome (IBS) is caused by the misfiring of nerve dendrites in the lining of the intestine. IBS is coming directly out of *anxiety and fear and insecurities.*

Colic

Colic can be from an *inherited spirit of fear.* Colic is a neurological manifestation in the child that is a direct result of a spirit of fear coming in at conception, in utero, or at birth. It's easy to deal with. Many times it's inherited from the mother.

Flu

The Bible seems to indicate that there are certain things that are "common to man." There is no spiritual root behind the flu necessarily. There are things that are common to man, but the Lord delivers us out of them all.

[19]**Many** *are* **the afflictions of the righteous: but the** Lord **delivereth him out of them all.** Psalm 34:19

There is another scripture that I was thinking about. The Bible talks about something called our "often infirmities" in 1 Tim. 5:23. Often infirmities are things that are common to man that are in the earth because of bacterium and other aspects of Adam's fall. They do not necessarily have a spiritual root as such, but are a part of the fall of man.

The exception: not taking care of your body, not getting enough rest, and enough good nutrition. You did not take care of the temple and have compromised your immune system and thus you are more open to viruses and flu.

Sjögren's Syndrome

Sjögren's Syndrome has an autoimmune mechanism attached to it. It's a chronic systemic inflammatory disorder of unknown etiology characterized by dryness of the mouth, eyes, and other mucus membranes. It is often associated with rheumatic disorders. *Sjögren's* shares certain autoimmune features such as *Scleroderma*. I am familiar with *scleroderma*. If *Sjögren's* is related to *scleroderma*, we have very obvious *extreme self-rejection and self-hatred coupled with much guilt*. The autoimmune component gives us the key. The inflammation indicates that there is a proliferation of white corpuscles, and so we know that we are dealing with a person *in conflict with self*.

When you have classes of disease, you find the spiritual roots to be the same. The faces and the names may change, and the open doors may change. You have to get involved in the person's life to find out where exactly that curse came in; how and why. That's part of our ministry and investigation. We find out where the devil came in, why he has a right to be in someone's life, where that curse came from, and what the cause was. That's all part of ministry.

Panic Attacks

Panic Attacks are a phobic, fear and anxiety disorder. Panic attack is an aggressive stage of a fear and anxiety disorder. The hypothalamus gland is the originating point and facilitator of the following life circumstances: *fear, anxiety, stress, phobia, phobic realities, panic attacks, rage, anger, and aggression*. All of these expressions in mankind are set into motion by one gland, the hypothalamus. In an anxiety attack there would be a rush of the hormone ACTH into the bloodstream. In a panic attack it goes directly to the receptor cells in the muscles of the heart causing an immediate respiratory rate increase, a pounding of the heart, automatic immediate hyperventilation, and over involvement of carbon dioxide retention in the brain. It causes fuzziness of thinking, a shutting down, and can even produce anaphylaxis and catatonic reality. It can go a full range just like that. It is caused by *the spirit of fear*.

Phobias

Phobias are a little different. Phobias are associative; panic is not associative. Panic can come out of nowhere. When you study what *phobias* are you will find that someplace in the person's life they have associated a geographical location or situation with a fear or unpleasant feeling. They immediately come to associate that location or situation and that feeling with the presence of a problem. *Agoraphobia* and *claustrophobia* are examples.

Phobic realities involve two mechanisms—projection and displacement, which constitute avoidance. It's a preconditioning of a phobic stressor that will reinforce itself by feelings and discomfort. To go near the stressor or even thinking about it will send a hormone into the bloodstream, via the hypothalamus, and produce the beginning stages of a panic attack in relationship to the phobia. It is nothing more than a *spirit of fear* and that's the first way you have to deal with it. How many times do we project things, then avoid them out of fear? *The battle is won or lost in the mind.*

Hypoglycemia

Hypoglycemia is low blood sugar. It is rooted in *anxiety and fear coupled with self-hatred and self-rejection coupled with guilt.* There is a neurological misfiring that does not allow the glucose to reach the brain. Glucose is the fuel that fires the brain cells. *Hypoglycemia* also involves an autoimmune component attached to it as a rider. So in effect, *hypoglycemia* can be the result of anxiety coupled with self-hatred and guilt. It is deeply rooted in lack of identity and insecurity. Performance orientation may also be implicated.

Hyperglycemia (Diabetes)

It involves high blood sugar and there is much evidence of an autoimmune component attached to it. *Hyperglycemia* is an autoimmune disease with an anxiety rider. In the case of *hyperglycemia,* which is *diabetes,* the white corpuscles attack the pancreas itself and interfere with its performance. On the other hand in *hypoglycemia,* there is a neurological misfiring that interferes with the glucose reaching the brain after it has been produced. Whenever your tissue is being attacked by white corpuscles, you have an autoimmune disease. Whenever you have neurological misfirings that interfere with the processes, you have stress, fear and anxiety. They are similar but there are two different spiritual roots behind it. (See diabetes.)

Hypothyroidism (Hashimoto's Disease)

Hypothyroidism in its advanced stages is called *Hashimoto's disease,* which is the manifestation of lowered levels of thyroxin being secretion by the thyroid. In the second stage of the General Adaptation Syndrome of the fear, anxiety and stress profile, the thyroid is directly affected by stress causing an under-secretion of thyroxin. The treatment programs provide for synthetic or animal derivatives of thyroxin to replace the deficiency. Many people have been healed through this ministry of anxiety disorders that included *Hashimoto's disease* as part of the profile. The majority of these people who have been healed of fear, anxiety and stress no longer have *Hashimoto's disease* today. *This disease is considered incurable in the medical community but I'm here to tell you that's not so.*

Just as the thyroid malfunctioned because of fear, anxiety and stress, when fear, anxiety and stress is eliminated through ministry, the thyroid kicks back into balance and begins to secrete thyroxin correctly again.

In *hypothyroidism*, which is the result of fear, anxiety and stress, there is an autoimmune component which kicks in involving white corpuscles which collect at the thyroid location causing nonbacterial inflammation and swelling. This advanced stage is called Hashimoto's disease. In this case self-hatred, self-rejection and guilt become the major root with fear/anxiety/stress becoming a rider component. In either case many, many people are well today because of our ministry programs for them concerning it in both of these manifestations. **This is a more excellent way.**

Hyperthyroidism (Graves' Disease)

Hyperthyroidism, which is an over-secretion of thyroxin, is called in many of its forms *Graves' Disease* and can produce goiters and swelling of the eyes and palpitations and tremors. There is an autoimmune rider attached to *Graves' disease* but I consider it to be primarily an anxiety disorder initially, then with the autoimmune component which would produce *Graves'* as opposed to *Hashimoto's* which is primarily an autoimmune disease with an anxiety rider. The root behind both these diseases is *anxiety and fear and/or self-hatred, self-rejection and guilt.*

I had a call from an individual who had just been diagnosed with *Graves' disease.* Their doctor, who happened to be a member of their church, suggested the immediate destruction of the thyroid through radioactive iodine. That was a pretty drastic solution, although *Graves' disease* left unattended is life threatening. The doctor's solution was to permanently erase the problem by destroying the thyroid. However, what the doctor did not tell this individual is that removal of the thyroid produces permanent *Hashimoto's disease.* So they would be exchanging one disease for another.

Now I want to tell you that on the phone as a minister, this insight that I had is really incredible. This individual wanted to know what I had to say first. So when I reviewed the medical information on *Graves',* I discovered something. The primary triggering point for *Graves'* can be the result of emotional shock or a prolonged period of anxiety. Now in my study I also read that *Graves disease* can have an autoimmune component attached to it.

Additionally when I looked at the therapy suggested in lieu of radioactive iodine, there was a drug that could be given for a period of 18 months. The drug would immediately arrest the forward motion of the disease and give a measure of time to try to solve the problem. With this information in hand, I asked this individual, "Did your doctor tell you that by destroying your thyroid you would have permanent *Hashimoto's disease?"*

They said, "No, it was never discussed."

I said, "Did your doctor tell you the findings of the medical community indicate that emotional stress could be a cause?"

The individual said, "No."

I asked, "Did your doctor tell you that over 18 months a drug could be taken and time allowed to resolve the issues?"

I was told, "Yes, but why go that route when we can solve the problem once and for all?"

I said, "Don't you think it would be maybe God's will that we go to Him and find out what your emotional conflict is? And is there any? And if there is any that would be a spiritual issue that God would be able to resolve in your life?"

In our conversation, we discussed many areas of emotional conflict and also the guilt and self-rejection that had come because of it. Those two scenarios are enough to produce *Grave's disease*. The final decision of this individual was to temporarily go on the drug and seek God to resolve the spiritual and emotional conflict. I'm happy to say today, the person still has their thyroid and is doing well. Don't you think keeping your thyroid and dealing with spiritual and emotional issues that can produce healing is **a more excellent way**?

Sometimes you need help to get well. If you could get yourself well by confession, if you could get yourself well by responsibility, recognition, renouncing and resisting, then why would we need the ministry gifts in 1 Corinthians 12? Why would we need to pray one for another? If you could do this all by yourself, why would we need to pray one for another? Why would we need ministry?

I have identified over 40 different statements in Scripture that show how God can be prevented from moving in His people's lives. Knowing the problem is not always the solution. *You're still going to have to line up with God all the way.* We cannot have our cake and eat it too.

God is a loving Father, and He is *not* going to share you with the enemy. You may want to cohabit with your enemy, but God does not like it and He is not going to compromise His position. Just because you are looking for a way out, or *a way to bypass the penalty of the curse* without going the extra mile, God will not allow that to happen.

I don't want God to leave me stranded. I want God to take me all the way into promise so that all the enemies of my land are defeated and I can stand before Him and know that we have done a wonderful thing in life. I'm still under construction. God is still working me over every single day and I love it. I love the convicting work of the Holy Spirit in my life. I love God molding me and making me into a vessel of honor. I cannot think of any greater honor than to think that God would care about me. I submit to Him as my Father, and I submit to the Word that He sent for me, and I submit to the Holy Spirit.

Editor's Note: Do not be confused with *Graves'* and *Hashimoto's disease* at this level because both represent a complete reality in their own right as being taught. However, as part of the profile of these two diseases, *hypothyroidism* or *hyperthyroidism* can exist in their own right and not be either *Graves' disease* or *Hashimoto's disease.* In these stages, both in *hypothyroidism* and *hyperthyroidism*, the sympathetic nervous system is implicated as the result of activity in the second level of the General Adaptation Syndrome of fear, anxiety and stress which would cause an over- or under-secretion of thyroxin.

Addictive Personality

Weight

There is both a genetic and a spiritual component to weight problems. The rate of your metabolism can be determined by how you think about yourself. The hypothalamus controls sleep, thirst, eating, and many other functions of our bodies. When you have lack of self-esteem, when you are in conflict with yourself and others, your hypothalamus gland in conjunction with your mind through the limbic system senses that you have spiritual and emotional problems.

One of the first things that the hypothalamus does in relationship to self-conflict is to reduce *serotonin* levels. Whenever you have a reduction in *serotonin,* you don't feel good about yourself. When you don't feel good about yourself, you go into insecurity. When you're insecure, you start "sucking your thumb." *The mouth is a contact place for love and security.*

People that smoke cigarettes have exchanged the thumb for something else. *All addictions are rooted in lack of self-esteem and insecurity and the need to be loved.* The mouth, and whatever you put in it, is designed to try to bring the person to emotional security. Excessive eating is a direct result of not feeling good about yourself.

When people do not feel good about themselves they will usually become involved in either *obsessive compulsive behavior* (OCD or Obsessive Compulsive Disorder) or an addictive behavior of some kind.

OCD is something that we have dealt with and we have seen great success. OCD always, without exception, involves a reduction in *serotonin* levels.

I did research involving the work of Dr. Sachs some years ago on *OCD, Anorexia,* and *Bulimia.* In reviewing his material and his conclusions, it was shocking to learn that the medical community had no real help. The best they could offer was a 12-Step program, synthetic *serotonin* derivatives to take as a supplement, and/or anti-anxiety drugs. That is the best they have available in America. As far as I'm concerned, that is a form of disease management.

I'm not into disease management, I'm into disease eradication and prevention at all times if at all possible so help me God. If you're being managed in your diseases then God bless you. I don't represent your management; I represent your freedom. The God that I serve doesn't represent your management; He represents your freedom.

I'm a minister of the gospel of Jesus Christ, and the gospel of the Father who sent Him, and I must hold out for **a more excellent way.** I will not teach a leavened gospel because of unbelief, doubts, fears, and the practices of mankind that hold people in bondage. I will be gracious and loving wherever and whenever I teach but I am going to help you confront your issues.

Recently the drug *Fen-Phen* was taken off the market. *Fen-Phen* is an upper. It was designed to build self-esteem. When you get so high, you have to take downers, then you have to take *more Fen-phen* to come back up. In these peaks and valleys, depression sets in. Depression, by definition, is the result of a chemical imbalance in the body. God created us chemically perfect.

An article in *Time Magazine* on July 21, 1997 said:

> It was the latest in a series of setbacks for the new generation of diet pills. They were initially seen as an improvement over the old "speed"-based pills because they were nonaddictive and worked more subtly, stimulating production of the brain chemical serotonin, which is associated with the feelings of satisfaction and satiety.

The problem with the drug *Fen-phen* is that there were incredible side effects that were dangerous to health, involving heart attacks, heart problems, depression, mood swings, and other aberrations of thought. *Fen-phen* would boost serotonin levels, which would make folks feel better about themselves. When you feel better about yourself, you don't put your thumb in your mouth. You don't put food in your mouth. This is the best that medical science has had to offer!

As we have discussed, *weight gain involves a lack of self-esteem*. This problem tends to grow every time the person looks in the mirror. When it does not tell you that you are the fairest of them all, your self-esteem suffers further. We are into comparing ourselves with others. You have taken your eyes off the living God who has created you and you have your eyes on others. Others have become your standard of acceptance and they have become your false god or idol.

Scripture says—judge no man; know no man after the flesh.

15Ye judge after the flesh; I judge no man. John 8:15

16Wherefore henceforth know we no man after the flesh: yea, though we have known Christ after the flesh, yet now henceforth know we *him* no more. 2 Cor. 5:16

I don't judge you by what your house looks like. I judge you by your spirit. I want to know who you are on the inside. God looks at the inner man. Sometimes we major in minors and minor in majors. I think relationships are important. If you are basing relationships on whether you smell good or not, we have a problem. We all have our moments of stench.

I want to cut through the facade of hypocrisy because we are so busy being rejected, and in fear of rejection, that we cannot be ourselves. The problem is that society has made everything anorexic desirable. In Russia, they have banned the Barbie Doll. They've got more spiritual sense than we have in America.

You know why they banned the Barbie Doll in Russia? Because it didn't represent the average Russian woman. There's nothing wrong, ladies, with a little meat with the potatoes. There's nothing wrong with being corn fed. We look at what Hollywood has presented to us as "normal" and we think we must all be like anorexic Barbie Dolls. There's something wrong with this picture.

One of the great blessings promised by God to His people is flesh to their bones. Flesh on our bones is a sign of health. Ladies, there is nothing wrong with you looking like a female should.

If you have weight increase that would be beyond the parameters of good health, there could be a genetic, biological or spiritual problem. The #1 psychiatric disease that produces death in America is *anorexia*. There are more people that die of *anorexia* in America than suicide.

If there has been an addiction to alcohol, another problem can develop. Alcoholics like sugar, carbohydrates, and desserts. Do you know why? Because the body converts the sugars and the carbohydrates into alcohol and you get your fix anyway. If we have a combination of OCD and addictive personality, not only do we have the satisfaction of putting something in our mouth but we also get the alcohol fix. Alcohol, to the basal ganglia, is a painkiller for emotional turmoil. It's an upper, so now you are getting a fix both ways.

These are the dynamics of addiction in OCD. If you're putting on weight, there could be a genetic component, but most weight increase that I deal with in ministry is coming out of *fear of man, fear of failure, fear of abandonment, fear of rejection, lack of self-esteem, and introspection where you look inside yourself and you don't like what you see.*

Shoplifting is the same thing as bingeing. Kleptomania is the result of *self-hatred, self-rejection and guilt.* People who take the credit card and spend thousands of dollars on a *spending binge* are exhibiting the same behavior as those who are bingeing on food. They are trying to increase the serotonin deficiency artificially and not only that, dopamine is also being secreted, which is the pleasure neurotransmitter because of the rush they get to fill the void.

Anorexia and Bulimia

Anorexia and *Bulimia* have the same profile but a different manifestation. In anorexia the person refuses to eat. In *bulimia* the person eats but purges themselves of the food just eaten. *Bulimia* also includes excessive eating in exchange for the void of not feeling loved. The roots are the same: self-hatred, self-rejection and guilt which effectively cause the *serotonin* levels to become deficient. Again, when you have lowered *serotonin* levels, the spiritual and emotional feelings of unloveliness are now reinforced by the chemical deficiency.

Teaching on Nutrition:

If you really want to work on excessive weight gain, first of all I would say you need to begin in your *nutrition*. I think you need to eat meals three times a day. America does not eat breakfast. Too much going on, you're either sleeping in, running off to work, or whatever. It's the morning meal that sets metabolism into motion for the rest of the day and burns the calories. If you eat lunch, and you haven't had breakfast, lunch becomes fat because the metabolism is overloaded when it should have been set in motion at breakfast. Eat something nutritious in the morning and drink plenty of water throughout the day. That is important for weight loss and metabolism. Remember one of the nine fruits of the Holy Spirit is temperance, which is moderation.

If you are concerned about the source of nutrition in today's society, I want to take you away from fear and put you back into wisdom. I tell people this in ministry—a one-a-day vitamin is all you need. All of this teaching on nutrition is not going to work if you are negating what nutrition represents by yielding to fear, anxiety and stress which will cancel the benefits by producing such diseases as malabsorption (leaky gut syndrome).

People are motivated by fear, and are trying to jump-start themselves into better health. If you feel like you need a little vitamin C, don't take 20,000 units of it at one swallow; rather, eat fruit or get it in a one-a-day supplement. I find people think more is better. They think that if a little vitamin C is what I need, then a whole bunch more will help me. Wrong! You can risk going into levels of toxic poisonings. You need to understand that when they tell you the daily required amounts that you need to exist as a human being, that's what you need. If you continue to put three, four, or ten times what you need into your body out of fear, you will risk throwing your body into chemical imbalance, injuring it, and ending up doing just the opposite of what you were hoping to do.

In high school, my best friend's father became obsessed with health. He became obsessed with nutrition and what was "clean" and what was "unclean." He thought that carrots and carrot juice were what he needed to be able to defeat all the problems of life. He became so obsessed, that he drank carrot juice by the gallon until his flesh started to change colors. He literally died of acute carrot juice poisoning.

In our ministry, proper nutrition is a valid consideration and we help people assess where they are in nutrition. I'm not out in left field. I'm in balance. Whatever you eat, if it is not of faith, it's sin. That's what Romans 14 says about food.

> **²³...for whatsoever *is* not of faith is sin.** Romans 14:23

In fact, in the area of vegetarianism and meat, I believe the Bible teaches in Romans 14, that those who are vegetarians are weak in the faith and those who are strong in the faith eat meat. However, if a person is a vegetarian and that is their conscience, then they eat vegetarian style unto the Lord and we are to leave them alone. If I eat meat unto the Lord, that meat is unto the Lord, and you are to leave me alone.

> **¹⁴:¹Him that is weak in the faith receive ye, *but* not to doubtful disputations. ²For one believeth that he may eat all things: another, who is weak, eateth herbs. ³Let not him that eateth despise him that eateth not; and let not him which eateth not judge him that eateth: for God hath received him.** Romans 14:1-3

In I Timothy 4 the Bible talks about the doctrines of devils: forbidding to marry and forbidding the eating of meat.

> **⁴:¹Now the Spirit speaketh expressly, that in the latter times some shall depart from the faith, giving heed to seducing spirits, and doctrines of devils; ²Speaking lies in hypocrisy; having their conscience seared with a hot iron; ³Forbidding to marry, *and commanding* to abstain from meats, which God hath created to be received with thanksgiving of them which believe and know the truth. ⁴For every creature of God *is* good, and nothing to be refused, if it be received with thanksgiving: ⁵For it is sanctified by the word of God and prayer.** 1 Tim. 4:1-5

I'm not going to tell you not to eat meat because the Word says that's a doctrine of devils. If you refrain from meat out of conscience, or out of your application, then God bless you. I honor you because you do it unto the Lord. I sanctify it with you.

Now, you may not be in agreement with that, and that's fine. However, as a student of the Word, and a teacher of the Word, I have to find my place in the midst of mankind without being a bull in a china closet. I have the right to teach truth as it is written, and what you do with it is up to you according to your own conscience.

Paul even dealt with long hair for a man. Although Scripture says in I Corinthians 11:14: "Doth not even nature itself teach you, that, if a man have long hair, it is a shame unto him?" Paul in dealing with the hair issue came to a conclusion in v.16 and said that he couldn't tell the Holy Spirit to be quiet in him, so let him prophesy before God and let his shame be his shame. In essence, Paul is establishing that even though long hair on a man according to Scripture would be a shame, that it would not be a basis for contention or strife and seems to indicate that anyone's hair (male or female) that seems to be different from someone else is to be left alone. I guess what Paul is saying is that what an individual is doing for the kingdom of God is more important than the physical appearance of a saint. Paul didn't get into it so why should you and I get into it?

> [16]**But if any man seem to be contentious, we have no such custom, neither the churches of God.** 1 Cor. 11:16

I want to release you to faith, because in the New Testament it says there is nothing evil in itself, but all things if taken with thanksgiving, are profitable because they are sanctified by the word of God and by prayer.

> [14]**I know, and am persuaded by the Lord Jesus, that *there is* nothing unclean of itself...** Romans 14:14

> [3]**Forbidding to marry, *and commanding* to abstain from meats, which God hath created to be received with thanksgiving of them which believe and know the truth. [4]For every creature of God *is* good, and nothing to be refused, if it be received with thanksgiving: [5]For it is sanctified by the word of God and prayer.** 1 Tim. 4:3-5

That's why, when we sit down to eat, we bless the food before God and then sanctify it so it will be made meet to our bodies. We do that because the Word tells us to do it, so that if there is anything unclean we are protected. In faith, with wisdom, we eat, sanctify it, receive it, and ask God to bless it and I believe He does.

Whatever God has created is for you, in moderation, without guilt and without self-rejection. You belong here just the way you are. There are ways to lose weight, and I'll be very honest with you. I believe that most diet programs are of the devil. I believe they are evil, and are rooted in fear, and rooted in self-hatred. I do believe that you can come before God and manage your lifestyle regarding food; and in ministry deal with *unloving spirits and self-hatred, guilt, and lack of self-esteem.* You can come to a place where you will be comfortable with your body.

Generational Blessings and Curses

Generational Sins and Genetically Inherited Disease

In Exodus 20, the Bible says—the sins of the fathers shall be passed on to the third and fourth generation of them that hate me.

> **⁵Thou shalt not bow down thyself to them, nor serve them: for I the Lᴏʀᴅ thy God *am* a jealous God, visiting the iniquity of the fathers upon the children unto the third and fourth *generation* of them that hate me;** Exodus 20:5

That scripture becomes the spiritual basis for all spiritual, biological, and genetically inherited diseases. In Nehemiah 9:2, we read about the children of the captivity—those that had come out of Babylon in the days of Nehemiah and Ezra. Ezra, the priest, brought the law and the Word of God and they stood there, the mommies and daddies and the children in Nehemiah 8:1-8—and Ezra the scribe gave cause and reason and understanding of the Word of God.

> **⁸:¹And all the people gathered themselves together as one man into the street that *was* before the water gate; and they spake unto Ezra the scribe to bring the book of the law of Moses, which the Lᴏʀᴅ had commanded to Israel. ²And Ezra the priest brought the law before the congregation both of men and women, and all that could hear with understanding, upon the first day of the seventh month. ³And he read therein before the street that *was* before the water gate from the morning until midday, before the men and the women, and those that could understand; and the ears of all the people *were attentive* unto the book of the law.** Neh. 8:1-3

> **⁷…and the people *stood* in their place. ⁸So they read in the book in the law of God distinctly, and gave the sense, and caused *them* to understand the reading.** Neh. 8:7-8

> **²And the seed of Israel separated themselves from all strangers, and stood and confessed their sins, and the iniquities of their fathers. ³And they stood up in their place, and read in the book of the law of the Lᴏʀᴅ their God *one* fourth part of the day; and *another* fourth part they confessed, and worshipped the Lᴏʀᴅ their God.** Neh. 9:2-3

They realized why mommy and daddy, grandma and grandpa had been in captivity. They had been disobedient to the Word of God. In Nehemiah 9:2, the children of the captivity stood and confessed their sins and the sins of their fathers.

> **²And the seed of Israel separated themselves from all strangers, and stood and confessed their sins, and the iniquities of their fathers.** Neh. 9:2

Why did they confess the sins of their fathers? They confessed them because they were the product of their parents' disobedience.

Family Tree of Abraham

I want to give you a family tree history. You'll be shocked, because where I am about to go is to the founding father of our faith. The founding father of the Jewish faith is Abraham. You can read this for yourself in Genesis. Father Abraham was called out of Ur of the Chaldees. God appeared to him, and he came with Sarai, his half sister and wife, and Lot, the son of Haran, into Terah (an area of Turkey). They hung out for awhile, went south, got into the land of promise but there was a famine in the land so they couldn't stay.

They went down into Egypt, the land of Pharaoh (Genesis 12). Abram (Abram's name was later changed to Abraham and Sarai's name changed to Sarah in chapter 19) said to Sarai, his wife, "You're the most beautiful woman in the whole world and I want you to tell the Pharaoh that you're my sister and I'm going to tell him you're my sister. If I say that you're my wife, he will kill me for you because you're that beautiful. Abram enticed his wife to lie and he also lied to the Pharaoh. The root problem behind people who lie is *fear of man, fear of rejection and fear of failure; primarily it is the fear of man.*

When you have children that lie, it's because they are afraid of judgment. The root behind all liars is *fear of man, fear of rejection and fear of judgment.* Father Abraham had a spiritual problem. First of all, *he had fear and he was a liar.* That's a good place to start. God came and dealt with that issue, and Abram had to repent. But Abram did not get the message.

He left the land of Egypt, and moved north into the land of the Philistines where Abimelech was king (Genesis 20). He came into the land of the Philistines, and told Sarai again that she was still very beautiful and he was afraid that he was going to lose her. He said, "Abimelech is a heathen king, so let's tell him that you're my sister." He told the same lie to Abimelech that he had told to the Pharaoh. He got in trouble all over again. He had to repent all over again. Now we've got Abraham caught in a double lie. He didn't learn the lesson the first time, or the second time. We find that Abraham continued to have *fear of man* and he had a *lying spirit.*

That's just the beginning. Then Abraham had a son, who was named Isaac. Isaac married Rebekah. Rebekah and Isaac, we're told in the book of Genesis, took a little vacation and went down into the land of the Philistines where Abimelech was still king forty years later (Genesis 26).

Forty years after Abraham had stood there before Abimelech, King of the Philistines, Isaac and Rebekah stood before King Abimelech. Isaac said to Rebekah, "You're beautiful, you're a real fox, and I'm afraid that if I say you're my wife, Abimelech will kill me and get you. Tell him you're my sister. *When you read it in Genesis, Isaac said word for word what his father Abraham had said forty years before* (Genesis 26). Now we have a second generation of fear and lying. It didn't stop there. We are just getting a good story going.

Isaac had two sons, Esau and Jacob. Rebekah comes along; she had already lied with her husband Isaac in the encounter with King Abimelech. She gets into a discussion with Jacob over the birthright and together they deceive Isaac and lie to him (Genesis 27). Now we have another generation of liars, Abraham, Isaac and Jacob. It doesn't stop there.

Jacob has twelve sons. Ten of the sons are jealous over Joseph, killed an animal, kidnapped Joseph, dipped his coat of many colors in the blood, took it back to Daddy and said, "Daddy, an animal just killed Joseph" (Genesis 37). They lied to Jacob. If it had not been for the intercession of Judah to sell Joseph into slavery, Joseph would have been killed.

Now we have 4 generations of liars. Not only that, Jacob's wife Rachel lied to her father, Laban, over the issue of idols (Genesis 31:35). Now we've got men and women and children lying.

That's where our faith begins—with a bunch of fear-filled, lying saints. Abraham, believe it or not, was called a "friend of God" (Isaiah 41:8, James 2:23). There's hope for you and me isn't there? Amen!

These biblical histories are the foundation to understanding inherited spiritual dynamics. They become a foundation of understanding and tell us why, in Exodus 20:5, God said—the sins of the father shall be passed on to the 3rd and 4th generation.

> ⁵**Thou shalt not bow down thyself to them, nor serve them: for I the L**ORD
> **thy God** *am* **a jealous God, visiting the iniquity of the fathers upon the children**
> **unto the third and fourth** *generation* **of them that hate me;** Exodus 20:5

The fathers are the holders of blessings and curses in the family. What about the females? They have a daddy, too, you know.

Numbers 30 says: if a man standing by hears his wife bind her soul with a vow and he standing by, holds his peace, and allows the words of his wife to stand, she's bound her soul to a curse.

If a man standing by hears his wife bind her soul to a vow and he disallows the words of his wife, he has released her from the curse.

The man standing by hears his daughter bind her soul with a vow with her words and standing by holds his peace and does not disallow the words of his daughter, she's bound her soul to the penalty of the curse.

If he, standing by hears his daughter bind her soul with a vow and he disallows it and says, "Daughter that's not cool" and she agrees, he has saved his daughter from the penalty of the curse. *There is no such provision for boys.*

The beginning of all healing in this planet is the salvation of all men. If you want to get this thing turned around, men, get right with God and tell every man you see to do the same. Get right with God, because the curse is upon us because of our failure.

Adam had a similar problem to Abraham. When it came time to choose between God and his woman, he chose his woman, and not God. He did not disallow her words concerning the eating of the fruit and the action. I firmly believe Adam could have changed the destiny of mankind and taught us obedience, not disobedience.

The Bible says the head of the woman is the man, the head of the man is Christ, and the head of Christ is God the Father.

> ³**But I would have you know, that the head of every man is Christ; and the head of the woman *is* the man; and the head of Christ *is* God.** 1 Cor. 11:3

I myself have had to get right with God, and I'm still working on it. We've got generations of bondage and entrapment behind us. The man is supposed to represent God the Father to his entire family, and the man is supposed to be to the woman as Christ is to the Church in all matters. It's amazing that we can talk to Jesus, but not to our husbands. Its amazing in church to say "Our Father," but we go to our earthly father and we're told to sit down, shut up, and be quiet. I think we've lost our way.

Each of you should build your own **family tree**. Were your family members in past generations Christians? Were they righteous or unrighteous? What were their personalities like? Were they filled with fear, hate, envy, strife, bitterness, etc.? What did they do for a living? Were they into alcohol, drugs, and pornography? Did their lives contain any of the elements that we are learning are the roots for disease? Go back as many generations as you can. This will give you an idea of what is in your family.

Every time you step outside of the covenant, you open yourself to the law and the penalty of the law. The good thing about the new birth and the provision of grace and mercy under Christ is that you're not dead by sundown. You have that time to maintain your forgiveness and your relationship with God in the area of sanctification.

All of the people in your family tree bring into the picture good and evil, blessings and curses. The reason I know this is because many Christians have disease that is genetically inherited. Where did you get that genetically inherited disease? You got it from whom? Your parents. If it's not dealt with before the Lord, you will pass it on to your seed. *Would you like to prevent disease in your children?* Wouldn't that be **a more excellent way?**

One thing I represent is disease prevention, not just the healing of disease. Do you think it is possible that inherited genetic disease can be prevented if the parents line up with God before conception? I do. Do you think that the unborn generation can be sanctified by believing parents that come before God, honestly and humbly, and know exactly what they are up against and why? Do we just shut our eyes, have children, and hope to God they turn out all right?

I'll tell you what the Word says—rebellion is bound up in the heart of a child.

> ¹⁵**Foolishness *is* bound in the heart of a child; *but* the rod of correction shall drive it far from him.** Proverbs 22:15

What does that mean? It means that a child is born with evil. I know mommies and daddies don't like to think about that, but you get them to about age 3 and then you know it's there. It does not go away at 15 either. In fact, it gets worse at 15.

King David said—in sin, my mother did conceive me.

> **⁵Behold, I was shapen in iniquity; and in sin did my mother conceive me.**
> Psalm 51:5

Did you ever meditate on that? King David was a man after God's own heart. He had a man murdered, stole his wife, lusted, tempted Israel, but he was called a man after God's own heart. You figure that one out. David's family was a tragedy; one son raped a daughter, and one son raised up in sedition, in anarchy, against him. One son died at childbirth because of the sins of the father, David.

The *male lineage* traces ancestry through your father, his father and his father's father. What do they have in common with you that could be considered sin? How many of you had parents that did not know God? You are a miracle if your parents did not teach you about God. Do you know anything about your family tree that isn't right? Did you ever hear rumors?

The *female lineage* traces ancestry back through her father and what he brought into it and then all the males before him. Your mother had a father, and this line channels right down through the male. Wherever you find a male, you find the curse channeling down through the female.

That's why you can inherit things from your mother, even though they were in the family tree of her father. Why is that? At any point, if there had been a man of God in that home, he would have taken every step to sanctify his wife and children. God holds the men responsible for all matters of the family, home and everything.

Do you have your family tree down on paper yet? We want you to be able to look at the inherited parts of your family tree. Start thinking about the desolation in the generations in your family. Mark down the characteristics: bootlegger, pirate, warlock, wife beater, molester, adulterer, fornicator, murderer—it's all there. Slanderer, division maker; do you think that's what God created? Do you think God created this mess that we have to unravel. NO!

There may be some things that you are dealing with in your life that you inherited. You say, "That's not fair." Well, it's not fair, but that's the price we pay for separation from God and opening ourselves to the devil and allowing him to be our father and our leader and our truth.

> **⁴⁴"Ye are of your father the devil, and the lusts of *your* father ye will do. He was a murderer from the beginning, and abode not in the truth, because there is no truth in him. When he speaketh a lie, he speaketh of his own: for he is a liar, and the father of it.** John 8:44

That's the price we pay.

Proverbs 26:2 says—as a bird by wandering and the swallow by flying so the curse causeless does not come.

> **²As the bird by wandering, as the swallow by flying, so the curse causeless shall not come.** Proverbs 26:2

In spiritually rooted diseases, there is always a spiritual defect. *That spiritual defect is an area of lack of sanctification.*

Generational Sins and Children

Fear can be inherited, allergies can be inherited, many of the things that we deal with can either develop in our lifetime or we can inherit it from our family tree. Now, when I see that happening in a child, I can go back to the father and mother, grandfather and grandmother—both sides and I'll find some abuse. I'll find victimization, I'll find rejection; I'll find somebody not being nurtured somewhere. That can be inherited, not only from a genetic standpoint, but also from a spiritually inherited standpoint. The Bible says in Ezekiel that the children do not have to die for the sins of the father. Exodus 20:5 says that the curse which is the result of that sin shall be passed on to the third and fourth generation.

We have a ministry to children, and we do minister to children. We come before the Lord and ask God to heal the child. But we have discovered something else very powerful. If we see that the child has a disease or problem that is the direct result of the parents, if we can get the parent to come before God and get that sin resolved, we have seen children instantly healed of diseases and prayer never even occurs on their behalf. When the curse is broken at that level, it is an amazing thing to see God's provision for children that are not yet at the age of understanding. It is amazing. The Bible says that the children are sanctified by the believing parents.

> **¹⁴"For the unbelieving husband is sanctified by the wife, and the unbelieving wife is sanctified by the husband: else were your children unclean; but now are they holy. 1 Cor. 7:14**

Yes, they can be healed. (See the story of the Syrophenician woman and her intercession for her daughter with Jesus in Mark 7.)

Forgiveness: What God Expects of Us When We're Forgiving Someone Else: 70x7

Peter and Jesus had an interesting conversation. Jesus was teaching and Peter asked the Lord how often should I forgive my brother? Seven times seven? Jesus said—no, I don't say seven times seven, I say to you seventy times seven.

> **²²Jesus saith unto him, I say not unto thee, Until seven times: but, Until seventy times seven. Matthew 18:22**

One day in my prayer time I asked the Lord, "What did you mean by that?" This came into my heart and into my understanding: Our days are 24 hours long, 8 hours for work, 8 hours for family and 8 hours for sleep. 8-8-8. If you take 8 hours of the day, whether it's business, family or yourself, this is the whole dimension of human existence, others, yourself and so on. If you take 8 hours, how many minutes are there to an hour? Sixty. Sixty times 8 is 480. What is 70 x 7? 490.

I felt that the Lord was saying it this way, "Every minute of your day, if your brother blows it regarding the same issue minute by minute, hour by hour, day by day, release him." But you say, "Lord, what if he does the same thing again?" Do you know how many people come to me and say, "I went to them, they repented, and then they did it all over again."

How often, Lord, should my brother sin against me, and repent to me, and I still be expected to forgive him? Minute by minute, hour by hour, day by day, release him. In releasing him you have released yourself. Besides when you go to other Scriptures, you quickly see that the Lord is his judge, not you.

> [7:1]**Judge not, that ye be not judged.** Matthew 7:1

> [10]**But why dost thou judge thy brother? or why dost thou set at nought thy brother? for we shall all stand before the judgment seat of Christ.** Romans 14:10

You forgive others because He has forgiven you. He has told you to forgive, and you are His obedient child. When you have forgiven your brother his trespass, then God releases you, because you have released your brother from his trespass.

You are now released from the spirit of bitterness, and that antagonistic high-octane ping on the inside goes away. When you think about your Aunt Sally and her trespasses tomorrow, or the next day, and when the work of the Holy Spirit has been completed in your life and you remember Aunt Sally, you don't feel her down here in your gut anymore and you don't have that high octane ping. You'll always remember the evil that was done to you, but you don't have to carry it as a sin in your own life.

You don't have to carry someone else's sin inside of you. That's their sin. God will be their judge. Your job is to release them, get back before God, get your heart right with God, and then keep on moving. *Your freedom does not depend on their resolution—it depends on your resolution.*

When you forgive others, you are not letting them off the hook but giving them to God still wiggling *on* the hook. *You* are now off the hook.

When you forgive someone, you continue to hate their sin, but you are commanded to love them. **To forgive, you don't have to condone their sin.**

Is that liberating? It was for me. God said to me, "Henry, when I forgave you, I did not condone your sin, son, I bore it. I took it." I said, "Thank You, Lord."

You see, you are not the judge. If you make yourself the judge, then you tell God to go sit down and shut up. I don't think that is what we want to do. God might want to save that person down the road, and you do not want to be in the way.

There are only two future judgments found in Scripture: the judgment seat of Christ and the white throne judgment of the Father.

> [10]**But why dost thou judge thy brother? or why dost thou set at nought thy brother? for we shall all stand before the judgment seat of Christ.** Romans 14:10

> [11]**And I saw a great white throne, and him that sat on it, from whose face the earth and the heaven fled away; and there was found no place for them.** Rev. 20:11

Scripture says one day we shall judge angels.

> [3]**Know ye not that we shall judge angels? how much more things that pertain to this life?** 1 Cor. 6:3

The only other judgment that I have found in Scripture is to judge yourself so you don't have to be judged by God.

> [31]**For if we would judge ourselves, we should not be judged.** 1 Cor. 11:31

That leaves judging others out. We are going to judge ourselves; we are going to judge angels. The Lord's going to judge the saints. The Father is going to judge the unrighteous and that's it! There is no provision for you to judge anyone. Paul said it—no man has judged me but God the Father has judged me.

> [4]**For I know nothing by myself; yet am I not hereby justified: but he that judgeth me is the Lord.** 1 Cor. 4:4

When we get right down to it, why are we judging someone to begin with? Because we want retaliation! Earlier, we taught you the seven factors of bitterness. The third was retaliation, that "I'm going to get even" mentality.

Whether that person responds to you in forgiveness or not, it's their problem and their sin. Walk away, keep your heart right, pray, and ask God to bring reconciliation. Do what you can to bring it about, and if you can't have your peace, keep on moving.

Teaching on the Gifts of the Spirit

Recognition, taking responsibility, repenting, renouncing, resisting may not be enough to produce your freedom. What then? You may need ministry. I'm looking for ministry teams all over America that can teach. We need teams that can teach churches how to heal the sick and cast out devils. Sometimes people just need a little help. Apart from simple prayer, in most churches today there are no ministry teams to heal disease, cure psychological problems, and cast out devils. In fact, lots of churches teach against it. They teach that it passed away a couple thousand years ago. I'm not here to debate or come into conflict with your theologies. I will tell you this: God has worked many healings, miracles, and deliverances at my hand and the hands of my staff. People all over America are suddenly realizing we've been "had." God can, and does, deliver and heal people today. The evidence is overwhelming that this is true.

The Five-fold Ministry

Ephesians 4:11-12 teaches us that the five-fold ministry, of which I am a member, was given by Jesus Christ to equip the saints for service.

> **[8]Wherefore he saith, When he ascended up on high, he led captivity captive, and gave gifts unto men...[11]And he gave some, apostles; and some, prophets; and some, evangelists; and some, pastors and teachers; [12]For the perfecting of the saints, for the work of the ministry, for the edifying of the body of Christ: Ephes. 4:8, 11-12**

Turn to 1 Corinthians 12; I want to lay a foundation for this teaching.

I Corinthians 12:27-30 says—you are the body of Christ and members in particular. And God hath set some in the church, first apostles, secondarily prophets, thirdly teachers, after that miracles, then gifts of healings, helps, governments, diversities of tongues. Are all apostles? (NO) Are all prophets? (NO) Are all teachers? (NO) Are all workers of miracles? (NO) Have all the gifts of healing? (NO) Do all speak with tongues? (NO) Do all interpret? (NO).

> **[27]Now ye are the body of Christ, and members in particular. [28]And God hath set some in the church, first apostles, secondarily prophets, thirdly teachers, after that miracles, then gifts of healings, helps, governments, diversities of tongues. [29]Are all apostles? are all prophets? are all teachers? are all workers of miracles? [30]Have all the gifts of healing? do all speak with tongues? do all interpret? 1 Cor. 12:27-30**

Because it says that not everyone does these things does not mean that there are not some that do these things. Some Christians claim, because it says that not everyone does these, that "Nobody does it anymore." That's not how that reads. It just says that it's spread out through the body and among specific members in particular. I'm a member in particular and you are a member in particular. Also the Scriptures indicate that it is God that has set these things in the Church. No one has the right or the authority to pick and choose, or add or delete, anything found in these scriptures. I'm a member in particular and you're a member in particular.

I Corinthians 12:7 says—but the manifestation of the Spirit is given to every man to profit withal.

> **⁷But the manifestation of the Spirit is given to every man to profit withal.**
> 1 Cor. 12:7

If I come, and I bring gifts of healing and deliverance and knowledge and discernment, what does that do for you? Does that bring profit to you?

To people that no longer have *lupus,* these gifts were to their profit. To people who no longer have depression, these gifts were to their profit. To people who no longer have fear and anxiety disorders, these gifts were to their profit. They were given to build them up.

Christ in heaven is not sick. His body in earth should not be either. Christ in heaven is not ignorant. His body in earth should not be ignorant.

I Corinthians 12:8-10 identifies the gifts of the Holy Spirit that are available to the Church today.

> **⁸For to one is given by the Spirit the word of wisdom; to another the word of knowledge by the same Spirit; ⁹To another faith by the same Spirit; to another the gifts of healing by the same Spirit; ¹⁰To another the working of miracles; to another prophecy; to another discerning of spirits; to another *divers* kinds of tongues; to another the interpretation of tongues:** 1 Cor. 12:8-10

These are gifts of God, through the Church, given to bring us to a place of health.

The gift of healing is a gift available from God to stop the forward motion of disease and bring the power of God in so that the body will heal.

There are parts of your bodies that do not heal. That's why we have organ transplants. Most nerve tissue does not regenerate, brain tissue does not regenerate, and organs do not regenerate. If God was going to regenerate something that could not be regenerated, then what kind of gift would it take? The gift of miracles.

If an evil spirit had gotten hold of your life, then you would need what? Discerning of spirits. What good is it to discern a spirit if you can't get rid of it? Discerning of spirits involves eviction of spirits from God's precious people.

So we have three dimensions of healing: (1) the healing of body tissue, (2) the regeneration of body tissue, and (3) the removal of things that are alien to us spiritually. Then we can stand before our God and give Him glory because we have just profited from His blessings. *God receives no glory from your disease.*

John 9:1-3 is the scripture about the blind man that the Lord healed. The disciples asked him if this was because of his sin or his parent's sin. Jesus said, "No this is for the glory of God."

> **⁹:¹And as *Jesus* passed by, he saw a man which was blind from *his* birth. ²And his disciples asked him, saying, Master, who did sin, this man, or his parents, that he was born blind? ³Jesus answered, Neither hath this man**

sinned, nor his parents: but that the works of God should be made manifest in him. John 9:1-3

Many people take that scripture and claim that this disease was for the glory of God. *Not at all!*

It was the *healing* of that disease that was for the glory of God. Jesus didn't stop and not heal him. If the disease had been for the glory of God, Jesus would have backed off and said, "Sorry, this disease is for the glory of God." He didn't say that; He healed him. That miraculous healing by the Lord was for the glory of God. *This healing is something called greater grace.* It was God's absolute mercy. I've seen people take this scripture and say that disease is for the glory of God.

The Word says that God receives no glory if we end up in the grave prematurely.

[18]**For the grave cannot praise thee, death can *not* celebrate thee: they that go down into the pit cannot hope for thy truth.** Isaiah 38:18

The grave can't praise Him, only you can praise Him in your generation (see the story of Lazarus in John 11).

Why do you think 1 Corinthians 12 says, "God has set some in the Church?" Why? Is it there for a reason? It is because sometimes recognition, taking responsibility, repenting, renouncing and resisting does not produce freedom in itself. It takes somebody coming along representing God, and using the gifts of God, to deal with it in ministry. That's why we need ministers back in the Church and saints ministering one to another under the oversight of the five-fold ministry.

We need people of God, who are anointed by God, raised up by God according to the Word of God, filled with the Spirit of God, to do the works of God, to edify the body of Christ and bring them back to health and sanity. That's what our ministry represents. This is our calling.

I am a gift of God to you. I'm a gift of God because I'm a member of the *five-fold ministry* of Ephesians 4. I am a pastor designed to equip, train, and bring to service the body so that it can start taking care of the body. God intended that you heal each other through the gifts and through the work of the Holy Spirit and you don't need me to do it. You should be doing it although the work of the pastor includes more than just equipping, training and bringing to service; and must include the care of those who will be used. *So many times we have directed our attention to only others who are in need to the expense of who we are in need.*

In James the question is asked and answered: "Is there any sick among you? Call for the elders of the church."

[14]**Is any sick among you? let him call for the elders of the church; and let them pray over him, anointing him with oil in the name of the Lord:** [15]**And the prayer of faith shall save the sick, and the Lord shall raise him up; and if he have committed sins, they shall be forgiven him.** [16]**Confess *your* faults one to**

another, and pray one for another, that ye may be healed. The effectual fervent prayer of a righteous man availeth much. James 5:14-16

1 Corinthians 12 teaches us that the body is supposed to take care of the body. The references given here in 1 Corinthians 12 to the gifts of the Holy Spirit are not just aimed at the church leaders, but are also directed to the lay people, the saints. The leadership is directed to set an example so that all believers can do the work of the ministry. That means the leadership and the saints are to be equally equipped. **It is very clear in 1 Corinthians 12 that the body is to take care of the body in all matters of health and sanity.**

Teaching on Romans 7

I want to take you into Romans 7, and give you a case history of a believer and a leader named Paul. Do you want to go past discernment into freedom? Paul is our example.

In Romans 7:15 Paul is speaking about himself. Paul is a believer. He's not only a believer—he's been an Apostle for at least 20 years. He's talking about his life and his challenges in living a Christian life.

In Romans 7:15 Paul says:

> **[14]For we know that the law is spiritual: but I am carnal, sold under sin. [15]For that which I do I allow not: for what I would, that do I not; but what I hate, that do I.** Romans 7:14-15

Does that sound familiar? The things that I want to do, I don't do. The things that I hate, that's what I do.

Do you think Paul was sinless? Do you think I'm being disrespectful to him? There is only one Man who was sinless, the man Christ Jesus. The rest of us are a bunch of sinners, saved by grace, working out our salvation daily, with fear and trembling.

> **[7]For he *is* our God; and we *are* the people of his pasture, and the sheep of his hand. To day if ye will hear his voice,** Psalm 95:7

> **[2](For he saith, I have heard thee in a time accepted, and in the day of salvation have I succoured thee: behold, now *is* the accepted time; behold, now *is* the day of salvation.)** 2 Cor. 6:2

> **[23]And he said to *them* all, If any *man* will come after me, let him deny himself, and take up his cross daily, and follow me.** Luke 9:23

> **[12]Wherefore, my beloved, as ye have always obeyed, not as in my presence only, but now much more in my absence, work out your own salvation with fear and trembling.** Philip. 2:12

Romans 7:16 goes on to say—if then I do those things that I wish I wouldn't do, I consent unto the law that it is good.

> **[16]If then I do that which I would not, I consent unto the law that *it is* good.** Romans 7:16

Now let me bring you to a point. Paul is saying if I do those things that are evil, I'm telling the law or the Word that this new law that I'm following which represents evil is good and the Word of God is evil. If then I do those things which I would not, I consent unto the Word that this new law that I'm following is the proper law.

Are we following a "different law" in our lives sometimes than the law of God? When the Word says, "Forgive your brother," and we don't, are we following a different law, a different gospel, a different way of thinking? Do you ever see Christians that don't forgive people? Have you ever seen any Christians gossip? Have you seen any Christians shun another Christian? Have you ever seen Christians do evil?

In other words, what Paul is saying is that when he does those evil things that he wished he would not do, he's consenting unto the law of God that this thing that he should not be doing is good and that automatically puts him under the authority of another gospel. Do you see what I'm saying? When we hate our brother, we are affirming a new gospel that overthrows the gospel of our God. The gospel of God says to forgive our brother. Then when instead we hold on to that unforgiveness and bitterness toward our brother, we are in fact following a different law, a different gospel, a different way of thinking from that of God. Do you know any Christians who gossip or have bitterness and unforgiveness toward another?

IT'S VERY IMPORTANT that you understand that sin involves the overthrowing of the government and the laws and precepts of God. By so doing, we are establishing another gospel in the earth for mankind to follow to their destruction, not to their benefit. There's not enough emphasis put on this dimension of sin in the Church today. We've become so anti-social around the issue of sin because we don't like to think that we have sin in our lives as Christians. I'm sorry, but it is in the Bible. I try to teach it in such a way that I don't hit you over the head. I hope you don't feel like I'm oppressing you with truth. If I am, I apologize; I'll cut your cabbage for a hundred years.

I want you to understand that when we allow fear to rule our lives, we are affirming the gospel of fear. Fear destroys faith, which is of God. When we are allowing guilt to rule our lives, we're affirming the gospel of guilt to the destruction of forgiveness by God. It's very important that you understand that we are setting up one gospel or another. We're either establishing the law of the kingdom of God or we are establishing the laws of Satan's kingdom. You can't have your cake and eat it, too! You cannot serve two masters; either you're going to love the one or hate the other. That has to be understood in this discussion. It has to be understood with regard to certain diseases before you can be healed. You cannot be healed of *lupus* and hang on to self-hatred. It's just not going to happen.

> [24]**No man can serve two masters: for either he will hate the one, and love the other; or else he will hold to the one, and despise the other. Ye cannot serve God and mammon.** Matthew 6:24

How do you figure that's possible? In 1 John 3:9, it says—whosoever is born of God cannot sin.

> [9]**Whosoever is born of God doth not commit sin; for his seed remaineth in him: and he cannot sin, because he is born of God.** 1 John 3:9

Does it mean we're not born again? "Whosoever is born of God cannot sin, and he that sins is of the devil." How do you reconcile that with the rest of the canon of Scripture dealing with grace and mercy?

This brings us to a place where we are working out our own salvation daily by faith, through grace and mercy. Our spots and our blemishes can be dealt with before the living God as the work of *sanctification*. God has taken the absoluteness of His position for us and He has shoved us back under the blood, grace, and mercy.

Now we are in a car wash called *sanctification*. Paul is describing himself in the car wash and he's not been cleaned up yet, and neither have you. If you tell me you are sinless, I'm going to tell you, you are a liar. The Word says—whosoever says he has not sinned is a liar.

> **⁵This then is the message which we have heard of him, and declare unto you, that God is light, and in him is no darkness at all. ⁶If we say that we have fellowship with him, and walk in darkness, we lie, and do not the truth: ⁷But if we walk in the light, as he is in the light, we have fellowship one with another, and the blood of Jesus Christ his Son cleanseth us from all sin. ⁸If we say that we have no sin, we deceive ourselves, and the truth is not in us. ⁹If we confess our sins, he is faithful and just to forgive us *our* sins, and to cleanse us from all unrighteousness. ¹⁰If we say that we have not sinned, we make him a liar, and his word is not in us.** 1 John 1:5-10

These scriptures are not addressed to unbelievers but are addressed to believers who sin after conversion. I heard someone say the other day that if you sinned after conversion, you were never saved. I guess there are no Christians in the earth today. We all fall short of the glory of God every day, don't we?

> **²³For all have sinned, and come short of the glory of God;** Romans 3:23

There are many who say this scripture only applies to unbelievers, yet I see many of the same sins in believers today that can be found in the unbeliever. *In both cases, saved and unsaved have fallen short of the glory of God. Both need to repent.* Let me ask you a question: why would God require the unsaved to repent for a sin and not require the saved to repent of that sin? That would make God unjust and He would condone evil in the name of salvation. But the Scriptures refute this position.

> **⁶:¹What shall we say then? Shall we continue in sin, that grace may abound? ²God forbid. How shall we, that are dead to sin, live any longer therein?** Romans 6:1-2

Have you ever struggled with any insecurities and fears? Do you ever doubt, have suspicions, even doubt your salvation from time to time? Do you ever get into a place where you wonder if your wife loves you? Ever get to a place where you think your husband doesn't love you? Ever get into those places where you think God is a million miles away? Do you ever go through those valleys of the shadow of death? Do you ever go into those dry places?

I had a cartoon of a guy driving down the highway on the interstate and the sun was shining, and then there was a line and there was a shaded area in the rest of the cartoon. It says, "Shaded area next 1460 miles." Have you ever been driving through life and you just drove into those shaded areas? The only thing you had going for you was that the sign said, "This will end some day."

Paul, in Romans 7:17, is talking about when he is doing things that are not right. "Now then it is no more I that do it (evil), but sin that dwelleth in me."

> **¹⁷Now then it is no more I that do it, but sin that dwelleth in me.** Romans 7:17

Wait a minute, Paul was an Apostle, born again, filled with the Spirit of God, teaching righteousness, and he's saying he's got sin within. Paul needed ministry.

If Paul needed help, what is our condition? These thoughts and blemishes, these "yucky-puckies," these "crispy critters," this stuff that I'm dealing with that produces disease involves the issue of *sanctification.* That is where the minister gets to come in and help you deal with it. It is in this ministry area where we confess our faults one to another that we may be healed.

> **¹⁶Confess *your* faults one to another, and pray one for another, that ye may be healed. The effectual fervent prayer of a righteous man availeth much.** James 5:16

We must separate ourselves from the sin that dwells within us, and that dwells within our neighbor. When you look at your neighbor, you are going to have to be able to separate them from their sin, to bring any kind of sanity into your Christian walk before God.

What happens when you see sin in your neighbor is that you make him the same as his sin. He's not sin, and if he's a believer, he's the redeemed of God. He may have sin, but he is not sin. He is the one that God saw from the foundation of the world. He's the one that the Spirit of God lives within. He's the one that's being redeemed. He's the one that God loves, but he's got some sin tagging along that needs to go. The sin needs to go; it's interfering with his sonship, interfering with his sanctification, interfering with his position before God, and that is the area we need to deal with.

Discernment unto freedom requires separation – seeing sin for what it is. What I am about to teach you right here is the foundation for your freedom – that's discernment and separation. You must be able to separate yourself from the sin that dwells within you. And you must be able to separate the sin that dwells within others from who they are as a person. The day that I got this insight from Paul in Romans 7 and saw that I needed to separate myself and my heart from the sin within is the day that *sanctification* began in my life and I was on my way to freedom. Our battle is not with flesh and blood, but with entities from another kingdom.

> **¹²For we wrestle not against flesh and blood, but against principalities, against powers, against the rulers of the darkness of this world, against spiritual wickedness in high *places.* Ephes. 6:12**

> **¹²For the word of God *is* quick, and powerful, and sharper than any twoedged sword, piercing even to the dividing asunder of soul and spirit, and of the joints and marrow, and *is* a discerner of the thoughts and intents of the heart. ¹³Neither is there any creature that is not manifest in his sight: but all things *are* naked and opened unto the eyes of him with whom we have to do.** Hebrews 4:12-13

We hear much quoting of verse 12, but seldom is verse 13 quoted along with it. Notice in verse 13 that the Word of God is making manifest those creatures that are within. That's those "yucky-puckies"/"crispy critters" that Paul is talking about in Romans 7. That's the stuff that I'm dealing with that produces disease. Dealing with this stuff for our healing and deliverance from these "yucky-puckies" that dwell within is the process of *sanctification*. No doctor of the physio can do this and no psychologist of the psyche can do this. This is in the realm of the spirit, where the pastor and THE CHURCH must deal with the spirit of man with the Word of God.

I can't forgive my brother unless I do separation. I can't forgive myself if I don't do separation. Without separation, I have become one with the sin; but that's not who I am; I'm not one with sin. I AM NOT SIN. I'm Henry, thank you! And I reserve the right to deal with sin and get it out of my life and remain Henry without it. When somebody victimizes me, I'm able to see the evil in them that they are now possessed with or under the control of, that is now making a victim of me and I see it's not them; it's the sin that lives within them so I can exchange the bitterness with compassion according to the knowledge of God. We must come to the place that we stop making ourselves, our brother, our children, or our neighbor one with the thought and blemishes, "yucky-puckies," "crispy critters," and all the sin that manifests within our hearts.

Now in your own life, you see that sin that dwells within, and you know it yields the fruits of self-hatred, bitterness, unbelief, doubt, fear, jealousy, envy, competition, and strife. Do you know that strife is found in the same verses as murder? Adultery? Fornication?

Romans 1:28-31, Mark 7, and Galatians 5 list many sins, all of which may be found in all Christians at one level or another.

> [28]**And even as they did not like to retain God in *their* knowledge, God gave them over to a reprobate mind, to do those things which are not convenient;** [29]**Being filled with all unrighteousness, fornication, wickedness, covetousness, maliciousness; full of envy, murder, debate, deceit, malignity; whisperers,** [30]**Backbiters, haters of God, despiteful, proud, boasters, inventors of evil things, disobedient to parents,** [31]**Without understanding, covenantbreakers, without natural affection, implacable, unmerciful:** Romans 1:28-31

> [15]**There is nothing from without a man, that entering into him can defile him: but the things which come out of him, those are they that defile the man...** [20]**And he said, That which cometh out of the man, that defileth the man.** [21]**For from within, out of the heart of men, proceed evil thoughts, adulteries, fornications, murders,** [22]**Thefts, covetousness, wickedness, deceit, lasciviousness, an evil eye, blasphemy, pride, foolishness:** [23]**All these evil things come from within, and defile the man.** Mark 7:15, 20-23

> [19]**Now the works of the flesh are manifest, which are *these;* Adultery, fornication, uncleanness, lasciviousness,** [20]**Idolatry, witchcraft, hatred, variance, emulations, wrath, strife, seditions, heresies,** [21]**Envyings, murders, drunkenness, revellings, and such like: of the which I tell you before, as I have also told *you* in time past, that they which do such things shall not inherit the kingdom of God.** Galatians 5:19-21

Why is that? Because we are not sanctified. That is what is causing our biological, spiritual, and mental diseases. That is what we are talking about. Paul is pointing the finger right back at himself.

When I get to heaven, I'm going to find brother Paul. I'm going to get hold of that boy. I'm going to hug him, and I'm going to say, "Paul, Chapter 7 of Romans saved my life." I could not separate myself from my sin and I felt yucky and pucky every way to Sunday and then I realized I had an enemy. I really had a heart for God, but I had an enemy that had to go. *The day that I learned to separate myself, and my heart, from my sin is the day that sanctification in my life began.*

Paul is saying in Romans 7:17-18:

> [17]**Now then it is no more I that do it, but sin that dwelleth in me.** [18]**For I know that in me (that is, in my flesh,) dwelleth no good thing: for to will is present with me; but** *how* **to perform that which is good I find not.** Romans 7:17-18

That is, in my flesh. Now here's a situation where "flesh" does not mean the human body. It's talking about something of the old man, the old nature, the unrenewed part of him; something within him was not of God. The word "flesh" has to do with the carnal nature. Paul is not talking about his human flesh.

Paul goes on to say in verse 18—for I know that in me (that is, in my flesh) dwells no good thing: for to will is present with me, but how to perform that which is good I find not.

Have you ever found yourself that way? Have you ever had a wonderful heart toward God, and the harder you tried the behinder you got? Have you ever had struggles in your Christian walk where it just didn't come together as fast as you wanted it to?

You see the prototype. You look into the mirror, the perfect law of liberty, and when you turn away you see the sin, don't you? Don't forget what you saw in the perfect law of liberty, but back over here is the real you. That's what Paul is looking at. He's looking with eyes of honesty.

Romans 7:19—for the good that I wish I would do, I don't do it and the evil that I wish I wouldn't do, that's what I do.

> [19]**For the good that I would I do not: but the evil which I would not, that I do.** Romans 7:19

What Paul said in verse 17, he repeats in Romans 7:20 which said as I do those things that I wish I wouldn't do, it is no more I that do it but sin that dwelleth in me (is doing it).

> [20]**Now if I do that I would not, it is no more I that do it, but sin that dwelleth in me.** Romans 7:20

He was talking about his carnal nature, that unrenewed part of him that doesn't match the nature of God within him. He has come to the realization that it is not him for he knows his heart before God is to do good, so he concludes that it is something else that is within him that is doing it, that is, the sin, yet the conclusion of this is that it is sin that dwells within causing an action through Paul that would become sin to him.

In this discourse of personal transparency of Romans 7, Paul has said more than once that his conclusion is that the evil that he is doing in his life as a Christian and apostle is *not him that is doing it, but that it is evil/sin that is dwelling in him that is doing it through him.* Do you think he was recognizing his own need for deliverance? I think so. He's looking at himself with eyes of honesty.

Have you ever found yourself that way? You know that you have a wonderful heart toward God and you want your nature to match His nature, but the harder you try, the behinder you get. The beginning of understanding is to be able to separate yourself from the sin that dwells within that is acting out its nature through you; thus the full meaning of Hebrews 4:12-13.

> **[12]For the word of God *is* quick, and powerful, and sharper than any twoedged sword, piercing even to the dividing asunder of soul and spirit, and of the joints and marrow, and *is* a discerner of the thoughts and intents of the heart. [13]Neither is there any creature that is not manifest in his sight: but all things *are* naked and opened unto the eyes of him with whom we have to do.** Hebrews 4:12-13

This is where healing of disease begins.

This sin that dwells within Paul is identified in Hebrews 4:13 as the creatures that need to be made opened and naked before Him with whom we have to do.

Romans 7:21-24:

> **[21]I find then a law, that, when I would do good, evil is present with me. [22]For I delight in the law of God after the inward man: [23]But I see another law in my members, warring against the law of my mind, and bringing me into captivity to the law of sin which is in my members. [24]O wretched man that I am! who shall deliver me from the body of this death?** Romans 7:21-24

Paul very clearly states that evil was present with him and that law (sin/evil) was in his members warring against the law of his mind and bringing him into captivity against the *law of sin* which was *in* his members. He's asking for deliverance right up front, and he tells us the answer in v. 25:

> **[25]I thank God through Jesus Christ our Lord. So then with the mind I myself serve the law of God; but with the flesh the law of sin.** Romans 7:25

Romans 8 is a continuation of Chapter 7. There should not be a new chapter. Before we go to Chapter 8, I want to give you a story of something that happened about 10 years ago.

I had a Christian man call me. He was a businessman, who had heard that I was helping people get straightened out in life. He had all kinds of problems in his business, and problems in his life and marriage. He called me and I listened to him for awhile and I said, "Brother, you've got sin in your life."

He said, "Brother, you err."

I said, "How do I err?"

He said, "Have you not heard the word of God?"

I said, "Yes. What do you have in mind?"

He said, "In Romans 8:1 it says there is therefore now no condemnation to them that are in Christ Jesus. So I'm a free man and I'm free of sin and the consequences of it."

I said, "Why don't you read the rest of that verse?"

He said, "There isn't any more."

He was reading from the <u>New International Version</u> (NIV) text. The NIV says this, "There is therefore now no condemnation to them that are in Christ Jesus." but the majority text (<u>King James Version</u>) says it a little different. I'll read it to you:

Romans 8:1—there is therefore no condemnation to them that are in Christ Jesus, who walk not after the flesh, but after the Spirit."

> **8:1*There is* therefore now no condemnation to them which are in Christ Jesus, who walk not after the flesh, but after the Spirit.** Romans 8:1

I said, "Brother you have blown it. You're on the wrong side of the road. I want you to notice that it says there is condemnation to them that walk after the flesh. And, yes, there is no condemnation to them that walk after the Spirit. You're following after the old nature, the old man. You're following after the lust of the flesh in your life, your business, and your family. Condemnation is here because the only place that you're free from condemnation under the law is if you're walking after the Spirit of God."

When you step outside those parameters, you're back under the law again and there is a consequence. Your freedom is directly related to your obedience. There is a consequence to sin and disobedience to God's word (Deuteronomy 28). That's not legalism; that's simply what Jesus meant when He said—if you love me, you'll keep my commandments.

> **15If ye love me, keep my commandments.** John 14:15

Keeping God's commandments is not legalism. Taking God's commandments and forcing them down someone's throat is legalism.

The letter of the law killeth but the spirit of the law giveth life (2 Corinthians 3:6).

> **6Who also hath made us able ministers of the new testament; not of the letter, but of the spirit: for the letter killeth, but the spirit giveth life.** 2 Cor. 3:6

If I could bring you the spirit of the law and let God the Holy Spirit convict you in your hearts and liberate you, and then let you keep your sin if you want to, would that be all right? NO, it wouldn't be all right.

Paul is dealing with an issue. He's saying I, myself, serve the law of God but I've got a problem. I have a problem in my life. I've got sin that dwells within me. Do you think he is just playing with us, or do you think he really meant that?

Fear is sin. Unforgiveness is sin. Strife is sin. Self-hatred is sin. Heresy is still sin. Adultery is still sin. Lasciviousness is still sin. Backbiting is still sin. Causing church splits is still sin. Jealousy and envy are still sin.

The disciples made a very serious mistake; they didn't wash their hands before dinner and the Pharisees caught them. Jesus is picking up this discussion in Mark 7:15—there is nothing from without a man, that entering into him can defile him: but the things which come out of him, those are they that defile the man.

> **[15]There is nothing from without a man, that entering into him can defile him: but the things which come out of him, those are they that defile the man.** Mark 7:15

It's not what goes in your mouth that defiles you; *it's what comes from within you, out of your mouth.*

Mark 7:16-23 says—if any man have ears to hear, let him hear. And when He was entered into the house from the people, His disciples asked Him concerning the parable, And He saith unto them, Are you so without understanding also? Do you not perceive, that whatsoever thing from without entereth into the man, it cannot defile him; Because it entereth not into his heart but into the belly, and goeth out into the draught, purging all meats? And He said, *That which cometh out of the man, that defileth the man. For from within, out of the heart of men,* proceed evil thoughts, adulteries, fornication, murders, thefts, covetousness, wickedness, deceit, lasciviousness, an evil eye, blasphemy, pride, foolishness: *all these evil things come from within, and defile the man.*

> **[20]And he said, That which cometh out of the man, that defileth the man. [21]For from within, out of the heart of men, proceed evil thoughts, adulteries, fornications, murders, [22]Thefts, covetousness, wickedness, deceit, lasciviousness, an evil eye, blasphemy, pride, foolishness: [23]All these evil things come from within, and defile the man.** Mark 7:20-23

Jesus was identifying the "yucky-puckies" within the spirit of man that defile the man. Paul recognizes this in Romans 7 and then we find Paul developing it as a spiritual principle of sanctification for THE CHURCH in 2 Corinthians 7:1.

Paul was talking about spiritual defects in the area of the human spirit.

2 Corinthians 7:1 says—having therefore these promises dearly beloved, let us cleanse ourselves from all filthiness of the flesh and spirit, perfecting holiness in the fear of God.

> **[7:1]Having therefore these promises, dearly beloved, let us cleanse ourselves from all filthiness of the flesh and spirit, perfecting holiness in the fear of God.** 2 Cor. 7:1

Paul is addressing the believer, not the unbeliever. Very clearly Paul is setting the stage for something called sanctification subsequent to salvation. In 1 Thessalonians 5:23, Paul again brings emphasis to sanctification as a very important first step to produce *wholeness.*

> **[23]And the very God of peace sanctify you wholly; and *I pray God* your whole spirit and soul and body be preserved blameless unto the coming of our Lord Jesus Christ.** 1 Thes. 5:23

Jesus is talking about what's in the heart of man that needs to be dealt with. Paul also picks up the topic in 2 Corinthians and 1 Thessalonians and in Romans 7 and says it applies not just to himself, but to every one of us.

I'm working out my salvation daily through grace and mercy, applying the love of the Father, the Word of God, and the work of the Holy Spirit, so that my heart, my spirit man, can be purged of all evil. My poor head gets the picture finally and I become *one* in my thoughts, spiritually (spirit) and psychologically (soul), so I can fulfill the Scriptures. I am in the process of putting on the mind of Christ. From glory to glory I am being changed into His image.

> [18]**But we all, with open face beholding as in a glass the glory of the Lord, are changed into the same image from glory to glory, *even* as by the Spirit of the Lord.** 2 Cor. 3:18

This is the process of *sanctification*, starting to remove spiritual, biological, psychological diseases of life, both generationally and personally. When we get before God and take an honest look at ourselves and when we survey our past generations and deal with the sin we find, we then come before God to let Him "work us over."

The Lord is saying to you today, "I'm here knocking, would you open the door of your heart? Would you let Me come in, with the Holy Spirit, and cleanse you, sanctify you, and remove the things that are separating Me from you. Could I heal you, could I deliver you, could I establish My heart for you; would you enter into that degree of covenant with Me? Could I be a God to you? Could I be a Savior to you? Could I be a healer to you? Could I be a redeemer to you? Could I be a husband to you? Would you fellowship with Me?

> [19]**As many as I love, I rebuke and chasten: be zealous therefore, and repent. [20]Behold, I stand at the door, and knock: if any man hear my voice, and open the door, I will come in to him, and will sup with him, and he with me.** Rev. 3:19-20

This scripture in Revelation is not addressed to unbelievers but it is addressed to a New Testament church at Laodicea and the Lord is not in their heart when they think He is but He is outside. I find this a tragic picture of the Church today. I do not want to hear these words being said to Him – "Yea Lord" and He saying to me "Depart from me, I never knew you."

> [20]**Wherefore by their fruits ye shall know them. [21]Not every one that saith unto me, Lord, Lord, shall enter into the kingdom of heaven; but he that doeth the will of my Father which is in heaven. [22]Many will say to me in that day, Lord, Lord, have we not prophesied in thy name? and in thy name have cast out devils? and in thy name done many wonderful works? [23]And then will I profess unto them, I never knew you: depart from me, ye that work iniquity.** Matthew 7:20-23

Fear, Stress and Physiology

There are many diseases that will fall under this category. One of the diseases is Multiple Chemical Sensitivities/Environmental Illness (MCS/EI).

Multiple Chemical Sensitivities/Environmental Illness (MCS/EI)

Most people that we deal with who have MCS/EI have been devastated for anywhere from 5 to 20 years. Most of them are "universal reactors." I want to give you an idea of just how extensive a healing can be by giving you a couple of folk's case histories. As I read these conditions, keep in mind that these people are totally healed today.

Case History One. This particular person had 17 peripheral diseases, and has been well for nearly 8 years. Prior to intervention by this ministry, their general prognosis was "guarded."

#1 Diagnosed with *multiple chemical sensitivity* as a universal reactor, this individual was allergic to all foods and chemicals, which caused an anaphylactic shock reaction, including throat closure. She was at one time naked due to the inability to wear any clothing, even white cotton clothing. She was down to only one least reactive food and had to live in foil lined rooms in the mountains or near the ocean. Oxygen and adrenaline were necessary for survival. This condition was ongoing for 10 years.

#2 *Electromagnetic Field Sensitivity* (EMF) was so bad that this person would have heart attack type symptoms, and at one point could not turn on a 20 watt light bulb or use heaters during winter months.

#3 Diagnosable Chemical Injury Exposure: Exposed for 1½ years to a 40% solution of formaldehyde left uncovered in the workplace.

#4 Immune Disorders:

    a) Helper/suppressor cells were inverted

    b) Abnormal elevated complement C-3 - 212 (normal is 70 to 176)

    c) Complement total Hem lower than 20 (normal is 70 to 150)

    d) Low B cell count of 176

    e) Low T cell of 700 (normal is 1000 to 2500)

NOTE: This person's immune system has been medically re-tested and is 100% normal.

#5 *Atypical Organic Brain Syndrome* (overall moderate to severe impairment).

    a) Mostly in the right hemisphere, affecting the limbic system/hypothalamus and right frontal lobe.

    b) Dyslogia—short-term memory loss/aphasias.

c) Had a drop of 25 points in IQ for 10 years.

d) Disequilibrium—loss of balance existed; this individual would fall several times a day.

Today, this person has tested totally normal in all brain functions.

#6 *Secondary Hypoparathyroidism*

#7 *Hypothyroidism* since 1957; now medically verified to be "totally well"

#8 Primary renal calcium leak (rare kidney disease)

#9 Secondary estrogen deficiency due to total hysterectomy, multiple fibroid tumors and pre-cancerous cyst – both ovaries

#10 Cervical and lumbar *Osteoarthritis* with narrowing of C5/C6/L5 – S1 interspaces – requiring braces, traction, *Demerol* and hospitalization

#11 *Leukopenia* and *neutropenia*

#12 Secondary kidney dysfunction due to previous renal shutdown and kidney dialysis (in coma for 1 month)

#13 Chronic high sedrate (indicative of inflammation in body) for 10 years – 60-80 (0-20 is normal)

#14 Positive IgE Rast test for traditional allergies (from childhood). Perennial allergic rhinitis (dust, molds, trees, animal danders, some foods, bee stings)

#15 Psychiatric Disease

a) *Schizophrenia*/paranoid catatonic episodes (began in 1962)

a) *Manic Depressive* – circular depressed (began in 1976)

a) Multiple personalities (14) from age 5 to the year 1992

a) Since childhood (age 8) had chronic suicidal ideation and attempts

a) *Anorexia nervosa/bulimia* – had to be hospitalized and tube-fed (began in 1964)

(All of the above included obsessive-compulsive behaviors, free-floating anxiety and panic disorders.)

#16 Chronic generalized *Myositis*, diffuse arthralgias, tendonitis and bursitis, requiring cortisone injections into joint spaces

#17 Chronic severe bladder infections

Case History Two. This person had 21 peripheral diseases brought on by MCS/EI.

General prognosis was "guarded." The illnesses started in 1973; the person was healed in 1993.

#1 Immune dysregulation deficiency syndrome included chronic fatigue, universal MCS, food allergy, pollen and mold sensitivity

#2 Marked allergy hypersensitivity producing chronic reactive airway disease

   a) Extrinsic asthma

   b) Obstructive sinusitis/laryngitis

#3 Organic brain syndrome with cognitive impairment

   a) Dyslogia – short-term memory loss/poor concentration and focusing

   b) Dyslexic dysfunction

   c) Disequilibrium

#4 Diffuse Arthralgias/myalgia/fibromyalgia syndrome

#5 Marked neuromyasthenia

#6 Chemical Injury

Significant heavy metal toxicity: Lead 132.6 (normal is below 57)

 Mercury 22.65 (normal is 0.63-6.72)

 Nickel 131.5 (normal is 18.5-53.8)

   a) Job-related in manufacturing plant (lead/solders and fluxes leading to nickel over-exposure)

   b) Deteriorating mercury silver amalgams in multiple dental restorations

   c) Elevated levels of polychlorinated biphenyls and organo-chlorine pesticide residues

   d) Heavy exposure to solvent-based marine paint

   NOTE: This individual has been re-tested since healing in 1993. Results: all levels are normal.

#7 Epstein-Barr Virus

#8 Hypothyroidism

#9 Marked posterior pituitary dysfunction

#10 Chronic blepharitis and lacrimal duct dysfunction (disorders of eyelids and eyes)

#11 Electromagnetic fields dysfunction (EMF)

#12 Chronic high cholesterol levels (both total and LDL)

#13 Bulimia and anorexia (dating back to adolescence)

#14 Significant candida antibodies

#15 Temporomadibular joint (TMJ)

#16 Diminished taste and smell

#17 Chronic cervical spine, thoracic spine as well as lumbosacral connective tissue dysfunction as a result of several auto accidents

#18 Increased susceptibility to viral infections

#19 Parasites: entamoeba Histolytica, entamoeba Coli, entamoeba Coli – precysts and trohozoites with inflammatory process

#20 Chronic uni-polar depression (free-floating anxiety and hyperirritability)

#21 Obsessive/compulsive disorder

> *(Art Mathias' note: I have met both of these people and have heard their testimony from them. They are both completely well today.)*

The depth of which God can move in your life is incredibly deep. God is still on the throne. He loves you, and He still answers prayer. You need to really let that be part of your heart.

I bumped into MCS/EI in 1990. I got a phone call from a person who said, "I hear God is really using you in people's lives, and I believe God can heal me through your ministry."

I said, "What do you have?" They said, "Multiple chemical sensitivity/ environmental illness, and I'm allergic to everything. I was exposed to pesticides about 10 years ago and since that time my immune system has been damaged and I'm allergic to everything. I'm living in a single room. I can't be with my family. I'm in a room where the floors are lined with foil. The walls are bare sheet rock; I'm sleeping on the dismantled springs of a box spring that has been wrapped in a material that has been specially conditioned for a year. I can eat hardly anything. I'm on oxygen and respirators. I cannot leave this room or be in the presence of one human being for too long."

I didn't know anything about the disease, and I told them I would pray about it. I had had some experience in the area of allergies and the healing of allergies. I was praying about it one day and I asked God what He wanted me to do. I had a release to get involved and I followed through. What a wonderful decision of obedience that was on my part!

There are close to 250,000 people who are suffering from MCS today. It is one of the most rapidly growing diseases in America along with *chronic fatigue syndrome* and *electromagnetic field sensitivity* (EMF).

I said, "OK, I'll go." I called the individual and I told them that I would give them 10 days of my life. I said, "I will leave the ministry and what I'm doing here and I will fly to where you are. I don't want anything from you." I made arrangements to go to that one person for 10 days.

I was on the plane flying across America to someone who did not know me and I did not know them. They were expecting to be healed of a disease, by God through me, that I knew nothing about. Would you like this assignment today? I just believed that God was in it and that He would talk to me and guide me through whatever I was supposed to do.

As I was on the plane with my Bible open, I had a conversation with my "Boss" about what I was supposed to do when I got there. Now the pressure was building. I would be expected to do something. I knew I could pray, but about what? I was letting my fingers do the walking and the Holy Spirit do the talking. I asked God, "Is there anything in here? Have you said anything about this situation?" I was flipping through my Bible and I bumped into one scripture. This scripture has been here since the day of Solomon, which was a little over 3,000 years ago. It's Proverbs 17:22—a merry heart doeth good like a medicine but a broken spirit drieth the bones.

> **²²A merry heart doeth good *like* a medicine: but a broken spirit drieth the bones.** Proverbs 17:22

I began to study that scripture, and right *there I saw a connection between the spirit of man and disease.* There are people who teach there is no connection between the spiritual and the physical. This scripture kind of blows that concept out of the water for once and for all. I realized that a broken spirit, or a broken heart, could have an impact on our health.

Then I started thinking about what is meant about being "dried up in the bones." It wasn't *osteoporosis* in this case, because this individual was too young for that. They didn't have an anemic problem. Drawing back to my college days as a premed student, I got to thinking about bones. What's in bones? Stuff. What kind of stuff? Red corpuscles and white corpuscles—the immune system. Part of the immune system is in the marrow of the bones. The other part is in the lymphatic system—the B and T cells. This scripture was talking about bones. I got to thinking about that and I said, "Wait a minute, it doesn't say that pesticides destroy the immune system."

The Word of God said that a broken spirit, or broken heart, can destroy the immune system. I said, "Is it possible that this individual was injured spiritually and emotionally at some point in their life?" I didn't know.

I got there and went to the house. The individual asked me, "Has God shown you anything about my disease?" I said, "I don't know, I'm not sure. I've got to ask you a question. I want to know who broke your heart. I want to know what happened that has put this kind of dread within you?"

From that point on, we had our hands full. I'm happy to tell you that 7 days later this individual was at the Sizzler eating everything on that smorgasbord, eating everything they could find. They were at the local yogurt shop eating hamburgers, French fries, and yogurt. I talked to this individual two Decembers ago by phone. I asked them if they were still well and they said that MCS/EI had never come back since that day.

That was the beginning of my journey into MCS/EI. Since 1990, we have literally had hundreds of people who have become healed from this disease all across America. From the extremes of being forced by severe allergies to go naked, not able to wear clothes, unable to eat almost every known food, allergic even to water, with multiple allergies, from EMF to exhaustion-type symptoms, these people today are living normal, productive lives with no relapse.

This ministry is considered "expert" in the healing of MCS/EI from coast to coast. There are people who specialize in the diagnosis, but they are not getting people healed. The environmental ecologist, the allergist with all modalities of Eastern mysticism, alternative modalities, allergy shots, rotation diets, sauna, supplements, and other treatments have produced no healings of MCS/EI long-term that I've ever been able to document during the past nine plus years although there are some reports of people doing better. But again this is just another form of disease management. I'm here to say that there are many, many people who are well today because of the involvement of our ministry in their lives. Hallelujah!

I'm going to mix the teaching of MCS/EI this afternoon with the teaching of fear, stress and physiology.

I have an article here about why females lose the emotional end of marital spats. The guys are over it as soon as it happens; the women do not recover for a long time. The damage to the immune system in a female that comes from strife in the home is incredible. Eighty-five to ninety percent of the people who have MCS/EI in America are female. The reason why the female is the one that gets sick is because she's more susceptible to the spiritual and emotional damage. God created the female to be a responder to good strong spiritual leadership, not to abuse.

My finding in thousands of cases across America in 9 years is that MCS or EI is the result of a breakup in the human relationship between the person who has the disease and someone else. The other person is usually a close family member, and one or more of four life circumstances is involved. I have found this in every person I've ministered to, without exception. Here are the four life circumstances that exist collectively or singly in MCS/EI:

1) Verbal and/or Emotional Abuse

2) Physical Abuse

3) Sexual Abuse

4) Drivenness to meet the expectations of a parent in order to receive love.

Concurrently, the individuals find themselves living in an atmosphere sterile of love and emotion, and it seems like they are in a straight jacket as far as relationships are concerned.

MCS/EI is an *anxiety disorder* that compromises the immune system to the degree that allergies, simple and complex, eventually develop. The only way to get

MCS/EI healed is to break the anxiety syndrome so the immune system can be healed. Then the allergies will fall away. Many of the peripheral diseases that have accumulated also go away. These include *candida, fibromyalgia, hypothyroidism,* and an ongoing list. These peripheral diseases are no big deal once you understand how they got a foothold to begin with. That's why once the root has been dealt with behind MCS/EI, these individuals are surprised to find that *candida, fibromyalgia, hypothyroidism* no longer exist in their bodies. If you have MCS/EI, and you're kind of scattered and smothered because of *candida,* don't worry about it. It'll go away. I don't minister to *candida* in people; I'm wasting my time.

If I find *fibromyalgia* in conjunction with MCS/EI, I don't bother to minister to it either. I'm wasting my time because it's the by-product of a root problem. *If you start chasing the fruit you are going to be just chasing a bunch of fruit. If you go to the root, and get the root problem solved, then you'll have good fruit one day.* This is **a more excellent way.**

I don't start on the outside. The allergist is starting on the outside. The allergist is trying to tell you that you have to avoid everything. God said that everything He made was not just good (Genesis 1:31). He said it was *very* good.

In our ministry, the first thing we want to do with people that are coming out of the food allergy profile is to get all the foods they ever wanted back into their lives. Do you like banana splits? Let's go for it. You want yogurt? Let's go for it. You like chocolate chip cookies? Let's go for it. What do you want? God only made good stuff!

This is from the *Dallas Morning News* (November 16, 1996) from an article called "Health and Science."

> **Hormonal reaction to stress is tied to disease, researchers say.** Stress and depression that send emergency hormones flowing into the bloodstream may help cause brittle bones in women, infections and even cancer, researchers say.
>
> A natural *fight or flight* reflex that once gave ancient humans the speed and endurance to escape primitive dangers is triggered daily in many modern people, keeping the hormones at a constant hyper-readiness, experts say. Even some forms of depression bring on a similar hormonal state.
>
> 'In many people, these hormones, such as cortisol, turn on and stay on for a long time' Dr. Philip Gold of the National Institute of Mental Health, one of the National Institutes of Health, said Friday. "If you're in danger, cortisol is good for you...but if it becomes unregulated it can produce disease."
>
> In extreme cases, this hormonal state destroys appetite, cripples the immune system, shuts down processes that repair tissue, blocks sleep and even breaks down bone, Dr. Gold said.
>
> He was among speakers of a two-day conference of the International Society for Neuroimmunomodulation, a group of experts who study the effects of stress and depression on physical disease.

Dr. Gold presented a study of bone density among 26 women, half suffering from depression and half with normal emotional states. The depressed women all had high levels of stress hormones, he said.

Although the women were about 40, he said those with depression uniformly "had bone density like that of 70 year old women. They were clearly at risk of fractures. The magnitude of bone loss was surprising."

What was the root? Fear, stress and anxiety. Continuing in the same article:

A study at Ohio State University showed that routine marital disagreements can cause the *fight or flight* hormone reaction.

Dr. Janice Kiecolt-Glaser, a psychologist, said a study of 90 newlywed couples showed that marriage arguments were particularly damaging to women.

In the study, the couples were put into a room together with blood sampling needles in their arms. The blood samples could be taken at interval without the subjects knowing it.

A researcher then interviewed the couples and intentionally promoted a discussion that aroused disagreement and argument.

"The couples were at a point in their marriage when they should be getting along well, when there should be little hostility," said Dr. Kiecolt-Glaser.

Yet, samples taken during the disagreements showed that the women experienced sudden and high levels of stress hormones, just as if they were in a *fight or flight* situation of great danger. The women also had steeper increases than the men.

The test continued through an overnight hospital stay and more blood samples were taken just before discharge. For the men, the blood hormone levels were back to normal, but the women still had high levels.

Remember what Ephesians 4:26 tells us—do not let the sun go down on your wrath.

²⁶Be ye angry, and sin not: let not the sun go down upon your wrath: Ephes. 4:26

Do you understand why that's in there now? Do you think God knows what can happen to us because of these spiritual dynamics of our life that go wrong? God is saying if you don't get this thing under your belt by sundown, you've got disease beginning to take hold in your body by the morning.

Medical science is telling you that also.

Romans 12:18 tells us to live peaceably one with another if at all possible.

¹⁸If it be possible, as much as lieth in you, live peaceably with all men. Romans 12:18

It's more fun living in peace don't you think? Isn't it more fun? They tell me it takes only about 17 or so muscles to smile and 30 or 40 to frown. Strife is considered a work of the flesh in the Bible. In fact, the Bible says—where there is strife there is every evil thing.

[16]**For where envying and strife *is*, there *is* confusion and every evil work.**
James 3:16

[19]**Now the works of the flesh are manifest...strife...of the which I tell you before, as I have also told *you* in time past, that they which do such things shall not inherit the kingdom of God.** Galatians 5:19-21

Would you consider strife to be a sin or a form of recreation? It's dangerous recreation!

Remember what Dr. Kiecolt-Glaser said: the stress hormone levels showed that the women were more sensitive to negative behavior than were the men.

> People with such high levels of stress hormones are at a much greater risk of getting sick, said Dr. Ronald Glaser, an Ohio State virologist and the husband of Dr. Kiecolt-Glaser.

> "If the hormone levels stay up longer than they should, there is a real risk of infectious disease," he said.

By the way, there is some evidence that the Gulf War Syndrome may be an *anxiety disorder*. From the *Houston Chronicle,* May 28, 1998, in studies concerning the Gulf War ills, the conclusion that is most rapidly happening right now is that it is a *stress disorder disease*.

Our ministry has been dealing with an individual in another state, female, who was in the Gulf War with her husband. She came down with a combination of what seemed to be CFS, MCS/EI, and Gulf War Syndrome. As we've been plowing into her case history, the evidence is that it is not bacterial, it's not poison, it's not chemicals, **it's fear** that is the cause of her disease. If I was a female in the Gulf War, I think I too would be afraid. If I was a guy, I think I would be afraid. It was a fearful (fear-filled) situation for everyone.

I also have an article taken from the World Wide Web from an organization that does research into MCS/EI. They've been tapping into something that we've been teaching for ten years. This article has to do with the limbic system. It is basically unfolding the mechanisms of the limbic system involving anxiety, fear, allergies, and a compromised immune system involving the hypothalamus. Dr. Iris Bell also has an article out supporting this insight into MCS/EI.

We're finding that, in order to get someone healed of MCS/EI, they have to be freed on two levels, spiritually and psychologically. Mankind is programmed on two levels. You think with your *spirit man* and you think with your *head*. It's your long-term memory. We taught you that already; that it involves protein synthesis, the RNA component, genetic component and long-term memory. Your long-term memory locks into your mind the objects of your fears, which are your stressors.

I'll never forget the time I was proving this to an individual who had come to us for ministry with MCS/EI. I told them, "I want to tell you that your EI reaction is based on the response of the hypothalamus gland, not a chemical." They doubted and didn't believe me.

Most people don't believe me because the medical community is telling you just the opposite, especially in the MCS/EI community. We're 180 degrees diametrically opposed to where the medical community is coming from because they are still chasing allergies.

We're chasing what causes allergies and they haven't even figured out there's a cause yet! They're calling it "chemical injury" or "chemical sensitivity." I want to tell you that people who have MCS/EI are, in fact, not reacting to any chemical. You've been had! You've been duped and deceived!

When you have a compromised immune system at that magnitude, when your killer cells and your B and T cells are compromised, when your lymphocytes are compromised at that level, you're going to react to everything.

How is it that the other 98% of our population living in the same environmental setting, going to the same stores, schools, churches and buildings don't have this problem? If the chemicals are causing the damage at that cellular level, we all would be down with some type of chemical poisoning.

What we found out is that it's not the smell that causes the reaction. The smell has programmed a response in you, i.e., fear. The smell is not what you are "allergic to" or "reacting to" and making you ill. The smell is the reinforcement of the mental and spiritual poisoning that keeps you in bondage, and makes that smell a stressor. If you are afraid of mice, I'll bring you a mouse and you'll be on the chair in a split second. If I say there is a mouse, you'll still be up on the chair lickety-split. The mass programming of the human mind has fear phobic realities.

I told this person that their EI reaction was coming out of a response to their hypothalamus gland, not an exposure to a chemical. They didn't agree with me. I bided my time, and one day in a ministry session when I had a team with me, I casually walked to the window and I said, "Oh! The bug man is here to spray." This individual went into an EI reaction just at the thought of it! They went catatonic and went into a massive EI reaction. They were not exposed to even one single chemical or smell. They came out of the EI reaction in about 10-15 minutes, and I looked at this person and said, "There was no bug man." They got mad at me at first. I can handle it. The important thing was that they got the message. The same EI reaction occurred without the chemical or exposure to it and this individual knew that they had been had! This same person is totally well today and praising God for their healing.

In a "**walk-out**" we help a person go back and take back every bit of ground they've lost. Every food, every building, every bit of clothing, everything they ever lost, they're going to take it back.

Well, we'd taken this particular person out to eat at a barbecue restaurant. You know how wood smoke is to some people with EI. It's a major stressor.

We got this individual a good meal and the restaurant had just cranked up the barbecue pit with smoke pouring out the chimney. We got in the car and were starting to pull out. This person saw the smoke and just at the sight of the smoke they were immediately staggering with an EI reaction. I looked at this individual and said, "Do you remember the bug man?" "Uh huh," they replied. I told this individual, "We're going to park this car and watch barbecue smoke out of a chimney for our dessert."

This individual said, "You can't do that to me." I wheeled that car around with my team and stopped that car at the base of the chimney, and we just sat there and watched barbecue smoke pile out of the chimney. That day this individual took back wood smoke and never lost it again. Why? They had been following the limbic system. This individual was following a stressor. They were following the mindset that had been built deep in anxiety and fear. They knew one more time that they had "been had."

Editor's Note: You must understand that the above story was in context of ministry with qualified ministers. I would not want anyone to think that this is simply a mind-over-matter situation. This was at a particular stage of **walk-out** in this person's ministry.

I have an article (from the World Wide Web) that is interesting because it confirms what we teach. It says that:

> The most vital component of the limbic system, the hypothalamus, governs: (1) body temperature via vasoconstriction, shivering, vasodilation, sweating, fever, and behaviors such as moving to a cooler or warmer environment or putting on or taking off clothing; (2) reproductive physiology and behavior; (3) feeding, drinking, digestive, and metabolic activities, including water balance, addictive eating leading to obesity, complete refusal of food and water leading to death; aggressive behavior, including such physical manifestations of emotion such as increased heart rate, elevated blood pressure, dry mouth, and gastrointestinal responses (Gilman, 1982).

> The hypothalamus is also the locus at which sympathetic and parasympathetic nervous systems converge. Many symptoms experienced by patients with food and chemical sensitivities relate to the autonomic (sympathetic and parasympathetic) nervous systems; for example, altered smooth muscle tone produces Raynaud's phenomenon, diarrhea, constipation, and other symptoms reported by these individuals.

> The hypothalamus also appears to influence anaphylaxis and other aspects of immunity (Stein, 1981). Conversely, antigens may affect electrical activity in the hypothalamus (Besedovsky, 19[Th]).

> **It is important to recognize that thoughts arising in the cerebral cortex that have strong emotional overtones also can trigger hypothalamic responses and recreate the physical effects associated with intense anger, fear and other feelings.** To implement its effects, the hypothalamus not only has a direct electrical output to the nervous system but also produces its own hormones, many of which stimulate or inhibit the pituitary's production of hormones (Gilman, 1982). Of interest in this regard, is that a disproportionate number of chemically sensitive individuals seem to have been treated for thyroid hormone deficiency at some time in their lives.

That's interesting, isn't it? It goes on and on about the biochemical mechanisms, the vascular mechanisms, and so on. This is a secular article coming out of the medical community, written by individuals that do research on some of the mechanisms of MCS/EI.

Fear, Stress and Physiology Continued

The Endocrine System

The endocrine system consists of the pituitary, the pineal gland, parathyroid glands, thyroid glands, thymus glands, adrenal glands, pancreas, ovaries, testes, and hypothalamus. I'm going to tell you where the hypothalamus gland is. How many of you have ever struggled with tension? When you have tension, do you ever have the back of your head hurt from tension? You remember which hand goes where? The hypothalamus gland is located in the third ventricle. This is where it starts to hurt. With tension, stress, and pressure, you start to rub your neck don't you? I check people for tension just by checking their neck out. That's the effect of stress and anxiety.

The hypothalamus gland is the "brain" of the endocrine system, and it sends out various types of chemical messengers to the endocrine system. There are many types of hormones involved in stress and anxiety. The hypothalamus gland is the facilitator for many things. We'll go over that with you.

Hormones travel to receptor sites in muscles or tissues where an action is produced. An EI reaction is a direct result of a combination of hormones being secreted by the hypothalamus, and the central nervous system being activated by fear and anxiety and stress. That's an EI reaction.

When you are subjected to your stressor, when you're exposed to the thing you think you're allergic to, sometimes people react. Sometimes they react, and don't even know they are around it, and that seems to reinforce their belief in their "allergy."

I have learned a lot about an invisible enemy called **"the spirit of fear"** which can see through walls and can see through you and knows exactly what's going on. You have a very intelligent enemy from the second heavens that may have gained access to your life.

FEAR IS NOT JUST AN EMOTION. The Bible calls fear at this level an evil spirit. I will be honest with you: in order to get a person healed of MCS/EI, *the spirit of fear has to be cast out of their life once and for all*. Now I don't know if that's part of your theology, and if you can get healed another way, then God bless you! All I know is that when the spirit of fear is gone, people are well. People are so afraid of the terms "demon" or "devil" or "evil spirit." Fear of evil is a national tragedy in the Christian Church.

I am saying that this is in a different dimension than the normal *fight or flight* response that God created you with. There is a natural fear that is part of your limbic system. *Fight or flight* is part of our creation, *but we have an enemy that would like to take that one step further and make that a permanent way of life. Yes, I'm saying your enemy knows you almost as well as your Creator does. He knows how to manipulate you and how to extend his kingdom to destroy you and manipulate you to bring his kingdom of oppression into your life.*

It is one thing to have *fight or flight* from playing in the traffic, or crossing the RR tracks. In MCS/EI the person is geared up in *fight or flight* all the time. When you gear up to face an invisible unknown enemy, parts of your body that are necessary for homeostasis shut down. Then we have the beginning of *candida, hypothyroidism, fibromyalgia, organic brain syndrome, exhaustion* and all the rest.

The parts of your body necessary for homeostasis are not required for *fight or flight. In fight or flight,* you need adrenaline. You are really just shadowboxing the invisible enemy all your life. It doesn't go away, it becomes progressive. *Like begets like, faith begets faith, fear begets fear, hate begets hate, love begets love, like begets like.* It's a crescendo of programming from the enemy to control our lives.

MCS/EI is rooted in *great insecurity, great mistrust, and great fear.* It has one other leg that it stands on which is *occultism.* I like to say MCS/EI, metaphorically, has two legs: one is fear and the other is occultism. **In fact, fear is occultism.** Why? Because it projects into the future something that is not true as it if were true.

Interestingly enough, most people that come to us for help don't come to us first; they come to us last. Pastors aren't supposed to know anything about disease. Yet these people have tried everything, spent all their money and it's not working. Then they hear there is some success with a pastor and his ministry teams *and then we get them.*

Before we get them, they have been to every which-way doctor for every which-way treatment that's known to man trying to become well. They have violated every scripture against the dark side in trying to get well. They have been to every New Age practitioner, every alternative practitioner, they've used every modality know to man, and they are still not well. You need to be careful when you go into that kingdom trying to get well; you open your spirit up to stuff that brings a tremendous consequence, and it brings more fear and more torment. I'm not trying to convince you at this stage. I'm sharing with you what I know. Without seeming presumptuous, with the Lord's help, this ministry has had many, many victories in healing disease. We speak with great authority, because of what God has done.

You know it's a matter of believing or not believing. I promise you that if you go into certain modalities of healing for MCS/EI, you can go in with 5 allergies and come out with 50 the first 24 hours you've been there. You can go into an allergist's office with 10 allergies and come out with 15-20 by the time you leave 30 minutes later. What I'm saying is that when you go into these modalities of healing, they don't have any solutions.

When you try to find a solution and it doesn't produce fruit, it produces more fear, hopelessness and despair, and by the time you come to this ministry, you don't believe us either. **We're the last resort.**

When you are geared up to fight a stressor, and that part of you inside is not feeling safe, there are all kinds of weird things happening inside your body and we're going to show them to you.

Limbic System

Now we're going to take a look at the *limbic system.* Have you ever heard of the mind/body connection? That's what science calls it, but in ministry we call it **the spirit, soul and body connection.**

> [23]**And the very God of peace sanctify you wholly; and *I pray God* your whole spirit and soul and body be preserved blameless unto the coming of our Lord Jesus Christ.** 1 Thes. 5:23

A principal gland in the limbic system is the hypothalamus. In fact, it's called the brain of the endocrine system and although it directly answers to the pituitary which is another gland involved in the limbic system, it is actually the hypothalamus which integrates the autonomic nervous system as well as the endocrine system.

Remember, psychology says that the soul is comprised of two compartments—conscious and collective unconscious. I don't find that in Scripture, but I do find *spirit, soul and body* as referenced in 1 Thessalonians 5:23 above. **What psychology is calling the collective unconscious is in fact the "spirit of man."**

Psychology says in the collective unconscious are the *archetypes and dark shadows* of our ancestral heritage. I say in the collective unconscious *(which is the spirit of man) is where the collective garbage of the "crispy critters" of our ancestral heritage resides.*

I'm reading now from the textbook *Principles of Anatomy and Physiology* by Gerard J. Tortora and Nicholas P. Anagnostakos, Harper & Row, 2nd edition, 1978:

HYPOTHALAMUS GLAND

1. It controls and integrates the autonomic nervous system, which stimulates smooth muscle, regulates the rate of contraction of cardiac muscle, and controls the secretions of many glands. Through the autonomic nervous system, the hypothalamus is the main regulator of visceral activities. It regulates heart rate, movement of food through the digestive tract, and contraction of the urinary bladder.

2. It is involved in the reception of sensory impulses from the viscera.

3. It is the principal intermediary between the nervous system and endocrine system – the two major control systems of the body. The hypothalamus lies just above the pituitary, the main endocrine gland. When the hypothalamus detects certain changes in the body, it releases chemicals called regulating factors that stimulate or inhibit the anterior pituitary gland. The anterior pituitary then releases or holds back hormones that regulate carbohydrates, fats, proteins, certain ions, and sexual functions.

4. It is the center for the mind-over-body phenomenon. When the cerebral cortex interprets strong emotions, it often sends impulses along tracts that connect the cortex with the hypothalamus. The hypothalamus then directs impulses via the autonomic nervous system and also releases chemicals that stimulate the anterior pituitary gland. The result can be a wide range of changes in body

activities. For instance, when you panic, impulses leave the hypothalamus to stimulate your heart to beat faster. Likewise, continued psychological stress can produce long-term abnormalities in body function that result in serious illness. These are so-called psychosomatic disorders. Psychosomatic disorders are real.

Let me say this to you: the hypothalamus gland is the facilitator and the originator of the following life circumstances: *all expressions of fear, anxiety, stress, tension, panic, panic attacks, phobia, rage, anger, and aggression.* These are all released and facilitated by this one gland. It only responds to you emotionally and spiritually. The hypothalamus is called the "brain of the endocrine system" but it is not a brain. It is a gland. It is a responder to thought. It is a responder to the environment of your life. It will only produce what is happening deep within the recesses of your *soul and your spirit.*

5. It is associated with feelings of rage and aggression.

6. It controls normal body temperature. Certain cells of the hypothalamus serve as a thermostat – a mechanism sensitive to changes in temperature. If blood flowing through the hypothalamus is above normal temperature, the hypothalamus directs impulses along the autonomic nervous system to stimulate activities that promote heat loss. Heat can be lost through relaxation of the smooth muscle in the blood vessels and by sweating. Conversely, if the temperature of the blood is below normal, the hypothalamus generates impulses that promote heat retention. Heat can be retained through the contraction of cutaneous blood vessels, cessation of sweating, and shivering.

7. It regulates food intake through two centers. The *feeding center* is stimulated by hunger sensations from an empty stomach. When sufficient food has been ingested, the *satiety center* is stimulated and sends out impulses that inhibit the feeding center.

8. It contains a *thirst center.* Certain cells in the hypothalamus are stimulated when the extracellular fluid volume is reduced. The stimulated cells produce the sensation of thirst in the hypothalamus.

9. It is one of the centers that maintain the waking state and sleep patterns.

(Principles of Anatomy & Physiology, by Gerard J. Tortora and Nicholas P. Anagnostakos, Second Edition, Harper & Row, 1978)

The *limbic system* is the connection between your cerebrum, where your brain is, down through to your hypothalamus. *It is the connection between psyche (thought) and physio (the body). It is the connection between soul and body.* Everything travels right down that connection that concerns thought. Good thoughts and bad thoughts. All of these parts are connected: the limbic lobe, the hippocampus, the amygdaloid, the hypothalamus, and the anterior nucleus of the thalamus. Everything is connected in order to process thought and give it expression in the physiological part of our lives. Just as fear can put you into *fight or flight,* peace can bring you into peace.

Jesus said this—peace give I unto you but not as the world gives, give I unto you.

[27]Peace I leave with you, my peace I give unto you: not as the world giveth, give I unto you. Let not your heart be troubled, neither let it be afraid. John 14:27

The Bible says in Jeremiah 6:13-14—the priest and the prophet have erred saying, 'Peace, peace' and there is no peace. In fact, it says the priest and prophet have erred and they have only healed the hurt of the daughter of my people slightly, saying peace, peace and there is no peace.

> **[13]For from the least of them even unto the greatest of them every one *is* given to covetousness; and from the prophet even unto the priest every one dealeth falsely. [14]They have healed also the hurt *of the daughter* of my people slightly, saying, Peace, peace; when *there is* no peace.** Jeremiah 6:13-14

Who is Jesus called? The Prince of Peace (Isaiah 9:6). He is the architect and He is the designer of our peace. AMEN.

> **[6]For unto us a child is born, unto us a son is given: and the government shall be upon his shoulder: and his name shall be called Wonderful, Counsellor, The mighty God, The everlasting Father, The Prince of Peace.** Isaiah 9:6

The Bible says—perfect peace belongs to those whose minds are fixed or stayed on the LORD.

> **[3]Thou wilt keep *him* in perfect peace, *whose* mind *is* stayed *on thee:* because he trusteth in thee.** Isaiah 26:3

The antidote to fear is fellowship with the Godhead. 2 Timothy 1:7 tells us—God has not given us the spirit of fear but of power, love and a sound mind.

> **[7]For God hath not given us the spirit of fear; but of power, and of love, and of a sound mind.** 2 Tim. 1:7

Power represents the Holy Spirit, love represents the love of the Father, and a sound mind represents the Word of God, Jesus. If you are filled with the fellowship of the love of God the Father, and of the Son, and of the Holy Spirit, fear does not have a shot at you. *If you're listening to fear, you're not listening to God.*

The limbic system functions in the emotional aspects of behavior related to survival. When you do not feel loved, when you have been victimized, when you don't feel secure, you fight for survival. When you've been rejected by a parent, or by anyone else, when you do not feel loved, when you feel violated, you are always looking over your shoulder for when the next hit is going to come. You are in *fight or flight.*

The limbic system also functions in memory. Although behavior is a function of the entire nervous system, the limbic system controls most of its *involuntary* aspects. One of the things about Environmental Illness is that it's all invisible (beyond conscious thought). It always involves everything deep within the person and we usually do not understand, by our intellectual processes, what's going on. That's why it is so difficult to see it. You can only see it if you understand the spiritual aspect from a Biblical perspective. You can only see it if you understand the enemy and his methods of attack.

This subject is called **stress and homeostasis**. *Homeostasis may be viewed as a specific response by the body to specific stimuli.* Homeostatic mechanisms "fine tune" the body. If the mechanisms are successful, our internal environment maintains a uniform chemistry, temperature and pressure. Homeostatic mechanisms are geared toward counteracting the everyday stresses of living. This is normal. This is what God created. We are going to show what happens when things aren't fine.

General Adaptation Syndrome (GAS)

If a stress is extreme or unusual, the normal ways of keeping the body in balance may not be sufficient. In this case, the stress triggers a wide-ranging set of bodily changes called *General Adaptation Syndrome* (GAS). Unlike the homeostatic mechanism, *General Adaptation Syndrome* (GAS) does not maintain a constant internal environment. In fact, it does just the opposite. For instance, blood pressure and blood sugar levels are raised above normal.

The purpose of these changes in the internal environment is to gear up the body to meet emergencies, known as stressors. The hypothalamus can be called the body's watchdog. It has sensors that detect changes in the chemistry, temperature and pressure of the blood. It is informed of emotions through tracks that connect it with the emotional centers of the cerebral cortex.

When the hypothalamus senses stress, it initiates a change of reactions that produce *General Adaptation Syndrome* (GAS). The stressors produce the syndrome. A stressor may be almost any disturbance, including strong emotional reactions. When a stressor appears, it stimulates the hypothalamus to stimulate the syndrome through two pathways. The first pathway is stimulation of the sympathetic nervous system and the adrenal medulla. This stimulation produces an immediate set of responses called the alarm reaction. The second pathway, called the resistance reaction, involves the anterior pituitary gland and adrenal cortex. The resistance reaction is slower to start, but its effects last longer.

The first part of an *Anxiety Disorder* is called the alarm reaction. The alarm reaction is *a fight or flight* response, and is the body's initial reaction to a stressor. It is actually a complex reaction initiated by hypothalamic stimulation of the sympathetic nervous system and the adrenal medulla. The responses of the visceral effectors are immediate and short-lived. They are designed to counteract the danger by mobilizing the body's resources for immediate physical activity. In essence, the alarm reaction brings tremendous amounts of glucose and oxygen to the organs that are most active in warding off danger. These are the brain, which must become highly alert; the skeletal muscles, which may have to ward off an attacker; and the heart, which must work furiously to pump enough materials to the brain and to the muscles. Hyperglycemia is associated with sympathetic activity. It is produced by epinephrine and norepinephrine from the adrenal medulla, fat mobilization, glucose sparing, and protein mobilization by the glucocorticoids.

The heart rate and strength of cardiac muscle contraction are increased. Blood vessels supplying the skin and the viscera, except the heart and lungs, undergo constriction. The spleen contracts and discharges stored blood. The liver transforms large amounts of stored glycogen into glucose. Sweat production increases. The rate of breathing increases; the production of saliva, stomach enzymes and intestinal enzymes decrease. This reaction takes place since digestive activity is not essential for counteracting the stress. This is what produces malabsorption. Sympathetic impulses to the adrenal medulla increase its secretion of epinephrine and norepinephrine. These hormones supplement and prolong many sympathetic nervous system realities.

A *fight or flight* stress creates the second stage—the *resistance stage*. The third stage is *exhaustion*. This can be progressive over years. It can come quickly, or it can come slowly. What happens is this: when you face the stressor, whether known or unknown, the first thing that gets stimulated is the hypothalamus gland. Nervous impulses are generated, the sympathetic centers in the spinal cord are activated, the sympathetic nervous system goes into motion, the adrenal medulla is affected, the production of epinephrine and norepinephrine occur and then begins the stress responses of an increased heart rate, constriction of blood vessels, contraction of spleen and on it goes.

General Adaptation Syndrome of Fear, Anxiety and Stress

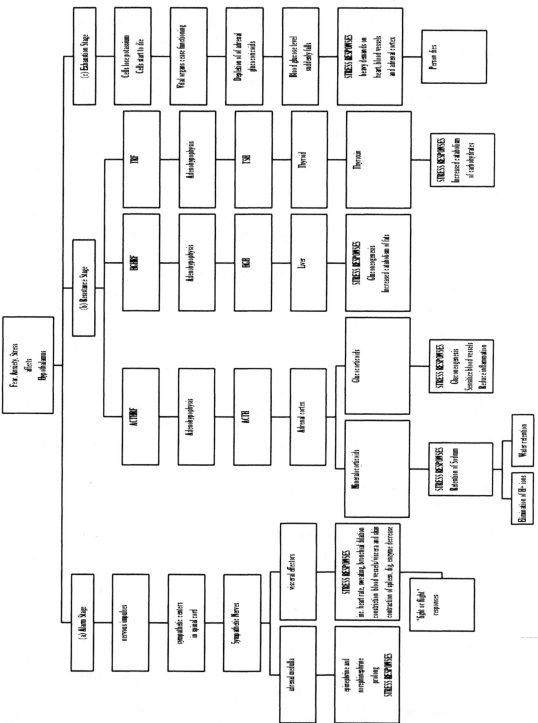

(a) Alarm Stage (called fight or flight); (b) Resistance Stage (being geared up to face the enemy long-term as a way of life); (c) Exhaustion Stage. This is how fear, anxiety and stress affects your body long-term. The final conclusion is all of the above.

MCS/EI Reaction Illustrated

Let's say we are up against our stressor, we have touched the 'forbidden food.' We're around the 'forbidden' smell, someone says the "bug man" is here and we are immediately programmed to think that he is the enemy. Instantly, there is a hormone generated by the hypothalamus that goes into the bloodstream. It docks at a receptor cell of the muscles of the heart. The heart and respiratory rates start to increase, rapidity of breathing begins, and it can go from slow all the way to panic. It can go so far that you reach a state of anaphylaxis, which is very dangerous because you can die from it. It can go to the extreme of catatonic realities. I have seen this happen in people's lives. *We've been very successful in breaking catatonic episodes, anaphylaxis and panic in every range of occurrence.*

In an EI reaction as we are exposed to our stressor, respiratory rate increases, and rapidity of breathing produces something called hyperventilation. In hyperventilation, two things are happening; you have either a reduction of oxygen in the upper level of the brain, or you have an increase of carbon dioxide levels. Hyperventilation interferes with getting the proper fuel to your brain cells; that's why, in the case of advanced EI reaction, individuals get fuzziness of thinking. They get "brain fog"; then they get diagnosed with organic brain syndrome. They have fuzzy thinking, and as they lose their concentration and brain fog develops, *their fear intensifies.* These people feel like they are literally losing their minds. They can't figure out what is happening; fear comes, it increases, more fears develop, more hormones are released, more fears, more hyperventilation, and they can reach the extreme of catatonic reality or anaphylaxis. It can go from calm to panic, just like that, with a massive rush of hormones. Once the stressors and their impact have passed, the fear subsides, the body returns to normal and the EI reaction is over.

An EI reaction does not last forever; however, what does last "forever" is the next stage of this disease—*the resistance stage.*

If a "normal person" is crossing the street in traffic and somebody blows their car's horn, the person would jump. If I were to lay my hand on a hot stove, the alarm stage would come, *fight or flight* would kick in, and I would quickly move myself out of the way. I would return back to normal, the parts necessary for homeostasis would kick back in, the parts for *fight or flight* would go away, my respiratory rate would come back to normal, my breathing would return to normal, and I would resume a normal life style.

In people with an *anxiety disorder* such as MCS/EI, they never leave *"fight or flight."* They move into the second level of this disease, *the resistance stage.* In the *resistance stage,* even though *fight or flight* is not so magnified, homeostasis never comes back to normal because the fear of the "enemy," "stressor" is always there. That's why you start getting all the various forms of malfunctioning. All the peripheral diseases start to develop.

The first thing that is affected in the *resistance stage* is the thyroid. That's why most people that are in advanced stages of MCS/EI also have *Hashimoto's disease* and/or *hypothyroidism* which is an under-secretion of thyroxin. Unless someone has messed with the thyroid through radiation, or through surgery, most people I have ministered to in the MCS/EI profile have been healed of either *hypothyroidism* or *Hashimoto's disease*, which the medical community would tell you is incurable. I'm here to tell you it's curable through the grace of God, when His conditions for spiritual healing are met.

Next to be affected is the liver. Right behind it is the adrenal cortex, and down here at the very ionic base of your body, elimination of $H+$ ions, water retention, and sodium retention. All kinds of things start to happen in here and your body starts to go out of whack, because the ionic base, the acidic levels, and the alkalinity levels are all messed up.

The next little creature that shows up on the marketplace in your life is *candida*. *Candida*, whether it is localized or systemic, is really a very painful disorder. It also does something else: it takes away your self-esteem. *Candida*, in a female, takes away her self-esteem because her sexual parts are usually affected first. Now, we have some more complications because of that.

As the fear intensifies, and as it becomes more and more obvious that this thing is not going away, then the rudiments and the roots of *fibromyalgia* set in and pain occurs that doesn't have any reason behind it. When you have that kind of pain, your faith is under attack. The next thing is hopelessness and despair, more fear, and more and more of you shuts down. When you go to the doctor, I promise you that you're going to leave with more fear.

This ministry is one of the few in the world that you can come to with respect to MCS/EI, *chronic fatigue syndrome* and *fibromyalgia* and be told that you can have a better day! The medical profession will tell you that you have to avoid this, and this, and this. You can go to various practitioners, spend $30,000 and more and eventually they will send you either to the desert in Arizona or mountains and oceans *with* your disease to live in isolation for the rest of your life.

Is there anyone here with MCS/EI today? I don't know if you will be healed today, but I will say this: there hasn't been a seminar since I've been in ministry on this disease where someone who has had MCS/EI, and listened to me teach, hasn't experienced release from this disease and total healing within 30 days.

Editor's Note: Since this seminar was taught, in the audience that day was a person extremely afflicted with MCS/EI. For three days they laid on the back floor with a face mask and listened to me teach about the roots of MCS/EI. This person is well today after years of devastation.

I will say something else to you:

- **Don't be afraid!**
- **Don't look at your symptoms—they are a lie.**
- **You're not alone in this disease anymore!**

We charge nothing for ministry—no cost to you. If you want to, you can get on our national ministry line and receive phone ministry and we'll start unraveling the mess. If that doesn't work, make arrangements to come to our facility. We do have a waiting list. When people come to Georgia, I tell them this: if you are coming for a quick fix, forget it. If you come here to get well then come prepared to get well. I would say to you today, if that's where you are at, don't be discouraged. We'd be happy to work with you and bring you to a place of healing.

Editor's Note: Part of our program now involves training churches, pastors and ministries across America to understand these diseases and the roots behind them. It is my goal within 5 years to have 7000 churches and/or ministries doing what we do so that the thousands of people who need help can be helped, and many of them in their local areas.

Editor's Note: If you are a pastor or the head of a ministry or an individual wanting to be trained to minister, please contact us as soon as possible so that we can get to know you and you can get to know us so that a network of individuals trained can be established.

Back to *General Adaptation Syndrome....*

The *resistance stage* of the *General Adaptation Syndrome* (GAS) allows the body to continue fighting a stressor long after the effects of the alarm reaction have dissipated. It increases the rate at which life processes occur. It provides the energy, functional proteins, and circulatory changes required for meeting emotional crisis, performing strenuous tasks, fighting infection, and so on. The *resistance stage* normally should carry you over to the recovery stage. But in MCS/EI there is no recovery. It just gets bigger and bigger. The body stays geared up to fight "the enemy" while the homeostasis needed for the bodily parts are still shut down. *The person is now geared up to fight this invisible threat all the time.*

At some point in this disease, it goes to the third and final stage of a fear/anxiety disorder, the *exhaustion stage*. Occasionally the *resistance stage* fails to combat the stressor, and the body gives up. In this case, the *General Adaptation Syndrome* moves into the stage of *exhaustion.* A major cause of exhaustion is loss of potassium ions. These are the biological, spiritual, and emotional mechanisms that surround MCS/EI.

I am still convinced that it is a disease of the broken heart.

> [22]**A merry heart doeth good** *like* **a medicine: but a broken spirit drieth the bones.** Proverbs 17:22

When you have a broken heart, you have *fear*. When you don't feel safe, you have *fear*. When you have anxiety, you have *fear*. MCS/EI is particularly difficult because it compounds itself upon a foundation of fear that continues to grow.

> [18]**There is no fear in love; but perfect love casteth out fear: because fear hath torment. He that feareth is not made perfect in love.** 1 John 4:18

From that standpoint of ministry, when dealing with MCS/EI, we bring a person to a place of safety. Safety first before God, secondly with themselves, and thirdly, with others. *There has to be a reconciliation in their heart at all three levels in order for healing to take place.*

Ultimately, the healing of MCS/EI is the removal of the *General Adaptation Syndrome* (GAS) in all three parts of its components. The more fear and anxiety decreases, the more the immune system starts to heal. *Let's say it this way: the more we increase in fear and anxiety, the more the immune system is destroyed. The more the immune system is destroyed, the more we have an increase of allergies.*

As fear, anxiety, and stressors go away, the reactions go away and that's why a person can take back 5 or 10 foods very quickly. It is amazing to them. Why is it that one day they are reacting to a particular food, and the next day they find they can eat it, and can eat it from that day on? What changed—the food? No, they did! The good news is this: you don't have the reaction, but you can eat the food!

> **Audience Question:** I heard a tape on MCS/EI, and your profile on the causes didn't fit me. My daughter says they do not fit her. I'm wondering if it's possible, in dealing with the concept of perfectionism and negativism, that MCS/EI could be the result of what is sometimes called church abuse, or legalism, rather than an early childhood situation involving a parent?

> **Pastor Henry's Response:** Yes, I would say that it probably could be. Again, we go back and look at verbal abuse, emotional abuse, physical abuse, sexual abuse, and drivenness to meet the expectation of the parent. As we begin to continue to understand this disease, anytime we get trapped in a relationship, or we come under the thumb of something that takes away our sovereignty and suppresses us, there could be a type of fear that would develop. I have seen a couple of cases where MCS/EI realities have not started in childhood, but came out of a marriage. I have seen situations where there has been oppressive legalistic abuse coming out of churches that has crushed people's spirits and has been very destructive.

That is something that I would be interested in talking further about. I certainly see that it has merit, and could be a root. *Anything that takes away our freedom produces fear.* Anytime we have been humiliated, or we have been suppressed, the situation has the potential to produce fear. It's a form of brain washing. It's a form of oppression, and it is a form of abuse. Legalism and church suppression that's abusive is as dangerous as sexual, physical, and verbal abuse. It's a tragedy and it's a horrible sin.

The elements of healing begin with trust. Healing of MCS/EI begins with having the ability to trust again, to be vulnerable. I find MCS/EI patients don't want to be vulnerable because they don't want to take the risk of more rejection. They withdraw in a world of protection mechanisms.

One of the things that I love to do in ministry is to make these guys and gals vulnerable and they are afraid to be vulnerable because they don't want to get trashed again. Could they dare believe? Could they dare love? Could they dare be vulnerable without being abused? Could I say then, that MCS/EI is a total result of some type of victimization? Could I say that and then could we not be so "black and white" as we are learning about the disease ourselves?

Let's move into the second part of fear, stress, and physiology. I want to begin with an incredible statement from the medical community. This part of the teaching will have to do with **fear and how it affects our lives**. America is plagued by fear. You are afraid of your mother, father, husband, wife, children, boss, disease, death, tomorrow, man, rejection, failure, abandonment, trains, planes, buildings, fear of this and fear of that. It's all over the place isn't it? Phobias: germ phobias, people phobias, food phobias.

What's the worst thing that can happen to you? Die and go to heaven, so what's your problem? God doesn't need you in heaven. You are of no earthly good if you go to heaven prematurely. The Lord doesn't need you there. If you get there too soon, He's going to ask you, "What are you doing here?" God says, "I wanted you down there in your generation to do something for Me. I don't need you here. I've got work for you. Everybody is so much in a hurry to get to heaven. You old lazy thing, you, get a grip!"

A stressor is anything that causes fear in your life. Let's see what parts of the body that one stressor can affect on a long-term basis. First of all, it directly affects the input to the central nervous system, including behavioral adaptations. The hypothalamus integrates the response to the fear. Then things start to happen; we have a releasing factor into the body with a hormone called CRF from the hypothalamus. Directly affected as the fear item begins to grow and progress, the Sympathetic Nervous System (SNS) becomes involved. The SNS is the part of the nervous system that makes you tick beyond your conscious thought. The voluntary nervous system is what I'm using to talk to you. My heart's beating, and that good lunch is moving around all over the place. That is happening in spite of my thoughts. That's controlled invisibly within me. That is what God created to make sure that I perk and function without me interfering with it.

So we have the SNS affected immediately in the Anterior Pituitary, the Posterior Pituitary, and then out of this the SNS, the norepinephrine from peripheral nerve endings, starts to get secreted. The adrenal medulla is affected and then we have the epinephrine release.

Because the norepinephrine is being released, we now have fear and anxiety being expressed. We have immune system breakdown effects beginning. We have increased contraction of the arterial smooth muscle; we have increased blood pressure, increased pupil dilation, and decreased gastric secretion.

Do you ever wonder sometimes why constipation goes with fear, or sometimes diarrhea goes with fear? *Diarrhea and constipation are fruits of fear/anxiety*. What I am teaching you is straight out of the medical community. This is what the medical community has found through years of research.

We have increased force of cardiac action, increased lypolysis of triglycerides, and increased circulation of fatty acids. There is a decreased degradation of cholesterol to bile acids. Serum cholesterol is increased. Over here, now, as this is beginning and increasing long-term, our liver is affected and so is our pancreas. In the liver, we have decreased glycogen synthesis, increased glycogenolysis, and increased gluconeogenesis. From the pancreas, we have decreased insulin, and increased glucagon, increased blood glucose, and decreased glucose.

The point of all this is that fear and anxiety are affecting your body behind the scenes; you don't even see it happening. Is that scary or what? This is just the beginning. All of that starts to affect the anterior pituitary and the posterior pituitary. We have vaso-suppression, ACTH being secreted, increased water retention, and from that, the beta-endorphins are affected. ACTH is a tremendous fear hormone. It sets everything into motion, and most of the EI advanced reactions are the result of the secretion of ACTH. ACTH, growth hormones, prolactin, and the adrenal cortex are effected by an increased release.

Cortisol

Now we come to cortisol. Cortisol is important in *fight or flight*, but if it's present on a long-term basis, it destroys your immune system. What God created for us to help fight an enemy has now turned on us, and has become the destroyer of our lives. (Pastor Henry begins reading from the <u>Pathophysiology</u> textbook again)

According to medical information, long-term over-secretion of cortisol has direct physiological effects on the following functions: carbohydrate and lipid metabolism; protein metabolism; inflammatory effects; lipid metabolism; immune reserve; digestive function; urinary function; connective tissue function; muscle function; bone function; vascular system and myocardial function; and central nervous system function.

"Cortisol directly influences immune responses to antibodies…cortisol inhibits the production of both macrophages and helper T cells. The diminished helper T cells cause a decrease in B cells and antibody production…"

Now begins the destruction of the immune system. What is destroying the immune system? Pesticides? No! According to the medical community it is fear, anxiety and stress. What did Proverbs 17:22 say—a broken spirit drieth up the bones.

> **²²A merry heart doeth good** *like* **a medicine: but a broken spirit drieth the bones.** Proverbs 17:22

The ongoing over-secretion of cortisol continues immunosuppression, decreased lymphocytes and monocytes, decreased circulating lymphocytes, and decreased macrophages. Right here, the negative effects begin. Right here, we have the breaking of the immune system and when you have the breaking down of the immune system, as we are about to show you, we have an interesting thing happen with the B cells.

When you have a reduction of B cells at that level, antigen-antibody relationships develop. Your body starts attacking everything. That's what an allergy is. That antigen becomes the enemy, but the antigen is the food you need. Now the body is eliminating what it needs to have in order to stay alive.

Could I say this, *"As the person disappears into fear and disappears into the self-rejection mode, the body takes on a profile of death."* Why? Because the person has been murdered. *Spiritually murdered.* Those are very strong words, aren't they? You say then, "How are they spiritually murdered?" When you deny your existence as God sees you and reject yourself in creation, a spirit of death comes to agree. *Numerous diseases are the result of this spiritual dynamic.*

The Power of the Tongue

The Bible teaches that if you gossip or slander about your neighbor, it is equal to murder. Do you know murder with the tongue is equally as damaging as killing someone with a gun?

Remember the saying, "Sticks and stones may break my bones but words will never harm me." Whoever wrote that was delusional. They were in denial.

The Bible says—words can pierce to the very penetrating of the human spirit.

> [8]**The words of a talebearer *are* as wounds, and they go down into the innermost parts of the belly.** Proverbs 18:8

They are arrows of destruction. There are words of death or words of life. The Bible says—life and death are in the power of the tongue.

> [21]**Death and life *are* in the power of the tongue: and they that love it shall eat the fruit thereof.** Proverbs 18:21

I'm either blessing you or cursing you with what I say. I'm either building you up or decreasing you. Has everybody always built you up? Has everybody always increased you? I thought we were supposed to be gifts one to another. I practiced being a gift to you because I practice being a gift to my wife and children. After I practice there, I come out and practice on you.

All of this stuff that I have shown you is what's affected by just *one area* of fear, anxiety and stress. Now let's add 15 dozen different areas at one time. Now we have a compounding of a major spiritual and biological problem.

As fear and anxiety is moving inside you, hormones are released to the α (Alpha) and β (Beta) receptors; and all parts of your body are affected. These are the physiological actions of the Alpha and Beta receptors: you've got muscles affected, blood vessels affected, the urinary tract affected, gastrointestinal tract affected, smooth muscle contraction, some vascular beds, increased insulin secretion, myocardial contraction, you've got all smooth muscle relaxation (bronchi, blood vessels, etc.); everything concerning your entire physiological body is now under attack. Gastrointestinal, cardiovascular, endocrine, neurological systems—everything that you are in creation is now taking a hit from fear and anxiety.

Catacholamines include epinephrine, norepinephrine, and dopamine. Let's take a look at the physiological effects of the catacholamines that are now being secreted because of anxiety and fear long-term, not to your benefit but to your harm. Look at the parts of the body that are affected: the brain, glucose metabolism, blood flow, cardiovascular, pulmonary, muscle, liver, skin, skeleton, gastrointestinal system, and lymphoid tissue. All the systems of your body are now being aberrated—are being attacked—and are changing and are being forced to do something that they were not designed to do.

Your whole physiological life is now under attack. That is why I gave you the case histories a while ago of those people who had 17-21 different peripheral diseases; because this is what comes. When we eliminated the foundational problem or root, then the rest of their body eventually—in a very short time—conformed to health as God intended. The diseases went away and the body snapped back into order and these individuals are well today.

Here is the problem: if you don't know this information and nobody tells it to you then you end up with 15 peripheral diseases, and you go to 15 different medical specialists. Not one collaborates with the other, and you end up chasing bad fruit with no regard to the originating root of the problem. You might end up on 15 different drugs seeing those 15 different specialists at 15 times the cost and with no solution ever in sight because the root problems have never even been discussed.

Continuing to read from <u>Pathophysiology: The Biologic Basis of Disease in Adults and Children</u>:

This is how cortisol effects cell-mediated immunity:

> Cortisol inhibits antigen-stimulated production of the peptide interleukin-1 macrophages, decreasing the initial recruitment of T lymphocytes. Cortisol also inhibits production of interleukin-2, reducing secondary proliferation of helper and suppressor T lymphocytes. Depending in part on the ratio of these two cell populations, production of antibody to the original antigen may be either facilitated or retarded. In some species, large doses of cortisol are lymphocytotoxic, causing cell death.

What we are looking at is the antigen and the macrophage and the progression all the way down as cortisol is increased—here's your T cells, here's cortisol, and here's cell death. Over here are T cells, helper cells, B cells, and when you have this happening and this over here suppressed and these suppressed you have antibodies to antigen and there's what an allergy is. (Wish we could watch Pastor Henry showing us the illustration as he speaks.)

When you can get your T cells and your B cells and your killer cells up to normal, and get the secretion of cortisol stopped, the immune system will heal itself. When the immune system is healed, the antibody to antigen no longer exists and that's why you can drink milk, when before you couldn't drink it. That's why you can be around certain smells today, when before you couldn't. It's because the foundational material that creates this mess is gone, and there is nothing to stimulate it. *That's exactly where we are in ministry. We want to remove the parts and pieces that allow the foundation of this disease to get a foothold.*

Let's go a little further. What causes the over-secretion of cortisol? *Fear/Anxiety/ Stress.*

These are the long-term problems relative to the *resistance* and *the exhaustion stage* of the fear/anxiety disorder. Carbohydrate and lipid metabolism are affected. Protein metabolism is affected. There are inflammatory effects. Lipid metabolism, the immune reserve, digestive function, urinary function, connective tissue function, muscle function, bone function, vascular system and myocardial function, and central nervous system function. Concerning the physiologic effects of cortisol there are many problems, for example: a decreased proliferation of fibroblast connective tissue (which delays healing and decreases bone formation) and somehow modulates perceptual and emotional functions.

Let's move away from something like an allergy, and let's see what they have to say about other diseases that are caused, in the long term by fear, anxiety and stress.

You were throwing diseases at me, and I was just saying this is the root and this is the cause. You're going "Wow, where did he get all that?"

I get it from many sources. I get it from the Word and I get it from studying what the medical community already knows about something. One thing I like about the medical community is they have done a nice job investigating and documenting our enemy. I want to thank the medical community and the psychiatric industry for their investigation and documentation of our enemy. It has saved me a lot of time and expense. I thank them for defining, showing, and demonstrating our enemy.

These are examples of fear, anxiety and stress-related diseases and conditions as documented in the medical community:

The target organ systems for fear, anxiety and stress:

Cardiovascular System

NOTE: Although this section of the teaching concerns cardiovascular disease that is a result of fear, anxiety and stress, I am going to cover the full spectrum of cardiovascular disease including three additional root areas and the diseases that come from these root areas so that you will have a complete picture of cardiovascular disease regardless of the root.

Spiritual Root: Fear/Anxiety/Stress

Angina (Pain)

Angina by definition in the dictionary is any disease in which spasmodic and painful suffocation or spasms occur. With respect to heart tissue, *angina pectoris* is more commonly known. The word in the Greek language literally means a strangling. The definition includes severe pain in the chest associated with emotional stress and characterized by feelings of suffocation and apprehension. From a physiological standpoint, *angina* occurs as three primary types: first, stable *angina* (or classic *angina*) is caused by luminal narrowing and hardening of the arterial walls. The second type is unstable *angina* and is often caused by a vasospasm that can cause inadequate oxygen supply. The third type is the variant *angina* which involves the entire thickness of the myocardial layer. Interestingly, it occurs unpredictably and almost exclusively at rest. Hyperactivity of the sympathetic nervous system produced by the hypothalamus in relationship to the mind/body connection is clearly implicated in the medical journals.

The Bible says—in the last days men's hearts shall fail them because of fear.

> **[26]Men's hearts failing them for fear, and for looking after those things which are coming on the earth: for the powers of heaven shall be shaken. Luke 21:26**

In the textbook <u>Pathophysiology: The Biologic Basis for Disease</u> under the heading "Examples of Stress-Related Diseases and Conditions," a primary target organ is the heart and/or the cardiovascular system. Diseases such as *angina, hypertension, arrhythmias, mitral valve prolapse* are listed and are considered fear, anxiety, and stress diseases by the medical community.

Not only does the medical community say the basis for these diseases is fear, anxiety and stress, but who else said it? In the scripture we just quoted from Luke 21:26, God said it—in the last days men's hearts will fail them because of fear. What good would it do for God to heal you, for example, of *angina* if you hold onto the spirit of fear and anxiety that is causing the stiffening, hardening, vasospasm, or hyperactivity of the cardiovascular system?

Do you think that God knows that fear and anxiety will produce *angina* pain and other cardiovascular problems? Do you think He knows that? If He knows that, don't you think He wants us to know it, too? That's why He told us, in His Word, exactly what would cause certain types of heart disease. He said that in the last days, men's hearts shall fail them because of fear.

Additional information found in the textbook <u>Principles of Anatomy and Physiology</u> under the section entitled "Blood Supply" states that most heart problems result from faulty coronary circulation. *The information continues to state that stress (fear and anxiety) which produces constriction of vessel walls is a common cause.*

High Blood Pressure (Hypertension)

What is *hypertension*? It is high blood pressure. High blood pressure is a result of a narrowing of the blood vessels so that there is a resistance to the flow, thus increasing the pressure because of the backup in the coronary vessels. What is the root for high blood pressure? Fear, anxiety and stress. Just as the Bible said in the last days that men's hearts shall fail them because of fear, statistics in America are that one out of every four Americans suffers from high blood pressure.

What I am teaching is not opposed to medical science. I'm not in opposition to medical science. In fact, what I see in the Bible only proves medical science and medical science only proves the Bible. I find no conflict. It's just that the third dimension of our existence (the spirit of man) is usually not recognized in the scientific and medical community. It is essential to understand that man is not just a soul and a body, but he is also a spirit and the problems are spiritual first, thus this is why a pastor is teaching this material.

Heart Arrhythmias

Heart *arrhythmias* are disturbances of heart rhythm or such things as arrhythmic problems. Many arrhythmic problems have as a root chronic fear, anxiety and stress. The first target organ for fear, anxiety and stress is the heart. Not only can the heart be stimulated by chemical messengers but through the involuntary nervous system is neurologically sensitive to thought via the mind/body connection.

Because of this reason, neurologically, the heartbeat can be interrupted. In the case of the speeding up or slowing down of heartbeat, this can be affected by the autonomic nervous system which is highly susceptible to thought via the mind/body connection. For example, when a person is startled or traumatized or victimized, the heart rate increases in response to the stressor. To help you understand this mechanism, it would be like cutting the electrical current off to something and then turning it back on.

Mitral Valve Prolapse (Heart Valve Disease)

Mitral valve prolapse can be caused by congenital defect, infections or damage by rheumatic fever, but in America today, *mitral valve prolapse* is a national epidemic and none of these possible causes can be found. Many people have been healed by God through this ministry of *mitral valve prolapse* over the past few years because we have discovered that the mitral valve and whether it stays open or closed can happen because of neurological misfiring. Very similar to arrhythmic problems, the reality of fear, anxiety and stress upstream in the spirit and the soul causes a whole sequence of events to go into motion through the mind/body connection so that the electrical connection to the valve is interrupted. When the fear, anxiety and stress of a person's life has been dealt with, we've seen *mitral valve prolapse* disappear out of a person's life quickly.

Self-Bitterness, Self-Rejection and Self-Hatred

Coronary Artery Disease

Coronary artery disease is the number one cause of heart attacks. Primarily, *coronary artery disease* involves blockage so that oxygen is prevented from reaching the heart muscle. *Coronary artery disease* involves hardening of the arteries which effectively leads to a narrowing of the arteries. Recent medical information now indicates that cholesterol is not necessarily the culprit, but there are other factors very spiritually rooted in nature that cause this problem in many people while many other people eating the same foods, living in the same homes, in the same environmental setting never have a problem.

A recent statement from one of the medical journals gave a sobering insight. Performing triple and quad bypasses does not eliminate *coronary artery disease* or blockage or hardening of the arteries because when they do the triple or the quad bypass, those new arteries will clog also. This indicates something very invisible and very consistent to spiritual roots. In reviewing case histories of people in ministry, we have discovered those suffering from *coronary artery disease* are filled with self-rejection and self-bitterness and self-hatred and have never overcome it.

Strokes

Strokes are the result of clogging of blood vessels so that the brain tissue is blood-starved and this is known as cerebrovascular insufficiency. In some cases there can be a hemorrhage that also interferes with the function by cutting off a part of its blood supply, but do not confuse this hemorrhagic stroke with what an *aneurysm* is. It has been my observation that individuals who have *strokes* also have self-rejection, self-bitterness and self-hatred. I suppose you could say that when you don't like yourself, that clogging of arteries is the immediate fruit physiologically. I guess it might be a good idea not to kill ourselves in our self-esteem because our body might conform to that image very quickly.

Diseases of Heart Muscle from Inflammation

This type of inflammation is non-bacterial inflammation and is not the result of a bacterial infection. This condition is part of a new disease class that we've been observing that is a combination of fear, anxiety, stress and self-hatred and the mechanism that produces this inflammation that is non-bacterial in nature, has an autoimmune component in which the white corpuscles are congregating in the heart muscle. When white corpuscles congregate there is non-bacterial inflammation as a by-product. This can be quite serious in heart tissue because the heart can quit beating. It's not quite as serious in other similar diseases of this nature such as prostatitis, interstitial cystitis, and asthma although asthma can be very life-threatening. Whenever I see white corpuscles congregating and/or white corpuscle activity that's abnormal, I find self-rejection, self-bitterness and self-hatred.

Anger, Rage and Resentment

Aneurysms

An *aneurysm* is an abnormal (often balloon-like) swelling on the side of an artery caused by a weakness in the arterial wall. There can be congenital brain *aneurysms* or there can be aortic *aneurysms*. In any event, an *aneurysm* involves either the swelling or the rupturing of blood vessels. Whenever I find exploding blood vessels or bulging blood vessels, I have found anger, rage and resentment in that person. Another observation is that this particular disease is highly inherited, not necessarily as a genetic defect disease but as an inherited spiritual disease. You see, anger, rage and resentment is not genetic, it is spiritual and it is sin.

> **[26]Be ye angry, and sin not: let not the sun go down upon your wrath:**
> **[27]Neither give place to the devil.** Ephes. 4:26-27

Varicose Veins

Varicose veins involve a swelling of blood vessel walls. In fact, they are a form of *aneurysm*. Again the root is anger, rage and resentment. Let me bring forth an important point: this anger, rage and resentment is not always externally explosive against others but can be internalized. Could I say the person is brooding, steaming, and deep inside they are filled with anger, rage and resentment. So, whether externalized or internalized, it is still sin and the result is the same.

Hemorrhoids

Hemorrhoids are varicose veins. The root is the same.

Thrombophlebitis (Vein Inflammation)

This type of *vein inflammation* primarily affects the body's superficial veins, those which are easily seen on the surface of the skin, especially in the legs. This condition is very common in persons who also have *varicose veins*. The root follows the rest: anger, rage and resentment.

Congenital, Inherited or Injury *in utero*

A defect of the heart or major blood vessels can be present at birth. Statistically in America, *congenital heart disease* is found in seven of every 1000 births. Genetic abnormality can be associated with heart defect so that the child is born with a heart disease problem. We would consider this the inherited genetic curse.

Other *congenital heart diseases* can have their origin *in utero* (in the womb). Such things as infections, German measles in the mother during early pregnancy, medications taken during pregnancy also increase the risk. In these cases of *injury in utero*, in ministry we simply ask God to do a creative miracle and restore the tissue that's been damaged.

Muscles

Tension Headaches

We started this teaching by discussing the hypothalamus. We talked about how you rub the back of your neck when you are under stress and tension. Fear, anxiety, and stress produce tension and tension headaches.

Muscle Contraction Backache

That is connected directly with the central nervous system, and to the sympathetic nervous system. It is coming out of *fear, anxiety and stress.*

The next target organ system for stress is the connective tissue.

Connective Tissue Disease

Rheumatoid Arthritis

I'm in a little disagreement with the medical community here. I'm wondering why the medical community has gone there, and I really don't agree with them on that although I can see where fear, anxiety and stress can play a part in it. Basically if I were to say it was fear, I would say the person was *afraid of themselves.* They just don't want to face themselves. Out of that comes *self-hatred*, out of that comes the *guilt*, out of that comes the conflict that causes the white corpuscles to attack the connective material of the bones and eat at it and produce rheumatoid arthritis.

Related Inflammatory Diseases of Connective Tissue

Prostatitis

In related inflammatory diseases of the connective tissue, you have two types of inflammation; you have bacterial and you have nonbacterial. In bacterial inflammation, you treat the person with antibiotics. The nonbacterial inflammation is caused by either an over-secretion of histamine (systemic or localized), or it's caused by a proliferation of white corpuscles that localize, producing the nonbacterial inflammation. A disease of record that would be a nonbacterial inflammation would be *prostatitis* in men or *interstitial cystitis* in females. These are a couple of diseases that kind of help you understand the roots that are in existence here.

Interstitial Cystitis

This disease is comparable to *prostatitis* (see definitions above).

Pulmonary System

Asthma (Called Hypersensitivity Reaction)

I've been teaching this for a decade and finally the medical community has agreed with me: that *asthma* has nothing to do with what you breathe. It has nothing to do with airway obstruction, has nothing to do with breathing such things as dander, dust, pollen and all the rest of it but something is happening deep inside the human person that's being triggered by something internally and we've known it to be caused by *fear, anxiety and stress* for over a decade.

John Hopkins University Research Team in 1996, confirmed this finding that will change conventional wisdom concerning *asthma* for the past 50 years. There is nothing that you breathe that is causing an asthmatic attack. It can be inherited, but it's coming out of *deep-rooted fear, anxiety and stress* and that is right here in this medical information. *Asthma* is now considered an anxiety disorder by the medical community. Now what do you think about that?

Editor's Note: Since this seminar was taught, Pastor Henry has identified a specific fear issue as a root for *asthma* and that root is fear of abandonment coupled with insecurity.

Hay Fever

Hay fever is also considered a hypersensitivity reaction. *Hay fever* meets the profile of antigen-antibody as discussed previously relative to a compromised immune system and is a fear/anxiety/stress disorder.

Immune System

Immunosuppression or Deficiency

We just went over what excessive secretion of cortisol produces and what the catacholamines do, and how they destroy the immune system and the resulting diseases. The autoimmune diseases are not the result of immunosuppression.

The autoimmune diseases are not the result of a lack of white corpuscles. The autoimmune diseases are when the white corpuscles attack living flesh and destroy it. *Lupus, Crohn's, diabetes, rheumatoid arthritis and MS* are examples, and on it goes.

The body attacks the body because the person is attacking themselves spiritually in self-rejection and self-hatred and self-bitterness. There is a spiritual dynamic that comes, in which the white corpuscles are invisibly redirected to attack living tissue while ignoring the true enemy which is bacteria and viruses. As the person continues to attack themselves spiritually, the body finally agrees in which the white corpuscles start attacking the body. That is a high price to pay for not loving yourself.

Autoimmune Diseases

Even though the medical community now associates autoimmune diseases (including lupus, Crohn's diabetes, rheumatoid arthritis, multiple sclerosis) with fear, anxiety and stress, I have come to the conclusion that most autoimmune diseases are primarily the result of an unloving spirit producing feelings of not being loved, not being accepted, self-rejection, self-hatred, self-bitterness coupled with guilt. In fact it could be said that autoimmune diseases are primarily a self-hatred disease with a fear, anxiety and stress rider attached to them.

Gastrointestinal System

Ulcers

I know what you have been reading about bacteria (H-pylori) causing ulcers. For years we have believed, and the medical community believed, that fear, anxiety and stress caused a flaring of dendrite activity in the lining of the stomach producing the irritation and finally the ulceration. Then they came along and said, "Well, we've diagnosed a bacteria so it's a bacterial problem."

People who have ulcers also have compromised immune systems. When you have a compromised immune system you don't have the firepower to defeat bacteria. Because they found the bacteria doesn't intimidate me about the original assumption of *fear, anxiety and stress.* I'm not convinced that the bacteria cause ulcers. I am convinced that the combination of both is the culprit. *I think the fear, anxiety and stress came first and the bacteria showed up after the immune system was compromised.*

There are a number of gastrointestinal problems that are caused by fear, anxiety and stress. They include *irritable bowel syndrome (IBS), diarrhea, constipation, nausea, vomiting, ulcerative colitis and malabsorption.* I agree with all of that but there are some more. There's *malabsorption,* and *leaky gut,* which I think, is probably close to *malabsorption. Much of the malfunctioning of the gastrointestinal tract is caused by not having peace in your heart regarding issues in your life,* with the exception of *Crohn's disease,* which is an autoimmune disease.

Irritable Bowel Syndrome (IBS)

Irritable bowel syndrome (IBS) is a fear, anxiety and stress disorder in which the dendrites are flaring in the lining of the colon, very similar to what's happening in the lining of the stomach that produces ulcers.

Diarrhea

Diarrhea again can be caused by a continual irritation in conjunction with liver malfunctioning as part of the profile of the *General Adaptation Syndrome* of fear, anxiety and stress.

Constipation

Constipation is similar to *diarrhea* in that the root is the same but the mechanisms of the activity of the liver and bowel are different so that *constipation* results rather than *diarrhea.* But fear, anxiety and stress can be a common restrictive reality.

Nausea and Vomiting

Nausea and vomiting also involve something that could be considered nervous stomach or as a result of fear, anxiety and stress. Excessive gastric activity in conjunction with the central nervous system can produce the nausea and, in extreme cases, result in actual vomiting.

Ulcerative Colitis

Ulcerative colitis is also considered a fear, anxiety and stress disorder in which the lining of the colon is irritated by excessive flaring of dendrites to the degree that the lining ulcerates and bleeds. This is in contrast to *Crohn's disease* which can ulcerate, not from excessive flaring of dendrites, but ulcerates because of the attack of the white corpuscles on the lining and in many cases, the entire gastrointestinal tract can be affected.

Malabsorption (Leaky Gut)

Malabsorption (leaky gut) has become a national plague in which the food being ingested and the nutrients from it never reach the cellular level through the bloodstream. In fact, a high percentage of the digested food just passes on through resulting in various stages of malnutrition. The root behind all of this activity is fear, anxiety and stress. The deceptive problem behind *malabsorption* in America is an attempt to compensate by heavy involvement in supplements and other health food products usually at a very high cost to regain the nutritional loss. *Unfortunately the expense of health food and supplements passes right on through just like the original food did.* What a deception!

Genitourinary System

Diuresis, impotence and frigidity are caused by fear, anxiety and stress. Isn't that amazing?

Diuresis

Diuresis or excessive bladder elimination can be a result of fear, anxiety and stress. Also incontinence may be found many times in fear, anxiety and stress disorders.

Impotence

Impotence affects many men in America. A recent statistic indicates as high as 30 to 40% of all men in America are impotent. Behind this is a spiritual root of fear, anxiety and stress coming out of self-rejection and lack of self-esteem.

Frigidity

Frigidity is a female disorder. Behind frigidity is fear, anxiety and stress and again a female's value system has been compromised and many times her sexual identity and her uncleanness in it can be implicated.

Skin

The next system that is under attack is the skin.

Eczema

Eczema is a skin disorder involving itching, redness, inflammation, and occasionally pustules that may or may not ooze. *Eczema* is considered to be a fear, anxiety and stress disorder. There could be some implications of excessive histamine secretion and/or excessive autoimmune activity. This particular disease is clearly identified in Deuteronomy 28 as a curse resulting from disobedience to God and His Word.

Neurodermatitis

Neurodermatitis is a chronic inflammation of the skin. The disease may have a strong psychogenic component that is a very definite spiritual root involving anxiety, mental tension and emotional disturbances. It is definitely a result of the mind/body connection and occurs more in women than in men. It is a fear, anxiety and stress disorder.

Acne

Acne is a skin disorder usually on the face, neck, back and shoulders. For many years it was considered to be strictly a result of excessive oil in the skin as a result of puberty. However, recent medical research has identified adolescent *acne* as fear, anxiety and stress that is a result of peer pressure. It is not a genetic, biologic problem by itself, but in most cases the kids are afraid of other kids. That level of fear and anxiety triggers increased histamine secretion behind the skin and also increases the secretion of oil in the epidermis and we have *acne*. Isn't that an amazing discovery? It is the result of fear, anxiety and stress.

Endocrine System

Diabetes Mellitus

This is an autoimmune disease like rheumatoid arthritis we mentioned previously as well as other autoimmune diseases even though the medical community has grouped these in the fear, anxiety and stress category. I am in agreement partially because in this disease the endocrine system is involved so that it interferes with the ability of the pancreas to produce enough insulin or interferes with the ability of the body to use the insulin that is produced. Again I still consider the root of this disease to be self-hatred and self-rejection coupled with guilt but with a fear, anxiety and stress rider attached to it. As in the case of the autoimmune diseases mentioned above, the medical community does see that fear, anxiety and stress is a root cause but they do not see a bigger root cause and that is the unloving spirit that allows self-hatred and self-rejection and guilt to come.

Amenorrhea

Amenorrhea is an interruption or stoppage of the menstrual cycle in females. Behind this is a very powerful root of fear, stress and anxiety and the medical community has defined the root as emotional stress or depression. It has been an incredible observation in this ministry that many females who had complete stoppage of menstrual cycles for years and upon dealing with the fear, anxiety and stress and being healed, one of the firstfruits of the healing was the resumption of a menstrual cycle.

Central Nervous System

Fatigue and lethargy, Type A behavior, overeating, depression, and insomnia are all caused by *fear, anxiety and stress.*

Fatigue and Lethargy

Fatigue and lethargy can be found as a third stage called *exhaustion* under the *General Adaptation Syndrome* of fear, anxiety and stress. Fear, anxiety and stress are great contributors to fatigue, lethargy and exhaustion.

It's amazing the number of people struggling with fatigue, exhaustion and lethargy in America today. The medical community does not attribute this necessarily to a virus, overworking or exposure to chemicals, but in the medical manuals they attribute it to fear, anxiety and stress. In fact, the third stage of *the General Adaptation Syndrome of Fear, Anxiety and Stress* is *exhaustion*. In the case of *hypoglycemia* which is a reduction in glucose levels, exhaustion is part of the profile. However, as discussed previously, *hypoglycemia* is primarily a fear, anxiety and stress disorder with an autoimmune rider attached to it of fear, self-hatred and guilt. But again, fatigue, exhaustion and lethargy are by-products of the root problem.

Type A Behavior

Type A behavior involves drivenness, performance and perfectionism. Many of them are recognizable as workaholics and many times a root can include fear of poverty and need to succeed in order to be loved, that is, to be accepted because of a success. Another is the expectation put on someone by a parent or a spouse can produce a type of anxiety.

Overeating

Overeating includes an addictive characteristic. Sometimes shades of obsessive/compulsive behavior can be found; but in short, fear of rejection, fear of man, fear of failure and fear of abandonment can be powerful forces that drive people and produce long-term fear, anxiety and stress. The overeating aspect is a pacifier to be a false calming reality, in other words, a false comforter. Also large amounts of fuel supply are burned by a person who is driven, thus producing also the chemical need for nutrition replacement beyond the normal scope of life.

Depression

Depression is many times dealt with by an antidepressant drug such as Prozac but clinically speaking depression is a result of a chemical imbalance in the body produced by conflict at the spirit and/or soul level in which the limbic system responds to this stress and the depression is a result of the chemical imbalance produced by the body in response.

Insomnia

Insomnia or the inability to sleep at night is a recognized fear, anxiety and stress disorder. The hypothalamus gland (Principles of Anatomy and Physiology p. 320) is one of the centers that maintain the waking state and sleep patterns. Sleep is regulated by the hypothalamus gland. If the hypothalamus gland senses conflict or fear, anxiety and stress in a person's life, it responds, thus interfering with the peace of the person. A result can be insomnia.

Our teaching continues on fear, stress and physiology. I think we need to pay attention to 2 Timothy 1:7 which tells us—God has not given the spirit of fear, but of power, love and a sound mind. Scripture also tells us—thou shall love the Lord thy God with all thy heart, with all thy soul, with all thy mind (Matthew 22:37) and Thou shall love thy neighbor as you love yourself (Matthew 22:39). John said it this way in 1 John 4:11—if God loved us, we ought to love one another.

> **¹¹Beloved, if God so loved us, we ought also to love one another. 1 John 4:11**

The Four Scriptural Aspects Behind Fear, Anxiety and Stress Disorders Including MCS/EI

1 John 4:18 is the foundational scripture for the healing of many fear, anxiety and stress disorders including MCS/EI.

Proverbs 15:13 and 17:22 are the introductory verses for the insight into the spiritual roots.

> **¹³A merry heart maketh a cheerful countenance: but by sorrow of the heart the spirit is broken.** Proverbs 15:13

> **²²A merry heart doeth good *like* a medicine: but a broken spirit drieth the bones.** Proverbs 17:22

It is quite obvious from these scriptures that our physiological wellness can be affected by victimization and by rejection by others.

In 1 John 4:18 there are four parts. Each of these four parts must be individually read, recognized and digested, and applied to our lives.

> **¹⁸There is no fear in love; but perfect love casteth out fear: because fear hath torment. He that feareth is not made perfect in love. 1 John 4:18**

Part (a): **"There is no fear in love."** If there is no fear in love, if you are not loved perfectly *then fear comes*. If I am loving you, are you going to be afraid of me? If I am not loving you, are you going to be a little skittish with me? 1 John 4:18 says, "There is no fear in love." What is the antidote to fear?

Part (b): **"...perfect love casteth out fear..."** If fear comes from not being loved or accepted perfectly, and if we've not been loved perfectly or accepted perfectly, then guess what comes into our lives? FEAR. How is your discernment? Can you tell me? If there is fear in not being loved, then if no love is there, there is a fear that comes. That's the fear that causes these diseases. The antidote then would be to receive perfect love, or could I say love casts out fear?

All spiritually rooted diseases that involve fear involve a breach in relationship at whatever level. It could be a breach in relationship between you and God. It could be a breach in relationship between you and yourself, because you won't forgive yourself for something you did in 1928. It may be a breach between you and others. Remember what I told you when we started two days ago:

> A spiritually rooted disease is a result of separation from God, separation from yourself, and separation from others.

The beginning of all healing of spiritually rooted diseases is:

- **reconciliation with God and His Love, receiving His Love, reconciliation with Him as your Father, and making your peace with Him**

- **reconciliation of you with yourself**

- **and reconciliation of you and others.**

Many people misunderstand the term "to fear the LORD" and are actually afraid of Him because of that word. They see the scriptures, "The fear of the LORD" or "the fear of God." There are 14 different Hebrew words that are translated into English and there are seven Greek words that are translated into English that are translated as "FEAR." The one specifically translated "fear" when referring to "fear of God" has to do with *reverential respect* because we honor Him for who He is.

You can respect somebody for who they are but it doesn't mean you have to be afraid of them. Let's get that word fear out of our Anglo-Saxon mentality, and do some word study on the Hebrew and the Greek and then we'll come back into a focus of the correct translation.

From that standpoint, if the breach is between God and ourselves and others, then the beginning of all healing is reconciliation with God, making peace with ourselves, and making peace with our brother. 1 John 4:18 says, "There is no fear in love. Perfect love casts out fear."

Part (c): **"...because fear hath torment..."** It is that fear-that-has-torment that produces *paranoid schizophrenia*. It is that fear-that-has-torment that produces MPD *(multiple personality disorder)*. It is that fear-that-has-torment that produces many mental and psychological diseases, either through the inherited component of genetics, or the inherited familiar spirits that come to produce it. Most of the things that happen upstairs (Pastor Wright taps on top of his head as he is teaching) occur because we are afraid. Psychoses, phobias, panic, fear, anxiety; it is a tormenting hell between the ears and in the depth of the heart. How do you get rid of the torment? Part (b) told you. *"Perfect love casts out all fear."*

Part (d): **"...He that feareth is not made perfect in love."** What that means is this: you have fear because you're in a breach somewhere in your relationships at some level with a parent, boss, teacher, pastor, spouse, or your church. This could be anybody that you didn't feel safe with, who did not cover you with perfect love, didn't nurture you, didn't forgive you, did not cover you in your weaknesses, drove you and made you attempt to be perfect; someone who put you down, wouldn't kiss you, wouldn't hold you, wouldn't tell you that they loved you, wouldn't give you support; everything that has happened on that level of "you are not made perfect in love" and then you have an unloving, unclean spirit that has attached itself to you and will stay there until you are delivered with perfect love. We know this because Scripture says, "Perfect love casts out fear."

If you are not able to give and receive love, then you have fear. Now I want to ask you, "How many people in here have difficulty receiving love, and how many people in here have difficulty giving love?" If you are unable to give and receive love, you have the fear that we are talking about that produces these diseases, all the way from autoimmune to stress-related diseases.

I think it is important that we pay attention to 2 Timothy 1:7—God has not given us the spirit of fear but of power, love and a sound mind. I trust that you have gained insight into the spiritual roots of many diseases that are coming out of fear, anxiety and stress.

Anti-anxiety drugs and antidepressant drugs are not the answer for fear. These are neurological blockers and calming agents with extremely dangerous side effects. That includes *Prozac, Paxil, Xanax, Klonopin* and all the rest of them. They are incredibly dangerous drugs, and they are given because we in the Church and those who are in the world are not in discernment about the spiritual dynamics and spiritual basis of our lives. Drugs are not the solution. They are a form of disease management and God would have you know with great authority that He wants you to be free of anxiety because He didn't give it to you. He would want you to be free to live a life of peace, spiritually, emotionally, and physiologically. If you just trust Him, and get away from the rudiments of the world in its thinking, you can come back before Him in simple trust. Drugs are a poor substitute for the peace of God.

There is **a more excellent way.**

> [27]**Peace I leave with you, my peace I give unto you: not as the world giveth, give I unto you. Let not your heart be troubled, neither let it be afraid.** John 14:27

> [14]**They have healed also the hurt *of the daughter* of my people slightly, saying, Peace, peace; when *there is* no peace.** Jeremiah 6:14

What's the worst thing that can happen to you? You can die and go to heaven. I encourage you to go before God and ask Him to reveal to you the strongholds in your lives.

Spiritual Blocks to Healing

The next subject that we will cover is the spiritual blocks to healing. We will look at spiritual blocks as taught in the Word, that will keep you from being healed by God even if you know the spiritual roots of disease. Just because you now have discernment doesn't mean you've lined up with Him to receive healing.

Sometimes people are not healed. If He doesn't heal you, I'm going to ask Him to start you on the highway of discernment so you can apply the principles that I have given you. I taught you previously that sometimes just discernment and repentance, renouncing, taking responsibility and resisting does not work. My ministry began when that failed. So we are looking deeper into this picture, looking deeper into our hearts, our souls.

We are looking for the roots and the blocks, looking for what is preventing you from receiving after repentance, so that renouncing and resisting can start to work in your life thus allowing God to sanctify you in a particular area of your existence. There has to be a heart change on the inside.

I believe that healing and deliverance comes as a direct result of sanctification; I also believe disease prevention can be a direct result of sanctification. A lot of times the people who believe in healing have done Christianity a disservice because they believe that we can have our blessings and keep our sins. It is just not going to happen long-term.

I come from a different perspective. When people find out a pastor is talking about disease and healing, they shudder and have visions of some of the excesses they have seen around healing. I hope that I have not increased that image, and I hope that we have been able to come and talk about real life and real things from a very practical Biblical perspective and also something that is very scientifically and medically accurate. I hope that we have achieved some of that in your lives.

I know many of you will never be the same after this study. God, through the Holy Spirit, will start to deal with you and many of you will not get the many diseases that would have come upon you because you had not heard. I trust the Holy Spirit deals with you, that God the Father loves you at that level, and the Word of God dwells richly within your hearts and not only your lives but the lives of your family, friends and enemies are enriched.

I teach in two dimensions. I believe in the traditional, fundamentalist position that God's grace is sufficient for us. I believe that when He said to Paul—My grace is sufficient for you

> **⁹And he said unto me, My grace is sufficient for thee: for my strength is made perfect in weakness. Most gladly therefore will I rather glory in my infirmities, that the power of Christ may rest upon me. 2 Cor. 12:9**

That is a scriptural, biblical principle and that includes us when we are in our problems as well as out of our problems.

If it were not for God's sustaining grace in our lives in disease, we would be most miserable in it. So I thank God that the principles of the **sustaining grace** of God are scriptural, are very Pauline. However, I have also come to **another understanding** in the Pauline teachings, that there is a **greater grace**.

> **⁴And my speech and my preaching *was* not with enticing words of man's wisdom, but in demonstration of the Spirit and of power: ⁵That your faith should not stand in the wisdom of men, but in the power of God.** 1 Cor. 2:4-5

> **¹¹And God wrought special miracles by the hands of Paul: ¹²So that from his body were brought unto the sick handkerchiefs or aprons, and the diseases departed from them, and the evil spirits went out of them.** Acts 19:11-12

> **⁸And it came to pass, that the father of Publius lay sick of a fever and of a bloody flux: to whom Paul entered in, and prayed, and laid his hands on him, and healed him. ⁹So when this was done, others also, which had diseases in the island, came, and were healed:** Acts 28:8-9

*The greater grace is **a more excellent** way with respect to sustaining grace.* The *greater grace* does not negate the *sustaining grace,* and the *sustaining grace* does not negate the *greater grace.* The *greater grace* is the absence of the problem and where God alone receives all the glory. The *sustaining grace* is His provision of grace and mercy in our lives at all times, including the problem. To Him, we give the glory in all things.

Now I have brought you a principle of my life. I teach both *sustaining grace* and *greater grace* and neither one is in opposition to the other. Both are scriptural, both are positionally correct and in it God meets all of us regardless of who we are and regardless of our circumstances in this journey as pilgrims. We are in a world that is going to be changed one day and is, even now, being changed through the Church.

> **³...they [Paul and Barnabas] speaking boldly in the Lord, which gave testimony *unto the word of his grace,* and granted signs and wonders to be done by their hands.** Acts 14:3

You and I are pilgrims, called by God, called by His name, and sealed by His Spirit. We are not as we shall be but in a twinkling of an eye we shall be changed and in that is our hope—the redemption of our bodies and establishment of the kingdom of God in righteousness which you and I one day, regardless of the curse, and the fall of Adam, and Satan, and sin will partake of that glorious promise that God through Jesus Christ has given us.

Scripture has said—eye hath not seen, ear hath not heard nor has it entered into the heart of man the things which God has prepared for those who love Him.

> **⁹But as it is written, Eye hath not seen, nor ear heard, neither have entered into the heart of man, the things which God hath prepared for them that love him.** 1 Cor. 2:9

I say to you, Father I love you. I think maybe I should have said that so you understand that I'm not trying to negate *sustaining grace.*

What if we know the spiritual roots of our problem? What if the root of our disease biologically or psychologically does, in fact, have a spiritual component and we now know that. We see it from the Word, and from medical science. The confirmation is there. Is there any guarantee that we will be healed of that malady or disease?

Even though you know the roots of the disease, there may be blocks to prevent God from moving in your life. You see discernment is just the opening of the door to understanding.

In Isaiah 5:13 God said—My people have gone into captivity because they have no knowledge.

> **¹³Therefore my people are gone into captivity, because** *they have* **no knowledge: and their honourable men** *are* **famished, and their multitude dried up with thirst.** Isaiah 5:13

Again, Hosea 4:6 says—My people perish for lack of knowledge.

> **⁶My people are destroyed for lack of knowledge: because thou hast rejected knowledge, I will also reject thee, that thou shalt be no priest to me: seeing thou hast forgotten the law of thy God, I will also forget thy children.** Hosea 4:6

So discernment brings us to a place of observation of spiritual principles.

In Hebrews 5:14 Scripture says—he who is able to handle strong meat (that's mature) is one who by reason of exercise of his senses is able to discern both good and evil.

> **¹⁴But strong meat belongeth to them that are of full age,** *even* **those who by reason of use have their senses exercised to discern both good and evil.** Hebrews 5:14

We come to a place of maturity that we take a look at all things, judge all things, on the basis of discernment. Does discernment alone produce freedom? Not necessarily, because there may be blocks.

You know, I still read in the Bible those words: **"If, then and but."** I also am reminded in many scriptures of the conditions of receiving God's promises. His promises are all yea and amen,

> **²⁰For all the promises of God in him** *are* **yea, and in him Amen, unto the glory of God by us.** 2 Cor. 1:20

but we have to *appropriate them through our obedience.* "Obedience is better than sacrifice."

> **²²And Samuel said, Hath the L**ord *as great* **delight in burnt offerings and sacrifices, as in obeying the voice of the L**ord**? Behold, to obey** *is* **better than sacrifice,** *and* **to hearken than the fat of rams. ²³For rebellion** *is as* **the sin of witchcraft, and stubbornness** *is as* **iniquity and idolatry. Because thou hast rejected the word of the L**ord**, he hath also rejected thee from** *being* **king. ²⁴And Saul said unto Samuel, I have sinned: for I have transgressed the**

commandment of the LORD, and thy words: because I feared the people, and obeyed their voice. 1 Samuel 15:22-24

We come to a place that we understand the words of Christ when He said—if you love Me, you'll keep My commandments.

¹⁵**If ye love me, keep my commandments.** John 14:15

In the keeping of the commandments of the LORD, we find that a provision in the Torah (the first five books of Moses) in Deuteronomy 28 is that blessings will come. The blessings are automatic when we are obedient to God.

We also taught you about the principles of blessings and curses. Blessings come from God. Curses come as the blessings of the devil in our life. We choose what we shall have, blessings or curses, life or death.

We talked to you about Mt. Gerizim and Mt. Ebal. We found that the mountain of curses was Mt. Ebal and Mt. Gerizim was the mountain of blessing. So in the type and shadow, we saw the separation of God's people as God taught them a very graphic lesson, He said this in the Torah, in Moses and the books of the law—bare this witness that of a truth our obedience to God brings the blessings and they are very close and near by, however, our disobedience to God will eventually bring the curse but it's a long ways off, but it will surely come (See Deuteronomy 28). In that, God has built the principles and the type and shadows in that His grace overextends His judgments and in that He gives us a measure of time that we may apply our hearts to righteousness and get this thing figured out. That even under the law, grace and mercy was a factor of God's nature.

Here we are today under grace and mercy, but *because we are under grace and mercy does not negate our responsibility for obedience to the living God and His Word.* I have to obey His commandments, but I don't do it because the law requires it. I do it because I love God and because I love the Lord Jesus and it's a small thing for me to be obedient to One I love.

It is teaching the blocks to healing that has allowed me to help more people get free, as well as knowing the spiritual roots.

The Spirit of the Lord is in the midst of us where two or three are gathered together in His name, there He is in the midst of us.

²⁰**For where two or three are gathered together in my name, there am I in the midst of them.** Matthew 18:20

The Holy Spirit within you bears witness with my spirit that we are sons of God and the Spirit of God bears witness to truth.

¹⁶**The Spirit itself beareth witness with our spirit, that we are the children of God:** Romans 8:16

> [13]**Howbeit when he, the Spirit of truth, is come, he will guide you into all truth: for he shall not speak of himself; but whatsoever he shall hear, *that* shall he speak: and he will shew you things to come.** John 16:13

I assume because you are still here in this seminar after three days is because the things that you have heard have borne witness. If it has not borne witness, then you should not be here. If it does not bear witness corporately, then I should not be here. We have come to a place of observation.

In beginning to understand the blocks to healing let me quote Proverbs 26:2—as a bird by wandering and the swallow by flying so the curse causeless does not come.

> [2]**As the bird by wandering, as the swallow by flying, so the curse causeless shall not come.** Proverbs 26:2

In other words, the enemy does not have the right to afflict your life just because he wants to. There must be open doors, both historically in your family trees and historically in your personal life, in which we have wandered outside the parameters of God's knowledge, His provision and His covenant.

We find ourselves opening the doors to many things. Some disease has a right to be on our lives because somewhere along the line we, or our ancestors, opened the door. Satan does not have the right to arbitrarily afflict us. If that were the case, he could have eliminated the body of Christ worldwide within one year. Because that has not happened, it indicates to me that the same parameters of protection are here today as were in the days of Job.

The open doors that were there for Job to be sifted by the devil first involved fear. Job said in chapter 3—the thing that I have feared most greatly has come upon me.

> [25]**For the thing which I greatly feared is come upon me, and that which I was afraid of is come unto me.** Job 3:25

The areas of spiritual pride and arrogance in his life can be seen in the description of Behemoth and Leviathan in chapters 40 and 41 of Job, and also in the great discourse in which God spoke to Job.

> [19]**He *is* the chief of the ways of God...** Job 40:19

> [34]**...he *is* a king over all the children of pride.** Job 41:34

> [40:1]**Moreover the Lord answered Job, and said,** [2]**Shall he that contendeth with the Almighty instruct *him?* he that reproveth God, let him answer it.** Job 40:1-2

The bitterness, fear, arrogance and the spiritual pride were *open doors* in Job's life, but he got the message and God restored to him double what he had lost.

Today, I still believe there are parameters that God has placed against the enemy. The way the enemy gets into our lives is that we have opened the door historically, genetically, through familiar spirits of ancestry, or we have wandered away from the main line of the path that God has called us to.

You may or may not agree with that, but that's my position. Proverbs 26:2 amplifies my position by saying that the curse without a cause does not come. Deuteronomy 28 says the curse involves all manner of disease and that the blessing involves all absence of disease.

As we begin our teaching on blocks to healing, I have listed 33 for the purpose of this teaching (and more can be found in Scripture). They must be considered because they reveal another dimension of separation from God. These blocks are very common to all men, including Christians. They hinder us from fully walking in the Spirit and receiving the blessings of God. Blocks need to be repented for with a heart change just as repentance is needed in dealing with the roots.

☐ 1. Unforgiveness

The first block to healing is lack of forgiveness (unforgiveness) and is the most important one. In fact, there is not one person that I ever minister to, or my staff ministers to, that we don't go here first. If we don't get this first block dealt with, *we are going no further in any dimension.* We are wasting our time with roots, or the other possible blocks. We are wasting our time even talking to God on the subject. I want to take you to Mark 11:22-24—and Jesus, answering, saith unto them: Have faith in God for verily I say unto you, That whosoever shall say unto this mountain, Be thou removed, and be thou cast unto the sea; and shall not doubt in his heart, but shall believe that those things which he saith shall come to pass; he shall have whatsoever he saith. Therefore I say unto you, what thing whatsoever ye desire when ye pray, believe that ye receive them and ye shall have them.

> [22]And Jesus answering saith unto them, Have faith in God. [23]For verily I say unto you, That whosoever shall say unto this mountain, Be thou removed, and be thou cast into the sea; and shall not doubt in his heart, but shall believe that those things which he saith shall come to pass; he shall have whatsoever he saith. [24]Therefore I say unto you, What things soever ye desire, when ye pray, believe that ye receive *them,* and ye shall have *them.* Mark 11:22-24

> [14]For if ye forgive men their trespasses, your heavenly Father will also forgive you: [15]But if ye forgive not men their trespasses, neither will your Father forgive your trespasses. Matthew 6:14-15

It is clear from the Scriptures that we are to ask and expect to receive the object of our prayers.

Now there are those in the body of Christ that build a doctrine around the first portion of this scripture saying that you can have all the blessings of God just by asking or just by confessing in faith. This position may become a presumptuous faith in that it does not take responsibility and accountability for sin, especially the sin of unforgiveness that is found in context of this promise. In fact, this position totally negates the conditions of receiving found in Mark 11:25-26.

When you read Mark 11, and you move into verses 25 and 26, there is a conditional scripture attached that never gets quoted when people are trying to make

God a bubble gum machine. It says—when you stand praying (in order to receive something from God), forgive, if ye have ought against any: that your Father also which is in heaven may forgive you your trespasses. But if you do not forgive, neither will your Father which is in heaven forgive your trespasses.

> **[25]And when ye stand praying, forgive, if ye have ought against any: that your Father also which is in heaven may forgive you your trespasses. [26]But if ye do not forgive, neither will your Father which is in heaven forgive your trespasses.** Mark 11:25-26

I say this to you, with the great authority of the Scriptures, that God's forgiveness for you is in direct relationship to how you forgive your brother. I know what it says in 1 John 1:9—if we confess our sins He is faithful and just to forgive us our sins and to cleanse us from all unrighteousness.

> **[9]If we confess our sins, he is faithful and just to forgive us *our* sins, and to cleanse us from all unrighteousness.** 1 John 1:9

I believe that, but at the same time I believe that forgiveness is in direct relationship to our own choice to be obedient in forgiving others following the example of Christ and being perfect as He is perfect in the area of forgiveness.

> **[34]Then said Jesus, Father, forgive them...**Luke 23:34

Many people struggle with a scripture quoted out of context that accuses them and makes them feel unworthy and that scripture is found in Matthew 5:48 which says—be ye perfect even as your Father which is in heaven is perfect. However this scripture has nothing to do with your perfection in relationship to the totality of God's holiness but is specific to having a nature like His in forgiveness. Could I say it this way: be ye therefore perfect in forgiveness towards others even as your Father in heaven is perfect in His forgiveness towards you.

> **[44]But I say unto you, Love your enemies, bless them that curse you, do good to them that hate you, and pray for them which despitefully use you, and persecute you; [45]That ye may be the children of your Father which is in heaven: for he maketh his sun to rise on the evil and on the good, and sendeth rain on the just and on the unjust. [46]For if ye love them which love you, what reward have ye? do not even the publicans the same? [47]And if ye salute your brethren only, what do ye more *than others?* do not even the publicans so? [48]Be ye therefore perfect, even as your Father which is in heaven is perfect.** Matthew 5:44-48

> **[36]Be ye therefore merciful, as your Father also is merciful. [37]Judge not, and ye shall not be judged: condemn not, and ye shall not be condemned: forgive, and ye shall be forgiven: [38]Give, and it shall be given unto you; good measure, pressed down, and shaken together, and running over, shall men give into your bosom. For with the same measure that ye mete withal it shall be measured to you again.** Luke 6:36-38

Jesus is saying that our forgiveness from God the Father is not a one-way street. Our forgiveness from God the Father begins vertically to the degree we make it work horizontally. This scripture in Mark 11:25-26 is one of the toughest scriptures in the Bible because it says that if you do not forgive your brother his trespass, your Father which is in heaven will not forgive you yours.

> **[25]And when ye stand praying, forgive, if ye have ought against any: that your Father also which is in heaven may forgive you your trespasses. [26]But if ye do not forgive, neither will your Father which is in heaven forgive your trespasses.** Mark 11:25-26

I've had many people come to me over the years in ministry that have had to go to the altar every service, every week, every year, every month, and still can't get free of their bondage. I have talked to people who have fasted and prayed and they have begged God to be free of certain vices, certain bondage, certain things in their life, and the harder they try, the more they pray, the more in bondage they find themselves. The skies of heaven seemed closed to their prayers.

When they came to me as a pastor, and they indicated that they have been begging God for something and it hadn't happened, the first thing I asked them was, "Who is it that gives you this high octane ping in your spirit when you think about their name or when you face them? Who is it?"

So you know what? I have found someone there, without exception. That high octane ping that goes off when you think about someone in the past who has wronged you or hurt you, and they may be already dead. You know how many people have unforgiveness against dead people? It's a tragedy.

How can you make it right with a dead person? How do you correct a wrong when the person is dead? You can't. The same is true even about people who are alive and you don't know where they are. Sometimes this applies to people who refuse to interact with you about past wrongs.

I believe this is how God judges it: He judges it by your heart attitude towards it. If you have something from your past and it is not possible for you to personally make it right with that person, then sincerely make it right with God and it is taken care of; you don't have to carry the guilt about this issue any longer.

The first block to receiving from God is you are going to have to make peace in your heart with every person that you have ever known and get that resolved before God. This does not mean that you have to make peace with them personally if they are not available. It does mean you have to get it right with God concerning them.

The Word of God says—those sins that you retain are retained and those sins that you remit are remitted.

> **[23]Whose soever sins ye remit, they are remitted unto them;** *and* **whose soever** *sins* **ye retain, they are retained.** John 20:23

I would say to you very carefully and very strongly: make sure that in your Christian experience you are a *remitter* of sins. That will make you perfect like your Father, which is in heaven (Matthew 5:48).

Forgiveness is an attitude of your heart toward others in love. The biggest problem that we have in the area of forgiveness is that when someone has sinned against us, we make the sin equal to them also. We have a perfect hatred for the sin and we have a perfect hatred for them in the sin.

You see, what you have to do is separate the person from their sin as God separated you from your sin when He saved you. When God saved you, He separated you from your sin in His heart. He sees the sin but He sees you without it. He is able to separate you from your sin. He has loved you from the foundation of the world.

> ³**Blessed** *be* **the God and Father of our Lord Jesus Christ, who hath blessed us with all spiritual blessings in heavenly** *places* **in Christ:** ⁴**According as he hath chosen us in him before the foundation of the world, that we should be holy and without blame before him in love:** ⁵**Having predestinated us unto the adoption of children by Jesus Christ to himself, according to the good pleasure of his will,** ⁶**To the praise of the glory of his grace, wherein he hath made us accepted in the beloved.** Ephes. 1:3-6

We need to have that faith and expectation of who we are in the Father because of Christ.

You don't forgive people that have wronged you because you feel like it. You need to forgive them because you're obedient to Christ and His commandments. You don't do it from an intellectual standpoint. You don't do it because it's a law. You need to do it because that's just the way you are. You are just a love bug that will forgive all manner of sin, and that makes you just like your Daddy, your Father in heaven.

You can do that because you are all indwelled by the Spirit of God and the Spirit of God gives you the ability to think like your Father, act like your Father, talk like your Father and to forgive like your Father whether you feel like it or not. I promise you God forgives whether He feels like it or not. Are you with me? *In the area of forgiveness it is an attitude of the heart, not a ritual of performance.*

Unforgiveness has to be dealt with. You are either a remitter of sin or a retainer of sins. I made up my mind that in my life that I am going to forgive all manner of sin to all men.

☐ 2. Ignorance or Lack of Knowledge

Ignorance or lack of knowledge, the second block to healing, can be found in Isaiah 5:13-14 and Hosea 4:6. In Isaiah we read—God said my people have gone into captivity because they have no knowledge.

> ¹³**Therefore my people are gone into captivity, because** *they have* **no knowledge: and their honourable men** *are* **famished, and their multitude dried up with thirst.** ¹⁴**Therefore hell hath enlarged herself, and opened her mouth without measure: and their glory, and their multitude, and their pomp, and he that rejoiceth, shall descend into it.** Isaiah 5:13-14

Hosea said—My people perish for lack of knowledge.

> **⁶My people are destroyed for lack of knowledge: because thou hast
> rejected knowledge, I will also reject thee, that thou shalt be no priest to me:
> seeing thou hast forgotten the law of thy God, I will also forget thy children.
> ⁷As they were increased, so they sinned against me:** *therefore* **will I change
> their glory into shame.** Hosea 4:6-7

One day I was dead in my trespass and sin and that was ignorance, but in *my* thinking
it was correct knowledge. **Ignorance is a form of knowledge.** People who are
ignorant do not know they are ignorant. The beginning of all wisdom begins with
knowledge. You cannot have wisdom unless you first have knowledge. You cannot
have wisdom if you do not preface it with knowledge. Knowledge apart from wisdom
is foolishness. It's vanity and it is humanistic in nature.

> **⁷The fear of the LORD** *is* **the beginning of knowledge: but fools despise
> wisdom and instruction.** Proverbs 1:7

> **¹⁰The fear of the LORD** *is* **the beginning of wisdom: and the knowledge of
> the holy** *is* **understanding.** Proverbs 9:10

How many of us have found ourselves ignorant in our lifetime, and we still are in
many areas? The Bible says very clearly that we still see through a glass darkly but
when He that is perfect has come we shall see and He shall be known and we shall be
known and we shall see Him as He is.

> **¹²For now we see through a glass, darkly; but then face to face: now I
> know in part; but then shall I know even as also I am known.** 1 Cor. 13:12

Knowledge ties the past to the present and wisdom ties the present to the
future. God wants you to understand your past, your present and your future. That's
why this teaching on spiritual roots of disease and blocks to healing is so important:
because it gives you knowledge, understanding and discernment so that the wisdom of
God for your future can include healing and prevention of disease. **This is a more
excellent way.**

☐ 3. No Relationship with God According to Knowledge

The third block is no relationship with God according to knowledge. In Mark
7:24-30, we see a difference between lack of knowledge and no relationship with God
according to knowledge. They seem to be similar, but they are different. Many times,
we come to a place in our relationship with God where we are not meeting Him
according to Scripture.

> **²⁴And from thence he arose, and went into the borders of Tyre and Sidon,
> and entered into an house, and would have no man know** *it:* **but he could not be
> hid. ²⁵For a** *certain* **woman, whose young daughter had an unclean spirit, heard
> of him, and came and fell at his feet: ²⁶The woman was a Greek, a
> Syrophenician by nation; and she besought him that he would cast forth the
> devil out of her daughter. ²⁷But Jesus said unto her, Let the children first be
> filled: for it is not meet to take the children's bread, and to cast** *it* **unto the
> dogs. ²⁸And she answered and said unto him, Yes, Lord: yet the dogs under the**

table eat of the children's crumbs. ²⁹And he said unto her, For this saying go thy way; the devil is gone out of thy daughter. ³⁰And when she was come to her house, she found the devil gone out, and her daughter laid upon the bed. Mark 7:24-30

You remember when Jesus was ministering on the border of Tyre and Sidon, He came across a certain woman whose young daughter had an unclean spirit and she had heard of Him and came and fell at his feet. The woman was a Greek and she looked for Him so He would cast a devil out of her daughter but Jesus said unto her: "Let the children first be filled, for it is not meet to take the children's bread and cast it to dogs" (Mark 7:27). What Jesus was saying to her is: you don't qualify. You are not in covenant. You are not with God according to knowledge, you are outside, and you are separated from God. You are asking for something that doesn't belong to you.

In Mark 7:28 she answered and said unto Him "Yes Lord, yet even the dogs under the table eat of the children's crumbs and He said unto her, for this saying go thy way. The devil is gone out of thy daughter. When she was come to her house she found the devil had gone out and her daughter laid upon the bed."

I struggle sometimes with people who are unsaved, who want God to heal them. For many years forty percent of our caseload nationally were unchurched and unsaved. People are coming from all over America; many of them are unchurched and unsaved or from New Age and false religions. They ask us, "Will God heal me if I don't accept Him? Do I have to accept Jesus in order to be healed?"

We tell them, "No, you can be healed without being in covenant" because we see this scripturally. You can be healed when you are not in covenant, but if you are healed outside of covenant it would behoove you to get into covenant quick because He who has healed you is He who you should follow the rest of your days. That's our position. After they are healed, they are grateful and they do come to the saving knowledge of the Lord and that's wonderful. God has healed people in our ministry and they weren't born again.

I don't know where you are theologically, but I do know they are not going to die first and be born again last. We try to get them healed first and born again before they do die. If they die, we can never get them saved. There is no provision for getting saved after death. There is no stopping off point, or reincarnation facility. It is appointed unto men to die and then judgment.

²⁷And as it is appointed unto men once to die, but after this the judgment: Hebrews 9:27

Sometimes people do not receive from God because they do not have a relationship with God according to knowledge. In Mark 7:6, Jesus said—He answered and said unto them; Well hath Isaiah prophesied of you saying that you honor Him with your lips but your heart is far from Him.

¹³Wherefore the Lord said, Forasmuch as this people draw near *me* with their mouth, and with their lips do honour me, but have removed their heart far from me, and their fear toward me is taught by the precept of men: Isaiah 29:13

> **⁶He answered and said unto them, Well hath Esaias prophesied of you hypocrites, as it is written, This people honoureth me with *their* lips, but their heart is far from me.** Mark 7:6

It also says in Hebrews 11:6 that you must believe that God is and that He is a rewarder of them that diligently seek Him.

> **⁶But without faith *it is* impossible to please *him:* for he that cometh to God must believe that he is, and *that* he is a rewarder of them that diligently seek him.** Hebrews 11:6

If you want to make God a slot machine, it's not going to work. Do you remember the scripture where the Bible says that sometimes we pray and God doesn't hear?

> **³Ye ask, and receive not, because ye ask amiss, that ye may consume *it* upon your lusts.** James 4:3

That really is referring to a prayer of vanity, and so we learn that when we're praying prayers of vanity, God is not interested in honoring them. God is not interested in answering prayers that are fraudulent.

The way I see it according to knowledge is that seeking after God is pursuing relationship. The first phase of relationship is fellowship with our Creator. Fellowship involves talking to God. Going to church and reading the Bible does not guarantee fellowship and relationship. Relationship involves going to church and Bible reading, but it also involves conversation with God, conversation with God about the desires, plans and purposes of His heart, not just yours. If I read the Bible correctly—and I could be wrong—I don't have all the answers—but I will say this to you...that the way I see it, according to knowledge, is the first thing that comes is fellowship with our Creator.

Draw nigh to God and He will draw nigh to you.

> **⁸Draw nigh to God, and he will draw nigh to you. Cleanse *your* hands, *ye* sinners; and purify *your* hearts, *ye* double minded.** James 4:8

Seek ye first the kingdom of God and His righteousness.

> **³³But seek ye first the kingdom of God, and his righteousness; and all these things shall be added unto you.** Matthew 6:33

The next thing that comes after *fellowship* is *worship*, because when you're in fellowship then you'll be in worship. And finally, and lastly, the *petition*. But if you come to petition first and you've not already come to fellowship and to worship, then your petition is fraudulent. And it's not according to knowledge. Are you with me? Many people begin with God and petition first and then don't understand why their prayers are not answered.

You have to reverse the order. You have to go back to fellowship first, don't skip worship, and petition is always last. What YOU want is last. The first thing you have to do is approach God because of WHO He is...and what He has done for you from the foundation of the world, whether He gives you anything or not.

[23]But the hour cometh, and now is, when the true worshippers shall worship the Father in spirit and in truth: for the Father seeketh such to worship him. John 4:23

The gift of salvation is enough. The rest of it is just icing on the cake, but the foundation is salvation. "Notwithstanding in this rejoice not, that the spirits are subject unto you; but rather rejoice, because your names are written in heaven" (Luke 10:20).

[20]Notwithstanding in this rejoice not, that the spirits are subject unto you; but rather rejoice, because your names are written in heaven. Luke 10:20

I find that many people come to this ministry from all over America wanting to get well from psychological and biological diseases, but they don't want my Boss. They don't want my Father. They don't want the Holy Spirit, who would seal them and do the work to begin with. They just want the "fix."

Well, they're really in for a rude awakening...because what they get from me first is that I take them to fellowship. They want me to go to petition. I go to fellowship and they gnash their teeth. They're trying to get the fix without the fellowship. It will never happen. *A hindrance in our healing, sometimes, is the attitude of our heart.*

Sometimes, part of this *"no relationship with God according to knowledge"* is that we are approaching God, not with what the Word has said about it, but by what some religion or man said we should do to get to it. So, if you're going to approach God, it's not from what some man teaches you; it's got to be on the basis of what you can prove in Scripture.

I do not believe that there is any canon available to us that cannot be found already written. I am not into advanced revelation that cannot be supported by Scripture already written. I have taken a firm stand on that as a minister and as a believer.

I say it this way: when you've mastered from Genesis to Revelation, then bring me your new esoteric knowledge and maybe I'll listen. But I haven't found anybody yet that has mastered Genesis to Revelation in its entirety. Maybe you have, but I haven't.

Every time I think I understand the Word, I go to read it some more and I see something new in there that I didn't see before. Did you ever have that happen to you? And I thought I had just mastered that thing...I go back and read it again and it's just fresh all over again. A whole new understanding just opens up to me. Oh, it's a wonderful thing to read the Word!

Now, we have dealt with the fact that sometimes people want something from God but they're not in covenant. But at the same time, we must always make provision for people that are not in covenant because they came to Jesus, not because they wanted to be in covenant, not because they wanted to repent and be baptized; they came to Jesus because they were sick. And then He taught the gospel. He never healed, He never delivered, until He first preached the gospel. Read it in Matthew, Mark, Luke and John. He preached first, healed second.

So, the first thing we do is that we must teach the ways of God. Now, in the meantime, if people come because they want to get healed, and Jesus heals them, great.

In Scripture, after Jesus healed, they followed Him. He was always telling people, "Follow Me." Paul said, "Follow me as I follow Christ" (1 Corinthians 4:14-16).

> **[14]I write not these things to shame you, but as my beloved sons I warn *you*. [15]For though ye have ten thousand instructers in Christ, yet *have ye* not many fathers: for in Christ Jesus I have begotten you through the gospel. [16]Wherefore I beseech you, be ye followers of me. 1 Cor. 4:14-16**

> **[11:1]Be ye followers of me, even as I also *am* of Christ. 1 Cor. 11:1**

And I say to you, follow Henry as he follows Christ.

☐ 4. Personal and Family Sins

The fourth block to healing is personal and family sins. In Isaiah 59:1-2 it says—behold, the LORD's hand is not so short that it cannot save; neither is His ear so dull that it cannot hear. But your iniquities have made a separation between you and your God, and your sins have hid His face from you, that He will not hear.

> **[59:1]Behold, the LORD's hand is not shortened, that it cannot save; neither his ear heavy, that it cannot hear: [2]But your iniquities have separated between you and your God, and your sins have hid *his* face from you, that he will not hear. Isaiah 59:1-2**

Editor's Note: This next sentence is a statement addressed to Wycliffe members at this live seminar.

I don't think it's God's perfect will that you precious people who are laying your lives down worldwide for the Word of God need to go out there and serve from the disadvantage of disease. I cannot see how that furthers the message and the mission that you've been called to. I don't think that it's God's will that your heart and your mission be hindered by disease. That's how I feel. And if I'm out of line, I'll repent to you.

Isaiah says that our sins can separate us from our God (Isaiah 59:1-2). Not only can our sins separate us from our God, the consequence of our ancestors' sins can transfer into us and we have evidence of that through genetically inherited disease. And not only do we have genetically inherited disease, but the psychiatric industry over the years has determined that certain non-genetic factors such as disposition, personality quirks, and idiosyncrasies can also be passed down through family trees without a genetic component being seen or known.

In Exodus 20:5 it says that the sins of the fathers shall be passed on to the children, on down to the third and the fourth generations. We also read this in Deuteronomy, so we have a confirmation of this in two different verses of the Bible.

> **[5]Thou shalt not bow down thyself to them, nor serve them: for I the LORD thy God *am* a jealous God, visiting the iniquity of the fathers upon the children unto the third and fourth *generation* of them that hate me; Exodus 20:5**

> **⁹Thou shalt not bow down thyself unto them, nor serve them: for I the LORD thy God *am* a jealous God, visiting the iniquity of the fathers upon the children unto the third and fourth *generation* of them that hate me,** Deut. 5:9

In Nehemiah chapter 8 and chapter 9:1-2, you find that Ezra, the scribe/priest, called all the people together—the mommies and the daddies and the children—it was one of the longest church services in the history of the Bible—it was twelve hours. For six hours they stood and heard the Word of God. The next six hours they worshipped and they confessed their sins and the sins of their fathers before God.

> **²And Ezra the priest brought the law before the congregation both of men and women, and all that could hear with understanding, upon the first day of the seventh month. ³And he read therein before the street that *was* before the water gate from the morning until midday, before the men and the women, and those that could understand; and the ears of all the people *were attentive* unto the book of the law...⁶And Ezra blessed the LORD, the great God. And all the people answered, Amen, Amen, with lifting up their hands: and they bowed their heads, and worshipped the LORD with *their* faces to the ground...⁸So they read in the book in the law of God distinctly, and gave the sense, and caused *them* to understand the reading.** Neh. 8:2-3, 6, 8

> **⁹:¹Now in the twenty and fourth day of this month the children of Israel were assembled with fasting, and with sackclothes, and earth upon them. ²And the seed of Israel separated themselves from all strangers, and stood and confessed their sins, and the iniquities of their fathers.** Neh. 9:1-2

As mentioned in Nehemiah 9:2, it says they stood there and confessed their sins and the sins of their fathers. Why? So that they could be freed from the curse of sin generationally.

God holds the fathers responsible for the spirituality of the family. The sins of the fathers are passed on to the third and fourth generations of them that hate Me (Exodus 20:5),

> **⁵...for I the LORD thy God *am* a jealous God, visiting the iniquity of the fathers upon the children unto the third and fourth *generation* of them that hate me;** Exodus 20:5

but blessings to thousands who love Me and keep My commandments. Thousands of what? Thousands of generations.

> **⁶And shewing mercy unto thousands of them that love me, and keep my commandments.** Exodus 20:6

So, we find that not only do we have this knowledge in Exodus and Deuteronomy but we also have it in Nehemiah. We also see the evidence today that the curse of the fathers is still here. So, we not only have to consider personal sins that separate us from our God, we have to consider inherited family tree sins.

It is amazing to me to see the rollover and the similarity between generations...and the bondages and the diseases that follow family trees, including insanity, including personality characteristics and all the rest. In fact, when people come to me for the first time for ministry and I sit down and just kind of listen to their personal case history for about 10 minutes, I can usually tell them (I don't know the people's names, I don't know their lifestyle and where they work) their spiritual dynamics back four generations of the family. Often, I can tell them about their mother, their father, their grandmother, their grandfather, and all the spiritual problems that they had, and I'm not usually wrong.

How do I know that? Is that some kind of esoteric knowledge? No, that's by pragmatic observation of the family tree and also what the Word has to say about generational curses that flow from family to family.

☐ 5. Not Having Faith in God

The fifth block can be found in Mark 11:22: not having faith in God. In Mark 11:22 it says: "And Jesus answering, sayeth unto them, Have faith in God.

> [22]**And Jesus answering saith unto them, Have faith in God.** Mark 11:22

The Bible also says that without faith, it's impossible to please God.

> [6]**But without faith *it is* impossible to please *him:* for he that cometh to God must believe that he is, and *that* he is a rewarder of them that diligently seek him.** Hebrews 11:6

Hebrews 11:1 says that faith is the substance of things hoped for, the evidence of things not seen.

> [11:1]**Now faith is the substance of things hoped for, the evidence of things not seen.** Hebrews 11:1

Matthew 21:21 says that if you have faith and doubt not...

> [21]**Jesus answered and said unto them, Verily I say unto you, If ye have faith, and doubt not...** Matthew 21:21

Hebrews 4 says the children of Israel, coming out of Israel under the leadership of Moses and Aaron, did not enter into promise, yet the same gospel preached to them was preached to us; preached to us, preached to them but they did not enter into promise because of unbelief and doubt.

> [2]**For unto us was the gospel preached, as well as unto them: but the word preached did not profit them, not being mixed with faith in them that heard *it...*[6]Seeing therefore it remaineth that some must enter therein, and they to whom it was first preached entered not in because of unbelief:** Hebrews 4:2, 6

When Jesus went back to His hometown of Nazareth and preached and tried to help the poor folk that He grew up with, Scripture says—He did no great miracles in Nazareth because great was their unbelief and doubt.

> [5]**And he could there do no mighty work, save that he laid his hands upon a few sick folk, and healed *them.* [6]And he marvelled because of their unbelief. And he went round about the villages, teaching.** Mark 6:5-6

In Mark 5:36-42, Jesus was about to raise a young lady from the dead, and there were a lot of people around because she had died and they were ready to have a wake, and He walked in and said, "but she's just sleeping" and they laughed at Him and scorned Him, and He put them out of the room, brought the family and His disciples into the room, and He raised her from the dead.

> [36]As soon as Jesus heard the word that was spoken, he saith unto the ruler of the synagogue, Be not afraid, only believe. [37]And he suffered no man to follow him, save Peter, and James, and John the brother of James. [38]And he cometh to the house of the ruler of the synagogue, and seeth the tumult, and them that wept and wailed greatly. [39]And when he was come in, he saith unto them, Why make ye this ado, and weep? the damsel is not dead, but sleepeth. [40]And they laughed him to scorn. But when he had put them all out, he taketh the father and the mother of the damsel, and them that were with him, and entereth in where the damsel was lying. [41]And he took the damsel by the hand, and said unto her, Talitha cumi; which is, being interpreted, Damsel, I say unto thee, arise. [42]And straightway the damsel arose, and walked; for she was *of the age* of twelve years. And they were astonished with a great astonishment. Mark 5:36-42

Why did He put them out of the room? Because their unbelief and doubt would negate His power and ability to heal.

Do you have hearts of belief, or am I casting seed on the stony, rocky ground? If I'm casting seed on good, fertile ground, then your faith is drawing my faith into a crescendo to move the hand of God.

But if there is unbelief and doubt in your hearts coming at me, I would stagger under it and I could do only a few things for you. As we mix our faith together before God, as we come here trusting Him to honor us, trusting Him to convict us, trusting Him to work with us, I am asking Him, in faith, to come to us.

> [8]I tell you that he will avenge them speedily. Nevertheless when the Son of man cometh, shall he find faith on the earth? Luke 18:8

☐ 6. The Need to See a Miracle

The sixth block is that you believe that you need to see a miracle in order to receive from God. Do you know how many people won't believe until they've seen a miracle? Well, what happened to the first person that saw a miracle? Who'd they look back at?

There were two thieves on the cross in Matthew 27:38-44—and those that passed by reviled Him, wagging their heads, and saying, Thou that destroyest the temple, and buildest it in three days, save Thyself. If Thou be the Son of God, come down from the cross.

> [38]Then were there two thieves crucified with him, one on the right hand, and another on the left. [39]And they that passed by reviled him, wagging their heads, [40]And saying, Thou that destroyest the temple, and buildest *it* in three days, save thyself. If thou be the Son of God, come down from the cross.

> **41Likewise also the chief priests mocking *him,* with the scribes and elders, said,
> 42He saved others; himself he cannot save. If he be the King of Israel, let him
> now come down from the cross, and we will believe him. 43He trusted in God;
> let him deliver him now, if he will have him: for he said, I am the Son of God.
> 44The thieves also, which were crucified with him, cast the same in his teeth.**
> Matthew 27:38-44

What did they want to see before they'd believe? They wanted to see Jesus come off the cross and that would have been the worst thing He ever did. You and I wouldn't be here today if He'd done that. You know what Jesus said to Peter when Jesus was preparing the disciples for His crucifixion: He said that He'd be going to Jerusalem and that He'd be betrayed and be crucified and Peter rebuked Him—remember that—and Peter rebuked Him and kind of told Him off and Jesus turned to him and told him what? Get behind Me, Satan. Thou savorest the things of men and not the things of God.

> **33But when he had turned about and looked on his disciples, he rebuked
> Peter, saying, Get thee behind me, Satan: for thou savourest not the things that
> be of God, but the things that be of men.** Mark 8:33

Well, do we have to see a miracle in order to believe that we can receive a miracle? The chief priest in verse 41 and 42 kind of echoed the same thing (Matthew 27:41-42): "Likewise also the chief priests mocking Him, with the scribes and elders, said, He saved others; Himself He cannot save. If He be the King of Israel, let Him now come down from the cross, and *we will believe Him*."

Wow! We will believe Him. Two classes of people would not believe until they could see some proof. Well, Jesus dealt with that issue with Thomas. Thomas said he wouldn't believe until he what? Until he saw the scars. And so Jesus showed him...the scars in His hands and in His side. And then Thomas said, "My Lord and My God" and Jesus said—blessed are those who do not see and yet believe rather than those who believe because they see.

> **28And Thomas answered and said unto him, My Lord and my God. 29Jesus
> saith unto him, Thomas, because thou hast seen me, thou hast believed: blessed
> *are* they that have not seen, and *yet* have believed.** John 20:28-29

Another great area of investigation of having to see a miracle to believe God...let's go to Matthew 4. You know, I'm in ministry and I want to tell you something. Because as a pastor I believe God heals and delivers today, do you know how many people ask me to prove it? Lots! I've had people come to me and say, do this, do that, do this, do that.

I can't do anything. I don't have any powers. I couldn't heal a fly with a toothache. I don't have any abilities. Who do you think I am? What are they doing? They are tempting me to tempt God. They come to me because they are sick but in their hearts they are saying, "Henry, if thou be the anointed son of God, do something," and in their heart they're also saying that, "If you can't, then you're not."

Let's see how Satan tempted our LORD Jesus in this area. Matthew 4:1-3—then was Jesus led up of the Spirit into the wilderness to be tempted of the devil. And when He had fasted forty days and forty nights, He was afterwards an hungered. And when the tempter came to Him, he said, *If Thou be the Son of God*, command that these stones be made bread.

> **⁴:¹Then was Jesus led up of the Spirit into the wilderness to be tempted of the devil. ²And when he had fasted forty days and forty nights, he was afterward an hungred. ³And when the tempter came to him, he said, If thou be the Son of God, command that these stones be made bread.** Matthew 4:1-3

Do you know what people say to me? "If thou be the anointed pastor, do something." *That is a hindrance to healing because you are NOT to look to me.* You're to look to Him, and the sanctifying work of the Holy Spirit, and the Word of God. All I am is His slave, His servant.

If you're looking at me and don't see Him behind me and the sanctifying work of the Word in your heart behind me, the love and purpose of the Father behind me, and if I don't become invisible and all you see is Him, then you've got a block.

So here we see the temptation of Jesus: *"do something."* How many of us have asked God? How many of us have put up fleeces? God, if you'll do this, then I'll believe You. Why couldn't we just believe Him to begin with? Because if He wanted to do it for us, He would anyway. Or He would come to us, and deal with us, so that He could.

☐ 7. Looking for Signs and Wonders

A seventh block to healing from God is that some are looking for signs. They are chasing signs and wonders rather than seeking the Word of God. I believe in signs and wonders, but I don't go chasing signs and wonders and I hope you don't either. But signs and wonders do follow them that believe. And there is a difference between chasing signs and wonders and having signs and wonders following you.

The issue is a matter of perspective. We must seek God and His Word, not the signs and wonders as the foundation of our faith. Disease is a fruit of the separation from God in some area of our life. The key is faith in God and His Word on the basis of relationship, not on the basis of signs and manifestations.

Romans 10:17 says that faith comes by hearing, and hearing by the Word of God.

> **¹⁷So then faith *cometh* by hearing, and hearing by the word of God.** Romans 10:17

Some people are looking for signs rather than the Word of God. John 4:46-48—so Jesus came again into Cana of Galilee where He made the water wine. And there was a certain nobleman, whose son was sick at Capernaum. When he heard that Jesus was come out of Judea into Galilee, he went unto Him, and besought Him that He would come down, and heal his son: for he was at the point of death. Then said Jesus unto him, Except ye see signs and wonders, ye will not believe.

> **[46]So Jesus came again into Cana of Galilee, where he made the water wine. And there was a certain nobleman, whose son was sick at Capernaum. [47]When he heard that Jesus was come out of Judaea into Galilee, he went unto him, and besought him that he would come down, and heal his son: for he was at the point of death. [48]Then said Jesus unto him, Except ye see signs and wonders, ye will not believe.** John 4:46-48

Matthew 12:38-39 — there's another scripture about an evil and an adulterous generation looking after a sign.

> **[38]Then certain of the scribes and of the Pharisees answered, saying, Master, we would see a sign from thee. [39]But he answered and said unto them, An evil and adulterous generation seeketh after a sign; and there shall no sign be given to it, but the sign of the prophet Jonas:** Matthew 12:38-39

The issue is that we're not seeking something like healing from God first—but we're seeking God first. Disease is a fruit of the separation.

☐ 8. Expect God to Heal on One's Own Terms

The eighth block to healing can be found in 2 Kings 5:8-14. Some people expect God to heal them on their own terms. They tell God exactly what He's going to do, when He's going to do it, and how He's going to do it and they expect Him to do it just that way on the terms they have set forth.

2 Kings 5:8-14 tells us the story about Naaman who had leprosy. I want to say something to you: this was a real important individual. Naaman was the captain of the host of the king of Syria. He was a great man, valued by his master, and honorable. And he had leprosy. He came a great distance to find this man of God that he'd heard could heal him, or fix him and get him right.

Now the real kicker of this story is that Elisha didn't go meet him at all. He sent his servant. That takes care of idolatry, doesn't it? You know, you have to be careful sometimes that you don't make your spiritual leaders an icon. You have to be careful sometimes that you don't make those who rule over you greater than they really are. I'm not greater than you. I'm a sheep just like you. I'm not greater than you. God doesn't love me more than He loves you. I don't have more of an edge with God than you do; He's no respecter of persons.

> **[34]Then Peter opened *his* mouth, and said, Of a truth I perceive that God is no respecter of persons:** Acts 10:34

What He has done for one, He will do for another. In my experience as a pastor, I'm just among equals. I'm just like you. I'm not greater than you—I'm with you. My only problem is this; I will get judged with a double judgment one day and you don't. Scripture also says that I'll get double honor, but I'll wait and see about that.

> **[17]Let the elders that rule well be counted worthy of double honour, especially they who labour in the word and doctrine.** 1 Tim. 5:17

It's that double judgment that bothers me.

³:¹My brethren, be not many masters, knowing that we shall receive the greater condemnation. James 3:1

You know that I have to stand before God one day in an area that you don't even have to. I have to give an account to God of how I conducted myself with the souls of men. I take this very seriously. I might have a little fun once in a while just to kind of lighten it up a little, but I consider this very serious business. My Boss is listening and watching every move I make.

In 2 Kings 5:10-12—and Elisha sent a messenger unto him, saying, Go and wash in the Jordan seven times, and thy flesh shall come again to thee, and thou shalt be clean." But Naaman was wroth, and went away, and said, Behold, I thought, He will surely come out to me (there you go—there's that pride) and stand, and call on the name of the LORD his God, and strike his hand over the place, and recover the leper (which is me).

> **¹⁰And Elisha sent a messenger unto him, saying, Go and wash in the Jordan seven times, and thy flesh shall come again to thee, and thou shalt be clean. ¹¹But Naaman was wroth, and went away, and said, Behold, I thought, He will surely come out to me, and stand, and call on the name of the LORD his God, and strike his hand over the place, and recover the leper. ¹²Are not Abana and Pharpar, rivers of Damascus, better than all the waters of Israel? may I not wash in them, and be clean? So he turned and went away in a rage.** 2 Kings 5:10-12

Well, Naaman had it all figured out how it was going to go. But what did Elisha tell the messenger to tell him? Go down to the river and wash seven times. What? You don't know who you're talking to. You don't know who I am. I want *you* to come out here, Elisha, call unto your God in heaven, strike your hand over the place, and that'd be a miracle. Now, I could go home and rejoice in that!

See, our subject is this: sometimes we expect God to heal us on our own terms and in the way that we think it should go. Well, do you think Naaman had a spiritual problem? Could you give me a spiritual root? Pride.

So he turned and went away in a rage. What was his next spiritual problem? Bitterness, resentment, unforgiveness, rage, anger. That's a good place to start receiving from God, isn't it? Verse 13 says—his servants came near and said, "My father, if the prophet had bid thee to do a great thing, would thou not have done it?"

> **¹³And his servants came near, and spake unto him, and said, My father, *if* the prophet had bid thee *do some* great thing, wouldest thou not have done *it?* how much rather then, when he saith to thee, Wash, and be clean?** 2 Kings 5:13

So who had the wisdom for the matter? His servants! And he went down and dipped himself seven times in the Jordan, according to the saying of the man of God and his flesh came again like unto the flesh of a little child and he was clean.

> **¹⁴Then went he down, and dipped himself seven times in Jordan, according to the saying of the man of God: and his flesh came again like unto the flesh of a little child, and he was clean.** 2 Kings 5:14

Well, that's God dealing with a Gentile guy again. Do you think God loves those unsaved, Gentile sinners? You say, well He loves the unsaved Gentile more than me it looks like, and I've been a saint for 48 years and I'm still waiting for my healing! Watch it now! Watch it now! *Sometimes, we expect God to heal us on our own terms.*

☐ 9. Looking to Man Rather Than God

The ninth block to healing is looking to man. We find this in Jeremiah 17:5. I want to say something to you very carefully. I am not against physicians. I am not against psychiatrists. However, we expect physicians to do something they are not qualified to do and that's to heal us of spiritually rooted diseases. They are not qualified to heal you of spiritually rooted diseases because you have to be born again to do that, first of all. And, secondly, as far as I can tell from Scripture, you have to be a spiritual leader to set it in motion.

I want to say something to you very carefully. I am not against physicians. I am not against psychiatrists. Don't you think for a minute that because I am in the healing business as a pastor that I automatically do away with the doctors and physicians. But what I do have to say to you is this: the Church has negated its role in the healing of disease and it has asked doctors to become spiritual healers and they are not qualified to do that. They are not listed in the five-fold ministry giftings of Ephesians 4. They are not qualified to heal you of spiritually rooted diseases. That has been ordained by God to be the role of the Church with the body healing the body as set forth in 1 Corinthians 12.

Doctors have their place, but in the area of spiritually rooted disease, they will not be able to bring forth the healing. The best they have to offer in these cases is disease management. I don't have a problem with you going and checking out your life. I am all for you getting a diagnosis. I don't play games with people's lives. I have to meet people in their faith and also in their faithlessness. What we need are doctors who understand there are spiritual components to disease and who will work with pastors who also understand the role of the Church in the healing of disease.

The point we are making in this block is that of looking to man, to doctors, for the healing before seeking God and without giving consideration to the spiritual dynamics behind the curse of disease.

In Jeremiah 17:5, 7, 9-10 it says—thus saith the LORD; Cursed be the man that trusteth in man, and maketh flesh his arm, and whose heart departeth from the LORD. Blessed is the man that trusteth in the LORD, and whose hope the LORD is. The heart is deceitful above all things, and desperately wicked: Who can know it? I, the LORD, search the heart, I try the reins, even to give every man according to his ways, and according to the fruit of his doings.

> [5]Thus saith the LORD; Cursed be the man that trusteth in man, and maketh flesh his arm, and whose heart departeth from the LORD...[7]Blessed *is* the man that trusteth in the LORD, and whose hope the LORD is...[9]The heart *is* deceitful above all *things,* and desperately wicked: who can know it? [10]I the

LORD search the heart, *I* try the reins, even to give every man according to his ways, *and* according to the fruit of his doings. Jeremiah 17:5, 7, 9-10

One of the great blocks to healing from God is to look to man to be your source. I am not your source. I am a road sign along the highway pointing out that this is the way you go.

I remember a joke I heard one time. I'm from Northern Maine; I was born and raised in Northern Maine, way up in Aroostook County where they grow potatoes. Down south of there, they have the "downeasters" and ya know they talk kinda funny. And they're a strange crew, them downeasters, down around Cherryfield and Machias and places like that. They told me a story one time about one of those city slickers from Boston who came up riding through Maine and got looking at stuff out there in the middle of nowhere, outside of Cherryfield and he came to a 4-way crossroads, and there were no signs. And up there was a house with an old guy sitting there, kinda rocking in his chair, surveying the situation.

The city slicker got out and walked up and said, "How are you doing, sir?"

The old guy said "Howdy."

Then he said, "I'm trying to get to Augusta. Can I take this road?"

And the old man looked over and said, "Yeah, yeah, I suppose you'd get there eventually."

And he said, "Well, how about this road over there?"

"Yeah, yeah I've been that way a couple of times and that'll eventually get you there."

"Well, how about this road over there?"

"Well, I've never been down that road too far but they tell me down that road you can get to Augusta too."

Well, by this time the city slicker has about had enough of it and he said, "You don't know much, do ya?"

And the old guy said, "Yeah, maybe so, but then again I'm not lost either!"

So, sometimes, I could be a road sign for you: this is the way you should go, but I am not your source. I'm just your friend. A lover of your soul. A lover of your life. Don't look to me, because if you look to me you need to understand that I'm looking to somebody else and that's my Boss—Jesus Christ—and the Father who sent Him.

In 2 Chronicles 16:7-12 is the story of Asa. Very clearly it says that he died, and one of the reasons he died was because he did not seek the LORD first, not only in war, but also in his personal life, when God had already proven Himself to be on his side in previous wars. His heart had hardened and in his apostasy and in his darkness, in his disease that was unto death, **Asa sought first not to the LORD but to physicians.**

> [7]And at that time Hanani the seer came to Asa king of Judah, and said unto him, Because thou hast relied on the king of Syria, and not relied on the LORD thy God, therefore is the host of the king of Syria escaped out of thine hand. [8]Were not the Ethiopians and the Lubims a huge host, with very many chariots and horsemen? yet, because thou didst rely on the LORD, he delivered them into thine hand. [9]For the eyes of the LORD run to and fro throughout the whole earth, to shew himself strong in the behalf of *them* whose heart *is* perfect toward him. Herein thou hast done foolishly: therefore from henceforth thou shalt have wars. [10]Then Asa was wroth with the seer, and put him in a prison house; for *he was* in a rage with him because of this *thing*. And Asa oppressed *some* of the people the same time. [11]And, behold, the acts of Asa, first and last, lo, they *are* written in the book of the kings of Judah and Israel. [12]And Asa in the thirty and ninth year of his reign was diseased in his feet, until his disease *was* exceeding *great:* yet in his disease he sought not to the LORD, but to the physicians. 2 Chron. 16:7-12

Wow! Let me say this to you. I am not against physicians. And I don't have a problem with you getting a diagnosis. And I don't have a problem with you going and checking out your life. I don't play games with people's lives. I have to meet people in their faith, but I also have to meet them in their faithlessness. In other words, I'm not sure where people are with God at any given moment in their life.

Why don't you take time out and seek the LORD first? Why don't we take time and go to the LORD? I want to say this to you: sometimes our diseases are unto death because we sought not the LORD first as His people. That's a hard word, isn't it? But it's a word I have to give you because Jeremiah 17:5 says "cursed be the man that trusteth in man."

> [5]Thus saith the LORD; Cursed be the man that trusteth in man, and maketh flesh his arm, and whose heart departeth from the LORD. Jeremiah 17:5

Although this is a hard word, it's hard because the Church has failed in its mission at this level to represent God and the people have nowhere to turn except to man. Granted, many churches teach their people to believe in God but they just don't understand disease and the cause for it which is, in 80% of all cases, spiritually rooted.

☐ 10. Not Being Honest and Transparent

The tenth block to healing is not being honest and transparent.

Two big reasons for not being honest and transparent are fear and pride. You would ask, "What do you mean by fear?" The answer to that would be fear of rejection, fear of man, fear of failure, fear of abandonment, fear of not being loved. The pride issue is very dangerous because it makes you appear holy when you're not and you're stuck with a real problem and that is an existence that is fraudulent. In other words, you're living a lie. It's a high price to pay because pride produces a fall and much disease.

> [18]Pride *goeth* before destruction, and an haughty spirit before a fall. Proverbs 16:18

Do you know how many people get nervous and jerky when I, as a minister, start probing into their personal life? What are they afraid of? God already knows. God knows everything. He knows you so well that the hairs of your head are numbered. He knows the secret thoughts of your heart. You "ain't" hiding nothing! Did you forget that God sees you? He hears every word I'm saying here tonight. He knows my thoughts; He knows your thoughts.

James 5:16 says this—confess your faults one to another that you may be healed.

> **[16]Confess *your* faults one to another, and pray one for another, that ye may be healed. The effectual fervent prayer of a righteous man availeth much.** James 5:16

It bears repeating: Confess your faults one to another that you may be healed.

> **[16]Confess *your* faults one to another, and pray one for another, that ye may be healed. The effectual fervent prayer of a righteous man availeth much.** James 5:16

Galatians 6:1 tells us—if a brother be overtaken in a fault, those of you who *"consider yourself"* spiritual, restore such a one in a spirit of meekness and consider yourself also lest you be tempted in like manner and fall away. Verse 2 says—bear ye one another's burdens and so ye fulfil the law of Christ.

> **[6:1]Brethren, if a man be overtaken in a fault, ye which are spiritual, restore such an one in the spirit of meekness; considering thyself, lest thou also be tempted. [2]Bear ye one another's burdens, and so fulfil the law of Christ.** Galatians 6:1-2

It's a scary thing to be transparent these days. I don't know if I can trust my life with you. Can you trust your life with me? Some of you have since I've been here, and I thank you for your transparency. Why is it so important to be transparent and confess our sins to God and each other? Proverbs 28:13 gives you a clue in that if you cover your sins you shall not prosper, but if you confess them and forsake them you shall have mercy.

> **[13]He that covereth his sins shall not prosper: but whoso confesseth and forsaketh *them* shall have mercy.** Proverbs 28:13

Isaiah said it in this way about God—the high and lofty one, He that inhabits eternity, dwelleth also with him that is of a humble and of a contrite heart.

> **[15]For thus saith the high and lofty One that inhabiteth eternity, whose name *is* Holy; I dwell in the high and holy *place*, with him also *that is* of a contrite and humble spirit, to revive the spirit of the humble, and to revive the heart of the contrite ones.** Isaiah 57:15

Do you know where God is? Right there in your mess, transparent one!

God can be found with a humble and a contrite heart. That made David a man after God's own heart, in spite of sin and in spite of inherited sin.

>⁵Behold, I was shapen in iniquity; and in sin did my mother conceive me.
Psalm 51:5

Because he had a perfect hatred for evil in the end, when he was convicted he repented, turned away from it (read Psalm 51—it's most beautiful). Sometimes I don't use the Romans Road to lead people to the Lord, I use Psalm 51. Psalm 51 to me is the best foundation for the sinner's prayer you can find. It just says it all. And then in the end David says, "and I will convert sinners" or something to that effect. In other words, when he's finished repenting he's out trying to get somebody saved! I love that guy. When I get to Heaven, I'm going to find Paul and David and give them bear hugs and say, I appreciate you guys. I am! They are fantastic!

>⁵¹:¹To the chief Musician, A Psalm of David, when Nathan the prophet came unto him, after he had gone in to Bathsheba. Have mercy upon me, O God, according to thy lovingkindness: according unto the multitude of thy tender mercies blot out my transgressions. ²Wash me throughly from mine iniquity, and cleanse me from my sin. ³For I acknowledge my transgressions: and my sin *is* ever before me. ⁴Against thee, thee only, have I sinned, and done *this* evil in thy sight: that thou mightest be justified when thou speakest, *and* be clear when thou judgest. ⁵Behold, I was shapen in iniquity; and in sin did my mother conceive me. ⁶Behold, thou desirest truth in the inward parts: and in the hidden *part* thou shalt make me to know wisdom. ⁷Purge me with hyssop, and I shall be clean: wash me, and I shall be whiter than snow. ⁸Make me to hear joy and gladness; *that* the bones *which* thou hast broken may rejoice. ⁹Hide thy face from my sins, and blot out all mine iniquities. ¹⁰Create in me a clean heart, O God; and renew a right spirit within me. ¹¹Cast me not away from thy presence; and take not thy holy spirit from me. ¹²Restore unto me the joy of thy salvation; and uphold me *with thy* free spirit. ¹³*Then* will I teach transgressors thy ways; and sinners shall be converted unto thee. ¹⁴Deliver me from bloodguiltiness, O God, thou God of my salvation: *and* my tongue shall sing aloud of thy righteousness. ¹⁵O Lord, open thou my lips; and my mouth shall shew forth thy praise. ¹⁶For thou desirest not sacrifice; else would I give *it:* thou delightest not in burnt offering. ¹⁷The sacrifices of God *are* a broken spirit: a broken and a contrite heart, O God, thou wilt not despise. Psalm 51:1-17

I want to give you a story that may shock you a little bit. It has to do with being honest and transparent without regard to pride, which is what we are talking about in this block. I was doing a seminar two years ago in Houston, Texas, teaching like I'm teaching you here now. I had an audience that was mixed which included about 30% New Age. And I was trying to tiptoe through the tulips. I was trying to be all things to all men, that I might win one or two to Christ in this seminar. About 30 minutes into it (and I'm not being funny when I tell you this) this voice came thundering into my head saying "Henry, cut the crap and shut up!" I staggered. I said out loud to the audience, "Excuse me! I think God's talking to me!" In my heart, God said, "Listen, I called you here to represent Me, not to appease the devil. Get off this thing and do what I told you to do!" I said, "What'd You tell me to do?"

In the audience, the people are watching me; I'm going back and forth—what? What? And God spoke to my heart and He said, "I want you to take yoga on for size."

I said, "God, leave me alone! You don't know what You're asking me. Half of these people are into yoga, Eastern mysticism, and meditation. And in my heart, God said, "Do what I tell you!"

I said, "God has said that I must deal with yoga." And as I started to reveal the foundation of kundalini and the divination principles of the Eastern mysticism of yoga, one-third of that audience got up and walked out. And as I watched them go, I thought, oh, I must have heard the devil; I'm trying to save them, Lord. And in my heart God said, "We've got work to do!" Things changed in the seminar and that first night we went until one o'clock in the morning; the second night until four o'clock in the morning; the third night, two o'clock in the morning.; the next Sunday went from nine in the morning until three in the afternoon. We had revival!

In the middle of this, as I was talking about yoga, and explaining the fallacies of yoga, a woman got up in the audience—a very, very ... how do I say this ... regal-looking woman that was Pakistani. She got up and interrupted me and she said, "Pastor, I practice yoga with my husband. I go to a Seventh Day Adventist church, but I practice yoga and Eastern mysticism with my husband and I am convicted." And she started to confess. Well, she also had five diseases! She had diabetes; she had diseases in her feet, I don't remember all the things that she had but she had five major diseases and she stood there and confessed with tears running down her face the sin of worshipping Satan through yoga. She stood there, humbling herself, this regal woman looking so majestic in her nationality, her pride, and the way she carried herself, and her stature. I'm listening to her just confess openly before a congregation just like this, and God spoke to me. He said, "Because she has humbled herself before Me and before you and this congregation, I am going to deliver her and heal her."

I waited until she finished, and when she'd finished I said, "Sister, God has spoken to me; He wants to deliver you and heal you. Would you come here?" And she walked to the front and I said, "You foul, unclean spirit of kundalini, of divination, come out of this woman in the name of Jesus Christ of Nazareth. That spirit of divination manifested in her and she told me later that it "wanted to tear you apart." But all she could do was just make a throat clearing/grunting noise and weakly pound her hands on my chest—and then it was gone!

God healed her, not only delivered her, but healed her of five "incurable" diseases! She came back to the next year's Houston seminar and gave her testimony. She is doing very well. And she is getting on with God! And she is free! Because she humbled herself and was transparent, God met her. Could it be that God stopped a service just to get and free one person that He loved?

So, sometimes you just have to be transparent, don't you? I love it when people are honest with me. You don't have to worry about me condemning you. Who am I to condemn you? My rap sheet is probably longer than yours is!

God hates pride, hypocrisy, and fraud. But we're so afraid of each other and have been so murdered by each other, we can't even trust each other any more. And that's in the Christian Church. God forbid we go to some of our pastors, we might hear about ourselves on Sunday morning!

Perfect love covers a multitude of sins.

> **⁸And above all things have fervent charity among yourselves: for charity shall cover the multitude of sins.** 1 Peter 4:8

> **¹⁸There is no fear in love; but perfect love casteth out fear: because fear hath torment. He that feareth is not made perfect in love.** 1 John 4:18

Aren't you glad He's our Father? AMEN!

☐ 11. Flagrant Sin or Habitual Sin

Number eleven is flagrant sin or habitual sin. Now there's a difference between temptation and falling into sin and repenting and getting out of sin and living habitually in it. *Temptation is not sin.* Jesus was tempted in all points such as we are, yet without sin.

> **¹⁵For we have not an high priest which cannot be touched with the feeling of our infirmities; but was in all points tempted like as *we are, yet* without sin.** Hebrews 4:15

So I know that temptation is not sin. But in Gal 5:19-21, in the great book against legalism and the great statement of grace and mercy, we find a real problem. It's right in the end of the great chapter of the book of Galatians that Paul uses to defeat legalism, and to establish our freedom from legalism, it says:

Now the works of the flesh are manifest, which are these; Adultery, fornication, uncleanness, lasciviousness, idolatry, witchcraft (that word witchcraft, by the way, is not the word that is used in the Hebrew; that word, witchcraft, is found only one time in the New Testament and it is the Greek word *pharmakeia*, Strong's number 5331, which means medication (pharmacy, sorcery) and is taken from the Greek root word 5332 *pharmakeus*, which means a drug, a druggist (pharmacist or poisoner, that is, sorcerer), hatred, variance, emulations, wrath, strife, seditions, heresies, envying, murders, drunkenness, reveling, and such like: of the which I tell you before, *as I have also told you in time past, that they which do such things shall not inherit the kingdom of God* (Galatians 5:19-21).

That's pretty emphatic, isn't it? The only way that we can survive and still maintain our freedom from legalism is to understand the context of God's grace and mercy. I believe I can quote Paul accurately to say in light of the word study done on the word "do" which translates as *those who habitually practice those things against God with a hardened heart as a way of life, they shall not inherit the kingdom of God.*

It is interesting to note that in Galatians, the English word "do" has three different Greek root words and three different meanings. It is important to understand that grace and mercy does not absolve us from responsibility for holiness.

> **⁶:¹What shall we say then? Shall we continue in sin, that grace may abound? ²God forbid...** Romans 6:1-2

In some quarters there are teachings that remove responsibility for sin because of grace and mercy, but I will tell you, Church, that the wages of sin are still death.

> **²³For the wages of sin *is* death...** Romans 6:23

If there is any doubt in your mind that there is no consequence to sin in the New Covenant, *just look around at the psychological and biological diseases that have engulfed the Christian Church,* especially in light of Deuteronomy 28 that clearly states that all disease is a result of separation from God, His Word, and disobedience to His Word.

Habitual, unrepented, flagrant sin is a major block to God healing you and meeting you in your life.

I've taken the position as a pastor—it may not be your position, and I'm not your pastor, so you don't have to believe a thing I say—but I've taken the position in dealing with people that I can have one person over here doing this sin, and one person over here doing the same sin, and one person is accepted before God in the sin and the other one over here is not accepted by God in the sin. I've observed it. Please understand that God does not condone sin in our lives, but my point is that grace and mercy seems to be extended to one person and not the other. How can that be?

The person over here that is not accepted before God, his heart is hardened toward God and he's just not going to change.

But the person over here, because of temptation has fallen into the sin—he still has a perfect hatred for it—his heart is right before God against the sin even though he is still in bondage, and God is dealing with that person, and He's still working him over. God does not condone sin but He has made a provision for it and a way out of the penalty because of it.

Are you with me? It's not the sin. It's your attitude of the heart toward the sin that God is looking at. But if you're into flagrant sin and your heart is hardened, then it keeps the hand of God from meeting you and healing you and delivering you.

☐ 12. Robbing God in Tithes and Offerings

The twelfth block to healing is in Malachi 3:8-11 and deals with robbing God in our tithes and offerings.

> **⁸Will a man rob God? Yet ye have robbed me. But ye say, Wherein have we robbed thee? In tithes and offerings. ⁹Ye *are* cursed with a curse: for ye have robbed me, *even* this whole nation. ¹⁰Bring ye all the tithes into the storehouse, that there may be meat in mine house, and prove me now herewith, saith the LORD of hosts, if I will not open you the windows of heaven, and pour you out a blessing, that *there shall* not *be room* enough *to receive it.* ¹¹And I will rebuke the devourer for your sakes, and he shall not destroy the fruits of your ground; neither shall your vine cast her fruit before the time in the field, saith the LORD of hosts.** Malachi 3:8-11

It says that you are cursed with a curse. Why? Because you've not brought the tithes and the offerings into the storehouse. You've robbed from God. How do you rob from God? Everything you have belongs to Him. You think your paycheck is yours? It's God's. He's just loaning it to you.

In fact, the Bible says that when you work for an employer, you're not working for him, you're working for the Lord. If he's an unjust employer, you're still working for the Lord. Everything we do is "unto the Lord," just or unjust. You do it unto the Lord. Is that how you're taught in your church? Everything we do is unto the Lord! Everything we have is His. He just loans it back to us. So robbing God is not just in tithes and offerings, but in the firstfruits of our substance, including our time.

If 10% is the gauge, then we have 168 hours a week that God has given us to exist. Ten percent of that is 16.8 hours a week and it belongs to God. You've got 90% for the rest. You've got 90% of that 168 hours for the rest so that in 8 hours for work, 8 hours for family, and 8 hours for sleep, God gets His share of our time.

Well, I don't become legalistic in that, but I just offer it as a point of challenge to challenge your hearts. Who we are and what we are involves a lot of things. I know you guys here give your time and more than a 10% tithe. I know. (This was addressed to the Wycliffe Bible-translating missionaries in the seminar.)

☐ 13. Some Are Just Not Saved

The thirteenth block to healing is because some are just not saved. They don't know Jesus or the Father. They perish because they received not the truth that they might be saved.

In 2 Thessalonians 2:10 it says: "And with all deceivableness of unrighteousness in them that perish; because they received not the love of the truth, that they might be saved."

> **[10]And with all deceivableness of unrighteousness in them that perish; because they received not the love of the truth, that they might be saved.** 2 Thes. 2:10

That's a tough scripture. God will give you over to a greater delusion. If you want to believe error, He'll allow more to come into your life.

> **[11]And for this cause God shall send them strong delusion, that they should believe a lie:** 2 Thes. 2:11

God says, "This is your party. Do what you want to do. You're a free will agent so 'go for it'." And some people go into greater delusion and greater separation from God and cannot be healed and delivered because they are not in covenant and they are not saved. They have a zeal – but not according to knowledge.

☐ 14. Sin of Our Parents

The fourteenth block is the sin of our parents. In 2 Samuel 12:13-14, there was a curse of death on David and Bathsheba's child. The child died because of the sin of adultery and murder.

In 1 Kings 14:1-13, there is a tremendous statement about God taking a child in death. It is the only scripture I can find where God has taken anyone through a disease just to preserve them for Himself. This is a tremendous chapter because this was a son of Jeroboam, and Jeroboam the king was very evil. God looked down from heaven, saw this child, and said if this child is allowed to live, his evil parents will pervert his heart and I will lose him from Myself forever. So God took him in disease to preserve him in the resurrection.

About the same time, Abijah son of Jeroboam got sick. Jeroboam told his wife: Disguise yourself so no one will know you're my wife, then go to Shiloh, where the prophet Ahijah lives. Take him ten loaves of bread, some small cakes, and honey, and ask him what will happen to our son. He can tell you, because he's the one who told me I would become king. She got ready and left for Ahijah's house in Shiloh. Ahijah was now old and blind, but the LORD told him, "Jeroboam's wife is coming to ask about her son. I will tell you what to say to her." Jeroboam's wife came to Ahijah's house, pretending to be someone else. But when Ahijah heard her walking up to the door, he said: Come in! I know you're Jeroboam's wife—why are you pretending to be someone else? I have some bad news for you. Give your husband this message from the LORD God of Israel: "Jeroboam, you know that I, the LORD, chose you over anyone else to be the leader of my people Israel. I even took David's kingdom away from his family and gave it to you. But you are not like my servant David. He always obeyed me and did what was right. You have made me very angry by rejecting me and making idols out of gold. Jeroboam, you have done more evil things than any king before you. Because of this, I will destroy your family by killing every man and boy in it, whether slave or free. I will wipe out your family, just as fire burns up trash. Dogs will eat the bodies of your relatives who die in town, and vultures will eat the bodies of those who die in the country. I, the LORD, have spoken and will not change my mind!" That's the LORD's message to your husband. As for you, go back home, and right after you get there, your son will die. Everyone in Israel will mourn at his funeral. But he will be the last one from Jeroboam's family to receive a proper burial, because he's the only one the LORD God of Israel is pleased with.

> [14:1]**At that time Abijah the son of Jeroboam fell sick.** [2]**And Jeroboam said to his wife, Arise, I pray thee, and disguise thyself, that thou be not known to be the wife of Jeroboam; and get thee to Shiloh: behold, there *is* Ahijah the prophet, which told me that *I should be* king over this people.** [3]**And take with thee ten loaves, and cracknels, and a cruse of honey, and go to him: he shall tell thee what shall become of the child.** [4]**And Jeroboam's wife did so, and arose, and went to Shiloh, and came to the house of Ahijah. But Ahijah could not see; for his eyes were set by reason of his age.** [5]**And the LORD said unto Ahijah, Behold, the wife of Jeroboam cometh to ask a thing of thee for her son; for he is sick: thus and thus shalt thou say unto her: for it shall be, when she cometh in, that she shall feign herself *to be* another *woman*.** [6]**And it was *so*, when Ahijah heard the sound of her feet as she came in at the door, that he said, Come in, thou wife of Jeroboam; why feignest thou thyself *to be* another? for I *am* sent to thee *with* heavy *tidings*.** [7]**Go, tell Jeroboam, Thus saith the LORD God**

of Israel, Forasmuch as I exalted thee from among the people, and made thee prince over my people Israel, ⁸And rent the kingdom away from the house of David, and gave it thee: and yet thou hast not been as my servant David, who kept my commandments, and who followed me with all his heart, to do *that* only *which was* right in mine eyes; ⁹But hast done evil above all that were before thee: for thou hast gone and made thee other gods, and molten images, to provoke me to anger, and hast cast me behind thy back: ¹⁰Therefore, behold, I will bring evil upon the house of Jeroboam, and will cut off from Jeroboam him that pisseth against the wall, *and* him that is shut up and left in Israel, and will take away the remnant of the house of Jeroboam, as a man taketh away dung, till it be all gone. ¹¹Him that dieth of Jeroboam in the city shall the dogs eat; and him that dieth in the field shall the fowls of the air eat: for the LORD hath spoken it. ¹²Arise thou therefore, get thee to thine own house: *and* when thy feet enter into the city, the child shall die. ¹³And all Israel shall mourn for him, and bury him: for he only of Jeroboam shall come to the grave, because in him there is found *some* good thing toward the LORD God of Israel in the house of Jeroboam. 1 Kings 14:1-13

That is a tremendous, tremendous insight. You can't make a big doctrine out of it, but it certainly helps you understand more about the people who die in disease. Sometimes, you just have to let God be sovereign. God wanted that child. What a tremendous statement!

Reflecting on this, I really don't believe that, as a rule, God uses or needs disease to get someone to heaven, but in observing human nature there is always a possibility that someone who God really wants for eternity could be lost to Him by falling away or things in life separating them from God totally.

☐ 15. Sometimes the Sickness is Unto Death

The fifteenth block to healing is that sometimes the sickness is unto death. In 2 Chronicles 21:4, 12-20 is the story of Jehoram. He once knew God and he turned away from Him. He killed his brothers and because of murder he got sick and died and the Bible says—it was a sin unto death. There are certain sins in the Bible that people will die from.

⁴Now when Jehoram was risen up to the kingdom of his father, he strengthened himself, and slew all his brethren with the sword, and *divers* also of the princes of Israel...⁶And he walked in the way of the kings of Israel, like as did the house of Ahab: for he had the daughter of Ahab to wife: and he wrought *that which was* evil in the eyes of the LORD...¹²And there came a writing to him from Elijah the prophet, saying, Thus saith the LORD God of David thy father, Because thou hast not walked in the ways of Jehoshaphat thy father, nor in the ways of Asa king of Judah, ¹³But hast walked in the way of the kings of Israel, and hast made Judah and the inhabitants of Jerusalem to go a whoring, like to the whoredoms of the house of Ahab, and also hast slain thy brethren of thy father's house, *which were* better than thyself: ¹⁴Behold, with a great plague will the LORD smite thy people, and thy children, and thy wives, and all thy goods: ¹⁵And thou *shalt have* great sickness by disease of thy bowels, until thy bowels fall out by reason of the sickness day by day.

> [16]Moreover the LORD stirred up against Jehoram the spirit of the Philistines, and of the Arabians, that *were* near the Ethiopians: [17]And they came up into Judah, and brake into it, and carried away all the substance that was found in the king's house, and his sons also, and his wives; so that there was never a son left him, save Jehoahaz, the youngest of his sons. [18]And after all this the LORD smote him in his bowels with an incurable disease. [19]And it came to pass, that in process of time, after the end of two years, his bowels fell out by reason of his sickness: so he died of sore diseases. And his people made no burning for him, like the burning of his fathers. [20]Thirty and two years old was he when he began to reign, and he reigned in Jerusalem eight years, and departed without being desired. Howbeit they buried him in the city of David, but not in the sepulchres of the kings. 2 Chron. 21:4, 6, 12-20

In 1 John 5:16 it also talks about a sin unto death. And what did John say? "I would not that you pray for it."

> [16]If any man see his brother sin a sin *which is* not unto death, he shall ask, and he shall give him life for them that sin not unto death. There is a sin unto death: I do not say that he shall pray for it. [17]All unrighteousness is sin: and there is a sin not unto death. 1 John 5:16-17

I don't know what that sin unto death is, but it is a sin that produced a disease unto death; it was a death sentence and praying for it to be healed was a waste of time.

I don't know personally, as a minister and a pastor, what that sin unto death is. This is a difficult scripture but this is how I understand it. If I see you sin a sin but it's a sin that won't produce a disease that will kill you, then I shall pray God for you that He may heal you. *But if I see you sin a sin that is a sin that produces a disease unto death, I shall not pray for you because it is a sin that is unto death. Of the many diseases that we have talked about in this seminar, many of them are unto death. Each one of them has a sin behind it. Unless that sin is dealt with, that disease will be a disease unto death. If I try to pray for that person without that sin being dealt with, I am wasting my time. So before I pray I get involved to deal with the "sin" issue first. Then I pray and minister not, understanding this is why many people are not healed after prayer.*

Diseases that are coming out of bitterness and unforgiveness are diseases unto death and those are the sins. Here is where we have missed it. Rather than praying healing for that disease, we must meet that person according to knowledge as we are instructed in 2 Timothy 2:24-26 and Galatians 6:1 and go to that person in love.

We must go because we want to remove the curse of death from their life. We must say to that person: according to the Word of God, I cannot pray for you. But because I love you, I have come to you and I want to instruct you from the Word to bring repentance to you, that you may recover yourself from the snare of this death penalty. Then when you have repented, I can come before God and ask His healing for you and He shall give it to you.

Sanctification for healing is the dimension that is not being taught in the Church today. The Church is not teaching why healing does not come. Cancer is a disease unto death that comes out of bitterness. Diabetes is a death disease coming right out of self-hatred. There is disease after disease that carries a death sentence. But it does not have to go that way, does it?

Do you know how tough it is for me as a minister not to just automatically pray healing just because I'm being asked to? I do not become presumptuous with the gift of healing. I promise you I operate in all nine gifts as the LORD wills, not as I will. I am very responsible when it comes to serving God and I take it very seriously. I am not a god; I am a servant of God. I am not greater than my master. If a person is not listening to God, why should they listen to me? And if I bring you truth which is truth from God and you don't listen to me, then why should I pray for you? Am I greater than my master? I can do no more for you as a minister of the gospel than you are already allowing God to do in your life. All I do is come along beside you and help Him and assist you in that victory. I cannot do it against your will. I cannot ask Him to dishonor His Word to do it for you and condone your sin. I could walk down through this congregation now and my success rate, if I didn't teach you properly, would be less than 10% and the other 90% of you would be mad at me and be mad at Him because you didn't get healed. The 10% would be rejoicing and the 90% would be sad. I want 100% of you to be happy. And I'm willing to take the time and the risk of offending you to bring you truth at this level. I don't like losing because my Boss never lost a battle. Jesus healed every single person that came to Him. And you say, "Pastor, why isn't that happening today?" Maybe God just gave you a clue to this question.

Somebody said the other day: well it's the HIV virus. I don't know if that's what it is. I have no idea. Nobody knows what it is. The point is this: sometimes there are sins and sicknesses that are unto death. 2 Kings 1:2-8 is the story of Ahaziah. He dabbled in sorcery and under the law of Moses, sorcery, witchcraft, and occultism brought a penalty of death. We find that this individual died because his sin was unto death.

> ²And Ahaziah fell down through a lattice in his upper chamber that *was* in Samaria, and was sick: and he sent messengers, and said unto them, Go, enquire of Baal-zebub the god of Ekron whether I shall recover of this disease. ³But the angel of the LORD said to Elijah the Tishbite, Arise, go up to meet the messengers of the king of Samaria, and say unto them, *Is it* not because *there is* not a God in Israel, *that* ye go to enquire of Baal-zebub the god of Ekron? ⁴Now therefore thus saith the LORD, Thou shalt not come down from that bed on which thou art gone up, but shalt surely die. And Elijah departed. ⁵And when the messengers turned back unto him, he said unto them, Why are ye now turned back? ⁶And they said unto him, There came a man up to meet us, and said unto us, Go, turn again unto the king that sent you, and say unto him, Thus saith the LORD, *Is it* not because *there is* not a God in Israel, *that* thou sendest to enquire of Baal-zebub the god of Ekron? therefore thou shalt not come down from that bed on which thou art gone up, but shalt surely die. ⁷And he said unto them, What manner of man *was he* which came up to meet you,

and told you these words? **⁸And they answered him,** *He was* **an hairy man, and girt with a girdle of leather about his loins. And he said, It** *is* **Elijah the Tishbite.** 2 Kings 1:2-8

King Saul died prematurely because of his sins. Saul first of all disobeyed God and secondly, he contacted the witch of Endor who had a familiar spirit. In Chronicles it says that when Saul committed suicide that Saul was judged in death because he disobeyed God and because he consulted with a familiar spirit. There are certain things that we have to pay attention to. In 1 Chronicles 10:13-14, there is a story about King Saul dying:

> **¹³So Saul died for his transgression which he committed against the Lᴏʀᴅ,** *even* **against the word of the Lᴏʀᴅ, which he kept not, and also for asking** *counsel* **of** *one that had* **a familiar spirit, to enquire** *of it;* **¹⁴And enquired not of the Lᴏʀᴅ: therefore he slew him, and turned the kingdom unto David the son of Jesse.** 1 Chron. 10:13-14

Many times in dealing with certain diseases, in order to get a healing from God for people, I have to bring people to a place of repentance before God for their involvement in occultism: that's contacting mediums, that's contacting witches, dabbling in sorcery and things of that nature. In fact, when I minister to somebody, I have a difficult time getting them healed if I don't get oujia boards dealt with because oujia boards are a means of contacting an evil spirit. What do you think makes that board move and spell those words out? It is the first medium of contact with Satan in children. Levitation, table tipping and spoon bending are all part of the kingdom and the power of Satan.

Many times occultism, involvement in spiritualism, involvement in mediumships, involvement in seances, involvement in this and that, will open us up unto the spirit of death. Under the law, dabbling on the other side carries a death penalty.

God said in His first commandment, "You shall have no other gods before Me" (Exodus 20:3) and you'd better get this one straight. Involvement in occultism is forgivable, but it can open the door to a curse of many diseases. Looking into the future or trying to control aspects of the future through any medium or person or mechanism as a replacement for consulting God and His Word is idolatry and makes that item or person a "god" to you in your life.

> **³⁴Take therefore no thought for the morrow: for the morrow shall take thought for the things of itself. Sufficient unto the day** *is* **the evil thereof.** Matthew 6:34

Sometimes insanity is because of dabbling in the occult. Oppression can be the result of dabbling in the occult or it occurs because someone sought the guidance of a witch doctor, a wizard, a warlock, or some other occultic practitioner to try to get healed of their disease. In matter of fact, they should have been seeking God and His Word from the very beginning and the spiritual roots.

Moses in Psalm 90 indicated that man's longevity would be 70-80 years as a promise. However, Solomon died prematurely at age 60 because of disobedience to

God and following the gods of his pagan wives. God appeared to him two times about this issue and he would not listen and he died losing one-quarter of his promised life expectancy.

☐ 16. Our Allotted Time in Life is Fulfilled

The sixteenth block to healing is simply that our allotted time in life is fulfilled. You know, sometimes we just have to be like the flower that fades away; it's time to go. Well, how soon should you go? I'll say this to you. In Psalm 90 God, by His Spirit through Moses, established the longevity of man as threescore and ten (70) comfortable years, or fourscore (80) with some trouble. Today, the average longevity of mankind in America is no more than 76 or so.

> [10]The days of our years *are* threescore years and ten; and if by reason of strength *they be* fourscore years, yet *is* their strength labour and sorrow; for it is soon cut off, and we fly away. Psalm 90:10

As far as I am concerned, until the coming of the Lord and the first resurrection, you won't find much extension as an average of what was declared by God in Psalm 90. This age will be over with before that happens. Psalm 90:12 says—so teach *us* to number our days, that we may apply *our* hearts unto wisdom.

> [12]So teach *us* to number our days, that we may apply *our* hearts unto wisdom. Psalm 90:12

Anything less than 70-80 years of longevity on this planet is a curse. God's promise is that we should have longevity in order to establish His righteousness in our generation and that we may number our days in righteousness and be part of His plan, His kingdom.

> [27]The fear of the LORD prolongeth days: but the years of the wicked shall be shortened. Proverbs 10:27

Eighty years of life, if the Lord tarries, should be the minimum you're looking for. That's how I see it in the Word.

When you find men whose lives were shortened, it was always a curse. Solomon died at age 60 and the reason he died at age 60 was because he was following the heathen gods of his thousand women. God appeared to him twice and basically said, "You'd better get it straight, boy." I don't know if you'll see Solomon in heaven or not. The man who was supposed to have the greatest wisdom to share with God's people was the dumbest concerning himself!

> [4]For it came to pass, when Solomon was old, *that* his wives turned away his heart after other gods: and his heart was not perfect with the LORD his God, as *was* the heart of David his father. [5]For Solomon went after Ashtoreth the goddess of the Zidonians, and after Milcom the abomination of the Ammonites. [6]And Solomon did evil in the sight of the LORD, and went not fully after the LORD, as *did* David his father. [7]Then did Solomon build an high place for Chemosh, the abomination of Moab, in the hill that *is* before Jerusalem,

and for Molech, the abomination of the children of Ammon. [8]And likewise did he for all his strange wives, which burnt incense and sacrificed unto their gods. [9]And the LORD was angry with Solomon, because his heart was turned from the LORD God of Israel, which had appeared unto him twice, [10]And had commanded him concerning this thing, that he should not go after other gods: but he kept not that which the LORD commanded. 1 Kings 11:4-10

Paul said it like this—what a tragedy that I win many to Christ and I myself am a castaway.

[27]But I keep under my body, and bring *it* into subjection: lest that by any means, when I have preached to others, I myself should be a castaway. 1 Cor. 9:27

☐ 17. Looking to Symptoms and Not to the Healer

Block number seventeen is looking to symptoms and not to the Healer. You know, when Peter was walking on the water, as long as he kept his eyes on the Lord, he was fine. When he took his eyes off the Lord, he went into unbelief and he started to sink. Before you throw stones at Peter, remember that at least he tried. At least he tried, which is more than the rest of us have ever done. So, we look to our symptoms and not to the healing.

I want to say something to you. If you're waiting for the symptoms of your disease to go away before you believe, you're going to be waiting a long time. *If you're waiting for the healing before you look for the Healer, you're going to be waiting a long time!*

You see, your symptoms of your disease are the fruit of the problem—not the root. Get your eyes off your pain; get your eyes off your disease; get your eyes back on the LORD and His Word and keep it there. Don't look at the symptoms!

I said to somebody the other day who was really struggling with physiological pain, and they were really dipping into it (and I'm not being insensitive—I really care—and even though I teach at this level does not mean that I'm insensitive) but I finally looked at them and said, "You and I need to cut through this, darling." I said, "Are you born again?" "Oh, yes, Pastor, I'm born again." "Where's the Spirit of God live in you?" "In my heart." "Wonderful. Is your human spirit a physical dimension or a spiritual dimension?" "Oh, spiritual." "Can your human spirit ever get sick from disease or feel pain?" "No, Pastor." "Then what's your problem?"

The Bible says that the spirit of man shall sustain him in his infirmity.

[14]The spirit of a man will sustain his infirmity; but a wounded spirit who can bear? Proverbs 18:14

You may have disease and you may have pain at this point but I will tell you that your human spirit is immune to it. Stay in the Spirit, stay before God, and let your heart be complete, and then ask God for His mercy as you are before Him about the roots and blocks of the disease.

The question is asked, "Then how can you stay in the Spirit?" The Scriptures teach that we are seated with Christ Jesus in heavenly places far above all principalities and powers. Remember who you are and where you are in the battle.

> [19]**And what** *is* **the exceeding greatness of his power to us-ward who believe, according to the working of his mighty power,** [20]**Which he wrought in Christ, when he raised him from the dead, and set** *him* **at his own right hand in the heavenly** *places,* [21]**Far above all principality, and power, and might, and dominion, and every name that is named, not only in this world, but also in that which is to come:** [22]**And hath put all** *things* **under his feet, and gave him** *to be* **the head over all** *things* **to the church,** [23]**Which is his body, the fulness of him that filleth all in all.** Ephes. 1:19-23

> [6]**And hath raised** *us* **up together, and made** *us* **sit together in heavenly** *places* **in Christ Jesus:** Ephes. 2:6

Remember that you are more than a physical body. Remember that you are more than a tormented soul. You must be born again and be a new creature in Christ Jesus, then your spirit must be alive unto God, you are alive unto God and the Spirit of God lives within you. The Bible says—let the same Spirit that raised Christ from the dead dwell in you; He shall quicken your mortal bodies.

> [11]**But if the Spirit of him that raised up Jesus from the dead dwell in you, he that raised up Christ from the dead shall also quicken your mortal bodies by his Spirit that dwelleth in you.** Romans 8:11

So we've got to keep our eyes off the symptoms and keep our eyes on the Lord.

☐ 18. Letting Fear Enter Your Heart

The eighteenth block to healing is letting fear enter your heart. *Fear will quench your faith, and faith will quench your fears. You can choose which will rule you. Faith and fear are equal in this dimension—both demand to be fulfilled and both project into the future.* Faith is the substance of things hoped for, the evidence of things not yet seen (Hebrews 11:1). The flip side of this scripture would be this: fear is the substance of things not hoped for, the evidence of things not yet seen.

Job had this to say:

> [24]**For my sighing cometh before I eat, and my roarings are poured out like the waters.** [25]**For the thing which I greatly feared is come upon me, and that which I was afraid of is come unto me.** [26]**I was not in safety, neither had I rest, neither was I quiet; yet trouble came...**[14]**Fear came upon me, and trembling, which made all my bones to shake.** [15]**Then a spirit passed before my face; the hair of my flesh stood up:** Job 3:24-26; 4:14-15

This is God's antidote to the spirit of fear:

> [15]**For ye have not received the spirit of bondage again to fear; but ye have received the Spirit of adoption, whereby we cry, Abba, Father.** Romans 8:15

> [14:1]**Let not your heart be troubled: ye believe in God, believe also in me.** John 14:1

²⁷**Peace I leave with you, my peace I give unto you: not as the world giveth, give I unto you. Let not your heart be troubled, neither let it be afraid.** John 14:27

²³**...for whatsoever *is* not of faith is sin.** Romans 14:23

☐ 19. Failure to Get Away in Prayer and Fasting

The nineteenth block to healing: failure to get away in prayer and fasting. This block has to do with a lack of closeness in personal relationship with Jesus and the Father. There is much confusion in the body of Christ regarding prayer and fasting and the reasons for it. I believe that this confusion exists because there is a misunderstanding that there is more than one kind of fast unto the LORD and their purposes are different.

Now, I want to say something to you: you don't pray and fast to receive from God—*you pray and fast to meet God.*

Now, I know what you've been taught from Isaiah 58:6, where it says that it's the fast that He's called you to that will break every yoke. But you'd better read that chapter in its context because it has nothing to do with fasting from food and water. Quite the opposite.

The fast of Isaiah 58 has to do with your service unto God on behalf of others. And in your service unto God, God will meet you and heal you of your diseases. For as you give unto others, God will give back to you. That is the "fast" He's called you to. Service unto others breaks the yoke. That's what Isaiah 58 teaches us.

The prayer and fasting issue that the disciples had to undergo was because they couldn't cast out the spirit of epilepsy. They got so involved in making a "science" out of this new ministry of healing in Christ that they forgot they were supposed to be in a tightly knit relationship with the Father and Jesus.

¹⁸**And Jesus rebuked the devil; and he departed out of him: and the child was cured from that very hour. ¹⁹Then came the disciples to Jesus apart, and said, Why could not we cast him out? ²⁰And Jesus said unto them, Because of your unbelief: for verily I say unto you, If ye have faith as a grain of mustard seed, ye shall say unto this mountain, Remove hence to yonder place; and it shall remove; and nothing shall be impossible unto you. ²¹Howbeit this kind goeth not out but by prayer and fasting.** Matthew 17:18-21

Let me say this to you about prayer and fasting—if you don't pray and fast in your lifetime, it will be a block to the hand of God because that means you're not setting yourself aside before God to let Him enrich you and bring you back into that place of fellowship where He's your priority.

A time of prayer and fasting is not for the purpose to get something from God. You pray and fast to meet God in relationship. This kind of fasting is not just the giving up of food as a sacrifice for so many days. This fast is that you set aside everything, including eating, so as to have a period of time where you are completely alone with God and His Word for relationship purposes. It is setting yourself aside before God to give Him the opportunity to enrich you and bring you into that place of fellowship where He is your priority.

I have come to this understanding about prayer and fasting out of these scriptures. One day some of the Pharisees came to Jesus and asked: "Why don't your disciples fast and pray like John's disciples do?" And Jesus said unto them, "Why should they? The reason for their prayer and fasting is here in the midst of them, but when I am gone, then they shall pray and fast (my paraphrase—He was saying that the relationship is right here in their midst). But when I'm gone back to heaven, they will enter into that relationship by faith again in prayer and fasting."

> [19]**And Jesus said unto them, Can the children of the bridechamber fast, while the bridegroom is with them? as long as they have the bridegroom with them, they cannot fast.** Mark 2:19

Do not confuse petition with fellowship when it comes to prayer and fasting. Prayer and fasting is primarily for fellowship out of which God blesses us, but many people go into petition only and have made prayer and fasting some type of spiritual mantra that automatically requires God to do something.

☐ 20. Improper Care of the Body

The twentieth block to healing is improper care of the body. You know, if you're asking me to get you well (and you're not, but if you were) and the disease is a result of your not taking care of the temple of the Holy Spirit, do you think God is going to answer my prayer for you? God's not going to answer my prayer for you if you are not getting good nutrition, if you are not drinking enough water, and getting enough rest and sleep. If you are not taking reasonable care of yourself, you are going to pay a high price. That is the consequence of negligence.

Now there's another area in this improper care of the body. In Philippians 2, there is a story about somebody serving the Lord who got sick unto death because they did not use wisdom in how much time they spent in ministry serving the Lord. Philippians 2:25-30 says—yet I supposed it necessary to send to you Epaphroditus, my brother, and companion in labor, and fellow soldier, but your messenger, and he that ministered to my wants. For he longed after you all, and was full of heaviness, because that ye had heard that he had been sick. For indeed he was sick nigh unto death: but God had mercy on him; and not on him only, but on me also, lest I should have sorrow upon sorrow.

> [25]**Yet I supposed it necessary to send to you Epaphroditus, my brother, and companion in labour, and fellow soldier, but your messenger, and he that ministered to my wants.** [26]**For he longed after you all, and was full of heaviness, because that ye had heard that he had been sick.** [27]**For indeed he was sick nigh unto death: but God had mercy on him; and not on him only, but on me also, lest I should have sorrow upon sorrow.** [28]**I sent him therefore the more**

carefully, that, when ye see him again, ye may rejoice, and that I may be the less sorrowful. [29]Receive him therefore in the Lord with all gladness; and hold such in reputation: [30]Because for the work of Christ he was nigh unto death, not regarding his life, to supply your lack of service toward me. Philip. 2:25-30

Do you understand what was just said? This guy was sick unto death because he was burnt out serving Paul and serving the LORD.

I work long hours. I'm not a pastor that shows up 2 days a week at a church service. We're very active. Our ministry is going 7 days a week, nearly 18 hours a day, 365 days a year. But I have to take it easy; I have to take time out. I have to measure my time and I have to allow my staff to measure their time because if we don't we'll die prematurely trying to save people's lives. It's a high price to pay. So, we're going to live, and you're going to live, but we're going to take time out to make sure that we do not end up in sin that becomes a block to our own healing, or even better, will prevent a disease from getting a foothold.

☐ 21. Not Discerning the Lord's Body

The twenty-first block is not discerning the LORD's body. 1 Corinthians 11:27-31 describes a situation where Paul is talking about a physical disease problem in God's people. Many are weak. Many are sickly. Many sleep—that means they died prematurely—because they did not discern the LORD's body. The term sleep refers to the death of believers.

[30]For this cause many *are* weak and sickly among you, and many sleep. 1 Cor. 11:30

It is the "LORD's body" we must discern. It is by His stripes we were and are healed.

[4]Surely he hath borne our griefs, and carried our sorrows: yet we did esteem him stricken, smitten of God, and afflicted. [5]But he *was* wounded for our transgressions, *he was* bruised for our iniquities: the chastisement of our peace *was* upon him; and with his stripes we are healed. Isaiah 53:4-5

[17]That it might be fulfilled which was spoken by Esaias the prophet, saying, Himself took our infirmities, and bare *our* sicknesses. Matthew 8:17

[24]Who his own self bare our sins in his own body on the tree, that we, being dead to sins, should live unto righteousness: by whose stripes ye were healed. 1 Peter 2:24

If we do not want to be sickly and die prematurely, then we must have faith in the healing that was/is provided by Christ as well as forgiveness.

[8]Jesus Christ the same yesterday, and to day, and for ever. Hebrews 13:8

Nothing will be impossible with such faith.

[22]And all things, whatsoever ye shall ask in prayer, believing, ye shall receive. Matthew 21:22

[23]Jesus said unto him, If thou canst believe, all things *are* possible to him that believeth. Mark 9:23

> [22]And Jesus answering saith unto them, Have faith in God. [23]For verily I say unto you, That whosoever shall say unto this mountain, Be thou removed, and be thou cast into the sea; and shall not doubt in his heart, but shall believe that those things which he saith shall come to pass; he shall have whatsoever he saith. [24]Therefore I say unto you, What things soever ye desire, when ye pray, believe that ye receive *them,* and ye shall have *them.* Mark 11:22-24

> [12]Verily, verily, I say unto you, He that believeth on me, the works that I do shall he do also; and greater *works* than these shall he do; because I go unto my Father. [13]And whatsoever ye shall ask in my name, that will I do, that the Father may be glorified in the Son. [14]If ye shall ask any thing in my name, I will do *it.* [15]If ye love me, keep my commandments. John 14:12-15

> [24]Hitherto have ye asked nothing in my name: ask, and ye shall receive, that your joy may be full. John 16:24

This scripture in 1 Corinthians 11 is talking about taking communion in unbelief, not realizing its true significance, and not discerning the LORD's body and blood to receive the benefits by faith. It also refers to the saved or unsaved man who takes communion with sin in his life, without making confession unto salvation and acknowledgment of personal needs, without judging himself so as to escape the chastening of God.

There are three facets to this block to healing. I really want you to pay attention, because this is very, very important.

Many do not discern the LORD's body correctly in communion. And there are three aspects. You will find them in 1 Corinthians 11:27-31:

> [27]Wherefore whosoever shall eat this bread, and drink this cup of the Lord, unworthily, shall be guilty of the body and blood of the Lord. [28]But let a man examine himself, and so let him eat of *that* bread, and drink of *that* cup. [29]For he that eateth and drinketh unworthily, eateth and drinketh damnation to himself, not discerning the Lord's body. [30]For this cause many *are* weak and sickly among you, and many sleep. [31]For if we would judge ourselves, we should not be judged. 1 Cor. 11:27-31

Let me give you the three aspects of why communion represents a block. These are the blocks in it:

Aspect #1: when you take communion, it's one of the sacraments of the Church. There are only three of them: water baptism, communion and foot washing. Only three sacraments are found in Scripture as commandments. And in communion you are celebrating the remembrance of Christ in two dimensions: His shed blood and His broken body. The cup for the blood and the wafer, or the bread, or the cracker, for His broken body.

When you unworthily partake of what forgiveness by God represents in communion, but do not repent unto Him, then you are guilty of fraud and you have cursed yourself with a curse. This is partaking unworthily. You have cursed yourself with a curse because you make what Jesus did at the cross of no effect for you. It's not the sacrament that saves you—it's the *obedience*.

Part of this aspect is not judging ourselves with regard to sin as the spiritual roots of disease to bring forth the repentance so the forgiveness, deliverance and healing can be appropriated to bring forth the full benefits provided in the LORD's Supper. Judging ourselves involves having the discernment to know specifically what is being repented for. Otherwise, we do not know what to stand against, what to change in our lives, and what to renounce out of our lives. Generic repentance and asking in a generic way for forgiveness of our sins without knowing what those sins are accomplishes very little. Many people say: "Father God, forgive me of all my sins." And He does forgive. But there can be no repentance without knowing specifically the sin area that needs to be sanctified out of our life.

Aspect #2: has to do with us "eating each other alive." This is "not discerning the LORD's body." In fact, it creates what we might call an "autoimmune disease" in the Church body. That is the body of believers attacking one another in relationships in like manner as an autoimmune disease attacks the physical body. The Church is called the body of Christ. We must learn to discern one another as part of our body.

> **27Now ye are the body of Christ, and members in particular.** 1 Cor. 12:27

> **2Bear ye one another's burdens, and so fulfil the law of Christ.** Galatians 6:2

This aspect has to do with fellowship and relationship with one another in the Church. If you say you love the LORD and you hate your brother, the love of God is not with you.

> **14We know that we have passed from death unto life, because we love the brethren. He that loveth not *his* brother abideth in death.** 1 John 3:14

When we partake of the LORD's Supper/Communion in remembrance of Him, we are saying to Him that because of what He did for us, we are ready to do that for each other. Not dying for each other's sins, but laying our lives down in service one to another. When we partake of communion and ignore our brother in his need and his disease, then we have negated that fellowship with him that communion represents and we are cursed with a curse. Communion is *koinonia* (#2842, Greek, Strong's Concordance), fellowship. We must focus on the horizontal relationship in the body of Christ which is our relationship with each other, as well as on the vertical relationship with each of the three persons of the Godhead.

> **16The cup of blessing which we bless, is it not the communion of the blood of Christ? The bread which we break, is it not the communion of the body of Christ? 17For we *being* many are one bread, *and* one body: for we are all partakers of that one bread.** 1 Cor. 10:16-17

> **7But if we walk in the light, as he is in the light, we have fellowship one with another, and the blood of Jesus Christ his Son cleanseth us from all sin.** 1 John 1:7

The cup/the blood is for forgiveness of sins on the vertical level from God and on the horizontal level with each other. The bread is the bread of life for healing of our bodies through helping one another deal with the spiritual roots of disease and blocks to healing. It is the Church being the Church ministering the life of God to each other. Then we can truly say:

> **¹⁷For the kingdom of God is not meat and drink; but righteousness, and peace, and joy in the Holy Ghost.** Romans 14:17

Aspect #3: the third aspect of the block to healing taught in 1 Corinthians 11 is even more serious. It is addressed to churches who do not believe that healing is for today. It is why, in many denominational churches, people are dying with insanity and disease, because the very thing—healing—that was provided for them at the cross, that the communion service represents, is negated by half; that is, one-half is rejected in unbelief and doctrinal positioning while still being celebrated in the actual communion service.

Here's how it works. The shed blood of Jesus was not for the healing of disease. His shed blood was for the forgiveness of sins. Scripture is clear that without the shedding of blood there is no remission of sins.

> **²⁸For this is my blood of the new testament, which is shed for many for the remission of sins.** Matthew 26:28

> **²²And almost all things are by the law purged with blood; and without shedding of blood is no remission.** Hebrews 9:22

So when we come into communion and we take the cup, we acknowledge that what He did for us allows us to be able to repent, have cleansing and forgiveness of all sin.

> **⁷But if we walk in the light, as he is in the light, we have fellowship one with another, and the blood of Jesus Christ his Son cleanseth us from all sin. ⁸If we say that we have no sin, we deceive ourselves, and the truth is not in us. ⁹If we confess our sins, he is faithful and just to forgive us *our* sins, and to cleanse us from all unrighteousness. ¹⁰If we say that we have not sinned, we make him a liar, and his word is not in us.** 1 John 1:7-10

However, the broken bread represents the stripes that were laid on Jesus. And the bread represents freedom from the curse and the curse is all manner of disease (Deuteronomy 28).

> **²⁴Who his own self bare our sins in his own body on the tree, that we, being dead to sins, should live unto righteousness: by whose stripes ye were healed.** 1 Peter 2:24

When we don't believe that healing is for today and we teach that it is not and we take the bread of communion which represents the freedom from the curse, but deny that that freedom is for today, we have brought that curse into our lives. We are cursed with a curse which is the disease that we now say we cannot be healed from, yet we celebrate the sacrament that provides for that healing. There is something wrong with this picture theologically.

This happens because we negate one-half of what Christ did at the cross. In partaking of the bread, we curse ourselves in our ignorance and our apostasy. For these three reasons, many of us are weak, are sick and die premature deaths—because we are cursed with a curse we have brought upon ourselves because of unbelief.

That's tough teaching, isn't it? But that's what I see. Those who are not rightly discerning the body of Christ personally, and what all the work He did at the cross represents correctly, open the door for sickness and disease and premature death. It's a spiritual block to healing.

☐ 22. Touching God's Anointed Leaders

The twenty-second block involves touching God's anointed leaders. If you have a pastor that's in sin, if you have a pastor that's in error, the elders ought to be able to straighten him out. I am not an island unto myself. What I teach, if you don't agree with me, come—we'll have a Bible study. *I can't afford to be wrong and neither can you.*

Don't touch God's anointed.

> ²²*Saying,* **Touch not mine anointed, and do my prophets no harm.** 1 Chron. 16:22

> ¹⁵*Saying,* **Touch not mine anointed, and do my prophets no harm.** Psalm 105:15

There is a major curse that comes with it. Many people get all upset about our president and I agree with you that he's got some squirrelly ideas. But I tell you what—he just represents the mores and morality of this nation. So what you have there is what you have here and you know it's true. *God has just given us what we are to convict us of what we're not.*

Touching God's anointed carries more significance than most Christians understand. God's anointed are all those set in place in leadership in the Church and it also includes their families. I don't care what you think about this man, Henry, who is speaking to you. But I do care for your sakes how you handle it. If you have anything negative to say, you had better say it to my face. If you don't say it to my face, you're cursed with a curse if you say it to anyone else.

You can read for yourself in the Bible about Korah and the 250 elders of Israel that went into sedition against Moses. You will find this in Numbers, chapter 16. Also read about Miriam, Moses' sister, being struck with leprosy because of her murmuring against the wife of Moses (Numbers chapter 12).

I use myself as an example, but I am not the only anointed one of God in your life. What you say about your pastor and church leaders is very important to your health and well-being. People do not understand the seriousness of the sins of the tongue and the sin of division against God's leaders and those who minister under them.

I want to make a bold statement to you because I see where the bridge is out in so many lives. Never be a part of a church split. You will not prosper and every church that is born out of a church split will not prosper. It will split and resplit and split and resplit until the coming of the LORD. Because there's a spirit that rules that is a curse. If you want to leave the church, don't burn bridges. Love that pastor even if you don't agree with him. Whatever reason, communicate and let him send you out in peace. And when you leave, don't be a division-maker and take others out with you. If you do, you will be cursed with a curse. Leave in peace, burn no bridges. Let God be God and stay out of it. Keep your mouth shut. Don't gather to yourself those who agree with you against God's anointed. If a church is not ministering to you and your needs, then find someplace where you can be fed; but don't murmur against that pastor. He is God's servant and God is the One who will deal with him.

☐ 23. Immoderate Eating

This twenty-third block involves not taking care of the body in nutrition. This ministry believes in temple maintenance and we believe in good nutrition and we believe all of that in moderation (temperance). You cannot expect to walk in health if you don't drink enough water and eat the proper mixture of food.

> [19]**What? know ye not that your body is the temple of the Holy Ghost** *which is* **in you, which ye have of God, and ye are not your own?** [20]**For ye are bought with a price: therefore glorify God in your body, and in your spirit, which are God's.** 1 Cor. 6:19-20

Our bodies belong to the LORD and we have a responsibility to give them proper rest, exercise, and good nutrition. You cannot expect to walk in health if you don't drink enough water and eat foods that nourish the body. These foods include whole grain cereals and breads, dairy products, protein and generous amounts of fruits and vegetables, especially the green leafy ones. The day should begin with a good breakfast. Many people have the idea that if I eat by faith and trust in God that I can eat anything I want with no regard to nutrition. Foolish presumptuous faith that negates the wisdom of God in good eating will not promote health of the body.

If you are concerned about excessive weight gain, first of all this is a spiritual problem rooted in self-hatred. Not eating breakfast is not the way to deal with the fear of gaining weight. It's the morning meal that sets metabolism for the rest of the day and burns the calories. If you eat lunch and you haven't had breakfast, lunch becomes fat because the metabolism is overloaded when it should have been set in motion at breakfast. If a person does not eat sufficient calories, then the metabolic fire goes low so as to conserve everything that is eaten and the body will actually hoard fat because of the slowdown in metabolism.

With regard to vitamin supplements we say if you are concerned then a one-a-day is all you need. Megadoses of vitamin and mineral supplements can unbalance body chemistry and even cause the body to go into levels of toxic poisonings. Meganutrition is only another of man's efforts to bypass the curse and maintain health artificially and unnaturally rather than the way God created it to be. Those who are caught up in mega amounts of vitamin, mineral and herb supplements are motivated by fear and are trying to jump-start themselves in health. Just because a little is essential and beneficial does not mean that a whole bunch more will help more. The chemical imbalance coming out of this can be a major block to God's health and wholeness. If you are doing megadoses of supplements, it is not wise to go off "cold turkey" and the body will not be able to handle the withdrawal shock. You need to take yourself off in a slow and gradual manner so as to give your body time to adjust back to normal. Good nutrition is absolutely important to our health, but nutrition cannot heal the defects that come from separation from God and His Word or deal with sanctification and sin issues that formulate roots to disease.

Another concern is the growing use of sugar substitutes being put in the foods we buy. We are finding these are contributing to depression, muscle spasms, headaches and chronic tiredness. Sugar in moderation is the better way to go. Get off these sugar substitutes and you will see the difference. It is not bondage to do a little label reading on the products you buy. This is wisdom to stay on top of the subtle effects of the marketplace in well-meaning efforts that through ignorance become man's attempt to bypass the curse. I find that God likes a little sugar Himself.

> **²³Thou hast not brought me the small cattle of thy burnt offerings; neither hast thou honoured me with thy sacrifices. I have not caused thee to serve with an offering, nor wearied thee with incense. ²⁴Thou hast bought me no sweet cane with money, neither hast thou filled me with the fat of thy sacrifices: but thou hast made me to serve with thy sins, thou hast wearied me with thine iniquities.** Isaiah 43:23-24

> **¹⁶Know ye not that ye are the temple of God, and *that* the Spirit of God dwelleth in you? ¹⁷If any man defile the temple of God, him shall God destroy; for the temple of God is holy, which *temple* ye are.** 1 Cor. 3:16-17

Our bodies are God's mobile homes. We must not take them for granted. If we will keep our spirits nourished with the Word of God and keep our lives free of devastating sin and occultism and exercise wisdom in the care of our bodies, we will enjoy greater and greater measures of divine health.

Moderation is the key, whether it be with regard to exercise, rest or what you eat. Moderation is one of the fruits of the Holy Spirit listed in Galatians 5:23 as temperance.

There is a movement even within the Church to selectably remove many foods from our diet and I consider this to be evil because what God has created to be taken with thanksgiving is now being eaten or not eaten out of fear. You can call what God created evil but I'm not going to because in Genesis in the creation, He didn't say it was good, He said it was very good. In fact, the Scriptures indicate it in the Word.

> **⁴:¹Now the Spirit speaketh expressly, that in the latter times some shall depart from the faith, giving heed to seducing spirits, and doctrines of devils; ²Speaking lies in hypocrisy; having their conscience seared with a hot iron; ³Forbidding to marry, *and commanding* to abstain from meats, which God hath**

created to be received with thanksgiving of them which believe and know the truth. ⁴For every creature of God *is* good, and nothing to be refused, if it be received with thanksgiving: ⁵For it is sanctified by the word of God and prayer. 1 Tim. 4:1-5

☐ 24. Pure Unbelief

The twenty-fourth block to healing is pure unbelief. Mark 6:4-6 refers to the unbelief in Nazareth. This is the story of Jesus being unable to do great works in His own hometown because of unbelief.

> ⁴But Jesus said unto them, A prophet is not without honour, but in his own country, and among his own kin, and in his own house. ⁵And he could there do no mighty work, save that he laid his hands upon a few sick folk, and healed *them.* ⁶And he marvelled because of their unbelief. And he went round about the villages, teaching. Mark 6:4-6

Paul, in Hebrews chapter 4, also addresses the issue of pure unbelief in those that came out of Egypt under the leadership of Moses and also the unbelief in those that he was addressing in these scriptures. Paul indicated that unbelief and doubt would keep us from our rest, and also when we find ourselves in that unrest, rather than belief and accept what God has said, we would then try to create that rest by our own labors. In fact, disease management is a form of that type of works designed to try and produce a rest apart from God.

> ⁴:¹Let us therefore fear, lest, a promise being left *us* of entering into his rest, any of you should seem to come short of it. ²For unto us was the gospel preached, as well as unto them: but the word preached did not profit them, not being mixed with faith in them that heard *it.* ³For we which have believed do enter into rest, as he said, As I have sworn in my wrath, if they shall enter into my rest: although the works were finished from the foundation of the world. ⁴For he spake in a certain place of the seventh *day* on this wise, And God did rest the seventh day from all his works. ⁵And in this *place* again, If they shall enter into my rest. ⁶Seeing therefore it remaineth that some must enter therein, and they to whom it was first preached entered not in because of unbelief: ⁷Again, he limiteth a certain day, saying in David, To day, after so long a time; as it is said, To day if ye will hear his voice, harden not your hearts. ⁸For if Jesus had given them rest, then would he not afterward have spoken of another day. ⁹There remaineth therefore a rest to the people of God. ¹⁰For he that is entered into his rest, he also hath ceased from his own works, as God *did* from his. ¹¹Let us labour therefore to enter into that rest, lest any man fall after the same example of unbelief. Hebrews 4:1-11

☐ 25. Failing to Keep Our Life Filled Up With God

The twenty-fifth block to healing is failing to keep our life *filled up* with God. Jesus said in John 5:14, after He had just healed someone—go your way, sin no more, lest a worse thing come upon you. What was He saying? Keep yourself *filled;* don't sin.

> ¹⁴Afterward Jesus findeth him in the temple, and said unto him, Behold, thou art made whole: sin no more, lest a worse thing come unto thee. John 5:14

There's another scripture that says this. Matthew 12:43-45—when the unclean spirit has gone out of a man, he walks through dry places, seeking rest, and finds none. Then he says, I will return into my house from whence I came out; and when he is come, he finds *it* empty, swept, and garnished. Then he goes, and takes with himself seven other spirits more wicked than himself, and they enter in and dwell there: and the last *state* of that man is worse than the first. Even so shall it be also unto this wicked generation.

> **[43]When the unclean spirit is gone out of a man, he walketh through dry places, seeking rest, and findeth none. [44]Then he saith, I will return into my house from whence I came out; and when he is come, he findeth *it* empty, swept, and garnished. [45]Then goeth he, and taketh with himself seven other spirits more wicked than himself, and they enter in and dwell there: and the last *state* of that man is worse than the first. Even so shall it be also unto this wicked generation.** Matthew 12:43-45

What is this saying? Bottom line: when God delivers you, you have an obligation to stay "filled up."

If I give you knowledge about how to get free, that same knowledge will keep you free. But if you fall back into the same roots of sin, then your chances of keeping your healing are not very good. However, if you keep yourself filled up, your chances of keeping your healing are excellent.

Many people say, well, they didn't "keep their healing." Did you ever ask God why? They probably fell back into their old sins all over again. So keeping ourselves filled up is essential; and if we don't, it's a block to keeping our healing and our well- being.

It is important to note that when the enemy is removed, he will come back to see if you're for real and if you are "filled up" with the knowledge of God and obedience to Him. The enemy is somewhat lazy in that he takes the path of least resistance. He needs you in order to be fulfilled. In fact, when the enemy is within you, he is at peace and you're in torment. And when the enemy is gone out of you, he is in torment and you're in peace. The enemy knows what it took to gain access to your life and he will try it again, but you have the knowledge and the tools that will keep you free.

□ 26. Not Resisting the Enemy

The twenty-sixth block to healing is not resisting the enemy. In Isaiah 38:1-5 is the story of Hezekiah the king. Remember that Hezekiah was sick unto death? And the prophet came and said, "boy, you're going to die." What did Hezekiah do? He had a disease unto death. Did he roll over against the wall and curse God? Did he roll over against the wall and go into abject bitterness? Did he roll over against the wall and have a pity party? Did he call the undertaker?

What did he do? *He prayed and he asked God for extended life.* Did God give it to him? Yes! Fifteen years! If you have a disease unto death, talk to God! Ask Him for fifteen more years. You've got a scripture to stand on!

> **38:1**In those days was Hezekiah sick unto death. And Isaiah the prophet the
> son of Amoz came unto him, and said unto him, Thus saith the LORD, Set thine
> house in order: for thou shalt die, and not live. **2**Then Hezekiah turned his face
> toward the wall, and prayed unto the LORD, **3**And said, Remember now, O
> LORD, I beseech thee, how I have walked before thee in truth and with a
> perfect heart, and have done *that which is* good in thy sight. And Hezekiah
> wept sore. **4**Then came the word of the LORD to Isaiah, saying, **5**Go, and say to
> Hezekiah, Thus saith the LORD, the God of David thy father, I have heard thy
> prayer, I have seen thy tears: behold, I will add unto thy days fifteen years.
> Isaiah 38:1-5

That's one aspect of not resisting the enemy – not asking.

The enemy is always trying to devour mankind through temptation, but the
Scriptures indicate that you can defeat him and he will flee.

> **8**Be sober, be vigilant; because your adversary the devil, as a roaring lion,
> walketh about, seeking whom he may devour: **9**Whom resist stedfast in the
> faith, knowing that the same afflictions are accomplished in your brethren that
> are in the world. 1 Peter 5:8-9

> **7**Submit yourselves therefore to God. Resist the devil, and he will flee
> from you. **8**Draw nigh to God, and he will draw nigh to you. Cleanse *your*
> hands, *ye* sinners; and purify *your* hearts, *ye* double minded. James 4:7-8

> **19**I call heaven and earth to record this day against you, *that* I have set
> before you life and death, blessing and cursing: therefore choose life, that both
> thou and thy seed may live: Deut. 30:19

☐ 27. Just Giving Up

The twenty-seventh block to healing is just giving up. You look at your
symptoms; you look at the prognosis; you look at the word "incurable"; and you come
into an agreement and acceptance of all this as the truth, rather than pursuing healing
in the face of what everything in the physical realm would indicate.

There are dozens of people walking around on this planet today who have come
to this ministry and who would have been dead if God and our ministry team hadn't
gotten involved. The doctors had given up on them. They are alive today, staying
"filled up"with God and His Word. Which is **a more excellent way?** Premature death
or a longer life in which to fulfill the will of God in your life? **The LORD is more
magnified in our healing than in a premature death.**

> **9**Mine eye mourneth by reason of affliction: LORD, I have called daily
> upon thee, I have stretched out my hands unto thee. **10**Wilt thou shew wonders
> to the dead? shall the dead arise *and* praise thee? Selah. Psalm 88:9-10

> **9**What profit *is there* in my blood, when I go down to the pit? Shall the
> dust praise thee? shall it declare thy truth? Psalm 30:9

What kind of mentality have we got that we're not prepared to live our 70-80
years in blessing? *God does not need a disease to get you to heaven.* Moses

prophesied in Psalm 90 (have you noticed that David did not write all the Psalms, the heading of this Psalm is: A Prayer of Moses) that the longevity of man would be threescore and ten (70) and if by reason of strength they be fourscore years (80), yet is their strength labor and sorrow, for it is soon cut off, and we fly away.

> [10]**The days of our years** *are* **threescore years and ten; and if by reason of strength** *they be* **fourscore years, yet** *is* **their strength labour and sorrow; for it is soon cut off, and we fly away.** Psalm 90:10

It doesn't say age 60 with some trouble. It doesn't say age 40 with some trouble. It doesn't say age 30 with some trouble. It says trouble doesn't start happening till you're age 80, then you've got some trouble. So I just really, really, really inside as a human being, get really irritated when somebody gives the devil credit for getting somebody to heaven. Are you with me? I just have to hang out for **a more excellent way.** Sickness and a disease are a curse and they do not have to be the way of life. We ought not to be dying prematurely. We are of no earthly good in heaven and God does not need us there before our allotted years on earth are fulfilled. God prophesied through Moses that He purposes for one's lifetime to be 70-80 years, so anything less than that would be a curse. Where did this term "retirement" come from? Moses was 80 years of age before he even started his ministry. What we should give consideration to is that when we retire from our livelihood jobs at age 60-65, that we would then spend the next twenty years devoted to the ministry of helping people get free of their diseases and preaching the gospel – the Good News!

☐ 28. Looking for Repeated Healings Instead of Divine Health

The twenty-eighth block to healing is looking for repeated healings instead of divine health. God's perfect will is not to heal you—*His perfect will is that you don't get sick.* Deut. 28 says that if we disobey the LORD our God, the curse comes upon us. If we obey the LORD our God, get all this stuff straightened out and keep working on it, He'll put none of the diseases of Egypt upon us. *God's perfect will is that you don't get sick.*

> [26]**And said, If thou wilt diligently hearken to the voice of the** Lord **thy God, and wilt do that which is right in his sight, and wilt give ear to his commandments, and keep all his statutes, I will put none of these diseases upon thee, which I have brought upon the Egyptians: for I** *am* **the** Lord **that healeth thee.** Exodus 15:26

> [23]**And the very God of peace sanctify you wholly; and** *I pray God* **your whole spirit and soul and body be preserved blameless unto the coming of our Lord Jesus Christ.** 1 Thes. 5:23

The same principles that I'm giving you that will move the hand of God to heal you, if you apply them to your life, will prevent the diseases from coming in the first place. Which is easier? Working this stuff out to get well or working this stuff out not to get sick? The same amount of work and the same amount of sanctification is involved. It requires the same amount of fellowship and the same amount of coming before God.

Why don't we start getting right with God now, not when we "have to"?
It is the more excellent way.

God is not interested in repeated healings for you. He is interested in you not getting sick to begin with. And if you're looking for repeated healings, you've missed the mark. 3 John 2 says—dearly beloved, I wish above all things that you prosper and be in good health, even as your soul prospereth.

> **²Beloved, I wish above all things that thou mayest prosper and be in health, even as thy soul prospereth.** 3 John 1:2

There it is; that's His will.

Do you think it's God's will to heal today? There it is. Do you think it's God's will that you be in good health today? There it is. Do you think it's God's will for your poor head to be straightened out today? There it is.

Oh, by the way, that's a New Testament scripture that is not found in Matthew, Mark, Luke and John or in the book of Acts.

☐ 29. Rejecting Healing in the Atonement as Part of the Covenant for Today

The twenty-ninth block to healing is rejecting healing in the atonement as part of the covenant for today. 1 Peter 2:24 tells us that by His stripes we are healed; Isaiah 53:5 says—by His stripes we were healed; Ps 103:3 says—I am the LORD thy God, the LORD who forgiveth thee of all thy iniquities and healeth thee of all thy diseases.

> **²⁴Who his own self bare our sins in his own body on the tree, that we, being dead to sins, should live unto righteousness: by whose stripes ye were healed.** 1 Peter 2:24

> **⁵But he *was* wounded for our transgressions, *he was* bruised for our iniquities: the chastisement of our peace *was* upon him; and with his stripes we are healed.** Isaiah 53:5

> **³Who forgiveth all thine iniquities; who healeth all thy diseases;** Psalm 103:3

I was at a pastors' meeting in my community a while back, and there was a pastor there who suggested we pray for some who were sick. So we all prayed for them. We prayed that they would get well. Later, outside, we were talking about a specific disease and I said that I believed God could heal and the pastor said, "I don't believe that's in the atonement today. I believe that passed away 2,000 years ago."

I said, "Just a minute. Weren't you just in the meeting praying for somebody to get well?" "Well," he said, "if He wants to...but it's not there....." I don't know where you're at in your theology—whether you believe that healing is for today or not – but I'm here to tell you that if it's not for today in *your* theology, then it's not. Healing will never happen!

☐ 30. Trying to Bypass the Penalty of the Curse

The thirtieth block to healing is trying to bypass the penalty of the curse without taking responsibility for the sin that causes it.

For example, if you have malabsorption because of anxiety, then taking a medication to block it is an attempt to bypass the penalty of the curse because the root is *fear and anxiety* which is sin. The fruit of it is the malabsorption and the drug is an attempt to manage it apart from dealing with it. We're always looking around for ways to get out of disease without dealing with the root that causes the disease.

It's like this: reincarnation is an attempt by mankind to bypass judgment—to get around it. Sometimes, we're trying to get well without going back to what God said – we're trying to get around what He has said.

An example is a cancer that is a result of bitterness against our mother or mother-in-law or sister(s) (which is sometimes what causes breast cancer). We do everything under the sun to try to get well, but what we should have done was gone back and made peace with our mother or mother-in-law or sister(s). Do you see what I'm saying?

Without coming before God and dealing with the sin in the situation and going back and dealing with the root cause, modalities of healings that we come up with to try to get well are an attempt to bypass the penalty of the curse by trying to get well without doing it God's way (in obedience to Him).

This does not mean that a person is never supposed to go to a doctor to find out what is wrong with them. What we are saying is that if your disease is spiritually rooted, the only way healing/wholeness will come is to deal with the spiritual root through repentance and sanctification. To do otherwise you are wasting your time and money seeking modality after modality for healing. If a disease is spiritually rooted, then no modality is going to do anything more than be an attempt to manage the disease. The modalities often further complicate the disease with drug side effects and oftentimes bring in occultism which become a block to healing. Many holistic practices are rooted in occultism.

What this block is saying is that you want your healing but you do not want to go through the right doorway to get it. You don't want to go the route of repentance and sanctification. You would rather put your trust in doctors and medicine as an attempt to bypass responsibility before God for the disease which is a curse in your life.

> [2]**As the bird by wandering, as the swallow by flying, so the curse causeless shall not come.** Proverbs 26:2

Editor's note: Proper medical care, including diagnosis, is highly recommended for everyone listening to this teaching and it should not be construed that I am against doctors and proper medical attention. This information is being offered as a spiritual insight to psychological and biological disease with regard to the etiology of various diseases that must be recognized in conjunction with the healing and/or prevention of these diseases.

□ 31. Murmuring and Complaining

The thirty-first block to healing is murmuring and complaining. Look at Numbers 12:1-15, and read about Miriam's leprosy.

> [12:1]And Miriam and Aaron spake against Moses because of the Ethiopian woman whom he had married: for he had married an Ethiopian woman. [2]And they said, Hath the LORD indeed spoken only by Moses? hath he not spoken also by us? And the LORD heard *it.* [3](Now the man Moses *was* very meek, above all the men which *were* upon the face of the earth.)... [10]And the cloud departed from off the tabernacle; and, behold, Miriam *became* leprous, *white* as snow: and Aaron looked upon Miriam, and, behold, *she was* leprous. [11]And Aaron said unto Moses, Alas, my lord, I beseech thee, lay not the sin upon us, wherein we have done foolishly, and wherein we have sinned. [12]Let her not be as one dead, of whom the flesh is half consumed when he cometh out of his mother's womb. [13]And Moses cried unto the LORD, saying, Heal her now, O God, I beseech thee. [14]And the LORD said unto Moses, If her father had but spit in her face, should she not be ashamed seven days? let her be shut out from the camp seven days, and after that let her be received in *again.* [15]And Miriam was shut out from the camp seven days: and the people journeyed not till Miriam was brought in *again.* Numbers 12:1-3, 10-15

1 Corinthians 10:10-11 tells us—neither murmur ye as some of them also murmured and were destroyed by serpents in the wilderness.

> [10]Neither murmur ye, as some of them also murmured, and were destroyed of the destroyer. [11]Now all these things happened unto them for ensamples: and they are written for our admonition, upon whom the ends of the world are come. 1 Cor. 10:10-11

That was about the time of Aaron. Murmuring and complaining are signs of ungratefulness and will block God's movement in our lives.

> [14]Do all things without murmurings and disputings: [15]That ye may be blameless and harmless, the sons of God, without rebuke, in the midst of a crooked and perverse nation, among whom ye shine as lights in the world; Philip. 2:14-15

□ 32. Hating and Not Obeying Instruction

The thirty-second block to healing is hating and not obeying instruction. Proverbs 5:11-14 says—and thou mourn at the last when thy flesh and thy body are consumed; and say how have I hated instruction and my heart despised reproof; I have not obeyed the voice of my teachers nor inclined mine ear to them that instructed me. I was almost in utter ruin in the midst of the congregation and assembly.

> [11]And thou mourn at the last, when thy flesh and thy body are consumed, [12]And say, How have I hated instruction, and my heart despised reproof; [13]And have not obeyed the voice of my teachers, nor inclined mine ear to them that instructed me! [14]I was almost in all evil in the midst of the congregation and assembly. Proverbs 5:11-14

For example, this teaching has come to instruct you in righteousness that you may experience **a more excellent way.**

In concluding this block to healing called hating and not obeying instruction, I would like to quote from Isaiah 28:8-18 and let the plumb line of God's conviction find its place in your heart. I suppose these verses sum up the entire problem of disease in the world and in the Church today.

> [8]**For all tables are full of vomit *and* filthiness, *so that there is* no place clean. [9]Whom shall he teach knowledge? and whom shall he make to understand doctrine? *them that are* weaned from the milk, *and* drawn from the breasts. [10]For precept *must be* upon precept, precept upon precept; line upon line, line upon line; here a little, *and* there a little: [11]For with stammering lips and another tongue will he speak to this people. [12]To whom he said, This *is* the rest *wherewith* ye may cause the weary to rest; and this *is* the refreshing: yet they would not hear. [13]But the word of the LORD was unto them precept upon precept, precept upon precept; line upon line, line upon line; here a little, *and* there a little; that they might go, and fall backward, and be broken, and snared, and taken. [14]Wherefore hear the word of the LORD, ye scornful men, that rule this people which *is* in Jerusalem. [15]Because ye have said, We have made a covenant with death, and with hell are we at agreement; when the overflowing scourge shall pass through, it shall not come unto us: for we have made lies our refuge, and under falsehood have we hid ourselves: [16]Therefore thus saith the Lord GOD, Behold, I lay in Zion for a foundation a stone, a tried stone, a precious corner *stone,* a sure foundation: he that believeth shall not make haste. [17]Judgment also will I lay to the line, and righteousness to the plummet: and the hail shall sweep away the refuge of lies, and the waters shall overflow the hiding place. [18]And your covenant with death shall be disannulled, and your agreement with hell shall not stand; when the overflowing scourge shall pass through, then ye shall be trodden down by it. [19]From the time that it goeth forth it shall take you: for morning by morning shall it pass over, by day and by night: and it shall be a vexation only to understand the report.** Isaiah 28:8-19

☐ 33. Past & Continued Involvement with Occultism

Past involvement or continued involvement in occultic practices, thinking, or modalities of healing and disease prevention that are not of God may prevent healing.

Often in following the various attempts by mankind to help himself or heal himself, we may have opened ourselves up to occultic intrusion and may be following a mind-set or action that is an abomination to God because these ways of thinking and actions do not even include him and do not match his Word.

In fact, many times these philosophies, mind-sets and various activities are merely an attempt to by-pass the penalty of the curse (which is the disease itself) without taking responsibility for the sin or spiritual defect that causes the disease. It would be God's will for you to be sanctified in these areas—not managed or manipulated in your spirit, soul, or body.

Ps. 90:12 says: "So teach us to number our days, that we may apply our hearts unto wisdom."

> **¹²So teach us to number our days, that we may apply our hearts unto wisdom.** Psalm 90:12

Our knowledge and wisdom comes from teaching which is based on the Word of God, not the study of creation such as the sun, moon and stars. God has given us the hours, days, months and years of time so that in time (sometimes just in time) we may understand what He has said concerning our thoughts and actions, not what a diviner, astrologer, soothsayer, false prophet or prophetess has said about the past, present, and future.

Even in the Church we have to be discerning in the application of the prophetic. Obedience is still better than sacrifice, and sanctification and righteousness including repentance from dead works (Heb. 6:1) is still the foundation, not what the future holds.

Today is the day of Salvation.....take no thought for tomorrow, the evil of today is sufficient unto itself.....Future revelation does not replace obedience to past revelation, yet in certain sectors I see an attempt to produce a better future through declaration and prophetic revelation. Yet the problems that these declarations and revelations are aimed at are the result of disobedience to past declarations and revelations of the Word. Recognition of this and repentance are in order, not more occultic motion to be gods unto ourselves in order to fix ourselves apart from repentance for sin.

When we exalt the wisdom of the gods (gods with a "little g" meaning the wisdom of this world or doctrine of devils as referred to in the New Testament), insanity and mental confusion often comes. Refer to Daniel 5:17-21 in regards to King Nebuchadnezzar and his insanity by suggesting that he was a god. Also when King Saul obeyed the voice of men and not God, and also consulted with a woman who had a familiar spirit....insanity came. When the Spirit of God departs, all that man has left is his own tormented mind or a spirit of insanity from the devil. The first evidence of this is fear and torment. 1 John 4:18 says "Fear has torment."

Occultism always projects a fear issue and the enemy's thoughts and mechanisms to seemingly solve the problem when, in fact, there is no real solution....just thoughts and actions and the accompanying torment that goes with it...you might say it's like a blind dog chasing his tail.....always in motion...but no ending.

The first line of defense against occultism is knowing the Word of God. Perfect peace belongs to them whose minds are fixed on the LORD....and the LORD is the Word of God. Many of the occultic modalities that are out there may offer various forms of spirituality but....are often missing the Word of God as a foundation and when Scripture is used, it is used out of context; or worse, is used to manipulate or create future promises of blessing without any regard to righteousness and holiness, and sanctification.

We are either establishing the Kingdom of God in the earth or we are establishing the Kingdom of Satan through men.

Some observable characteristics of occult bondage and influence are:

Deep, deep confusion
Hatred of God
Distrust of God
Unable to sleep, night torment, night terror
Hostility, Aggression, and Conflict
Fear of Authority
Fear of Relationships
Impatience
Control of Others
Suspicion
Frustration
Insanity
Depression
Oppression
Tormenting thoughts
Certain types of pain, especially in relationship to the central nervous system
Feelings of isolation
Out of Body experiences
Feelings of accusation against others and oneself
Division makers and trouble makers
Fear
Obsessions
Inability to hear God's voice
Falling asleep in church
Falling asleep while reading the Bible
Rebellion
Stubborness
Disobedience To God's Word…chronic activities
Losing interest in attending church and reading God's Word
Inability to develop a prayer relationship with God

In conclusion, occultism always offers itself as the real thing from God when, in fact, the real thing is obsured and hidden.

Satan always wanted to be like the Most High God and will guise himself in order to accommodate himself to men. The Scriptures do say that Satan is the god of the world.

What I have given you are some ideas from the Word and some examples that should challenge you that sometimes knowing the root is not always the only solution. Sometimes there may be blocks.

Closing Remarks

Hopefully your hearts are challenged by the insight of roots of disease and blocks to healing so that in your lives you can come before your God according to knowledge, not according to ignorance. Then the Holy Spirit can convict you, work with you, so that your lives can be better lives because God is working in your midst according to knowledge that His good will may be performed in your lives. Amen.

I've finished my teaching. We're going to come back together and come before the Lord and I'm going to lead you in prayer and we're going to ask the Lord to do some things in your life.

I would like to read from Nehemiah chapter 8, to prepare your hearts, beginning at verse 1:

> 8:1And all the people gathered themselves together as one man into the street that *was* before the water gate; and they spake unto Ezra the scribe to bring the book of the law of Moses, which the LORD had commanded to Israel. 2And Ezra the priest brought the law before the congregation both of men and women, and all that could hear with understanding, upon the first day of the seventh month. 3And he read therein before the street that *was* before the water gate from the morning until midday, before the men and the women, and those that could understand; and the ears of all the people *were attentive* unto the book of the law. Neh. 8:1-3

> 4And Ezra the scribe stood upon a pulpit of wood, which they had made for the purpose; and beside him stood Mattithiah, and Shema, and Anaiah, and Urijah, and Hilkiah, and Maaseiah, on his right hand; and on his left hand, Pedaiah, and Mishael, and Malchiah, and Hashum, and Hashbadana, Zechariah, *and* Meshullam. 5And Ezra opened the book in the sight of all the people; (for he was above all the people;) and when he opened it, all the people stood up: 6And Ezra blessed the LORD, the great God. And all the people answered, Amen, Amen, with lifting up their hands: and they bowed their heads, and worshipped the LORD with *their* faces to the ground. 7Also Jeshua, and Bani, and Sherebiah, Jamin, Akkub, Shabbethai, Hodijah, Maaseiah, Kelita, Azariah, Jozabad, Hanan, Pelaiah, and the Levites, caused the people to understand the law: and the people *stood* in their place. Neh. 8:4-7

> 8So they read in the book in the law of God distinctly, and gave the sense, and caused *them* to understand the reading. 9And Nehemiah, which *is* the Tirshatha, and Ezra the priest the scribe, and the Levites that taught the people, said unto all the people, This day *is* holy unto the LORD your God; mourn not, nor weep. For all the people wept, when they heard the words of the law. Neh. 8:8-9

> 10Then he said unto them, Go your way, eat the fat, and drink the sweet, and send portions unto them for whom nothing is prepared: for *this* day *is* holy unto our Lord: neither be ye sorry; for the joy of the LORD is your strength. 11So the Levites stilled all the people, saying, Hold your peace, for the day *is* holy; neither be ye grieved. 12And all the people went their way to eat, and to

drink, and to send portions, and to make great mirth, because they had understood the words that were declared unto them. [13]And on the second day were gathered together the chief of the fathers of all the people, the priests, and the Levites, unto Ezra the scribe, even to understand the words of the law. [14]And they found written in the law which the LORD had commanded by Moses, that the children of Israel should dwell in booths in the feast of the seventh month: Neh. 8:10-14

And it goes on... So now let's come to Chapter 9 and verse 2:

[2]And the seed of Israel separated themselves from all strangers, and stood and confessed their sins, and the iniquities of their fathers. [3]And they stood up in their place, and read in the book of the law of the LORD their God *one* fourth part of the day; and *another* fourth part they confessed, and worshipped the LORD their God. Neh. 9:2-3

This is what happens when conviction comes. We get the engrafted Word of God, we come before the LORD, we worship Him, our hearts are circumcised, and we stand and take responsibility not just for our sins but for the failures of our ancestors.

Why? So that genetically inherited disease can be broken and the familiar spirits of our generations that rule us in our souls can also be defeated.

I want you to take whatever time you think is necessary for you personally, if you want to get down on your knees, or just sit quietly in your chair, and if you want God to move in your life because of what we've been teaching. We have been giving you the Word—and the understanding—if you want God to heal you and deliver you from something, or to set something in motion so that thing will change in your life, if God is dealing with your heart and we've taught you something that bears witness, I want to take a little time here and I want you to come before the LORD and I want you to confess your areas that you're dealing with and if you see it in your family tree, I want you to bring that to the LORD and say, "forgive my fathers also." And when you have your little checklist done in your heart, then you'll be done.

So I want you just to take this time now, until most of us are finished, and then I'll bring you together for a prayer—then—and I'll bring you into a prayer now. And then I'm going to pray another prayer at the end where I'm going to ask God to honor you and to heal you where you sit, corporately and individually.

That's what I saw in 2 Chronicles Chapters 29 and 30...that after this type of thing was done, *the LORD heard the voice of Hezekiah and He honored the voice of Hezekiah and He healed the people.*

[5]And said unto them, Hear me, ye Levites, sanctify now yourselves, and sanctify the house of the LORD God of your fathers, and carry forth the filthiness out of the holy *place*. [6]For our fathers have trespassed, and done *that which was* evil in the eyes of the LORD our God, and have forsaken him, and have turned away their faces from the habitation of the LORD, and turned *their* backs...[10]Now *it is* in mine heart to make a covenant with the LORD God of Israel, that his fierce wrath may turn away from us...[15]And they gathered their

> brethren, and sanctified themselves, and came, according to the commandment of the king, by the words of the LORD, to cleanse the house of the LORD...[31]Then Hezekiah answered and said, Now ye have consecrated yourselves unto the LORD, come near and bring sacrifices and thank offerings into the house of the LORD... 2 Chron. 29:5-6, 10, 15, 31

I'm not Hezekiah; I'm Henry. But I'm going to ask the LORD to do that tonight, and match the integrity of your hearts and ask Him to heal you in the areas you are asking Him for healing, or to set in motion those things that will bring the conviction necessary to get you out of that bondage into a place of freedom.

Could we do that now, please? Let me pray...

> Note: At the end of the seminar Pastor Wright led the people to a place of repentance before the LORD. It was a powerful time. We have tried to maintain that Spirit as we repeat it in writing.

> **Father, I consider this a very sovereign time; I ask that You sanctify these people in the name of the Lord Jesus Christ, where they sit and as they come and where they're at...**

> **I ask that You'll meet them in the integrity of their hearts and as they come before You, having heard the Word of God, mixing it with their faith, I ask that You hear them and receive their petitions unto You and forgive them their trespass and release them from the curse of their generations. I ask You this, Father, in the name of our precious Savior, our Lord Jesus Christ, as the work of the Holy Spirit, I release it, Amen.**

> (Pastor Henry goes to the piano to pray and play some beautiful music while folks are praying...he plays "Have Thine Own Way, Lord"...)

> **Thank You, Father....**

> **Lord, hear our hearts; hear our prayers...receive us. Hide not Thy face from us. Forgive us; release us from the sins of our fathers; forgive us of our sins and our trespasses as we forgive those who trespass against us. Lord, heal us; heal our families. Save us, oh God, save our families. We pray for our enemies and those who spitefully use us. Lord, regard not the iniquities of Your people. May Your mercy and Your grace overshadow us. Heal us personally. Heal our marriages; heal our children. Heal our churches. Heal our political leaders. Heal our nation. God, let your salvation be spread to the islands of the sea from the rising of the sun to the setting of the sun. Let the earth be filled with the knowledge of the living God. God, we pray that this planet shall be inhabited in righteousness. Let Your Spirit move in our midst; convict us of sin; deliver us from all evil. Heal our land. Father, I thank You tonight for being in our midst. Lord, be Lord of our hearts. We are Your people, the sheep of Your pature. Your mercy endureth forever. Blessed be the Name of the Lord. Thank You, Father... Hear our prayer, oh God. Send Your Spirit. Thank You, Father. We give You thanksgiving, Lord; we have not made ourselves, but You have made us. You are He that forgiveth us of all our iniquities and You are He that healeth us of all our diseases. You are He that daily loadeth us with benefits; yeah, even the Elohim of our salvation. Lead us not into temptation, but deliver us from evil. Thank You, Father... In Jesus' Name... AMEN**

(Music plays for about 10 minutes...soft, beautiful hymns...)

Did you make some peace with God in that private time? Good.

I'm going to bring this meeting to a close with a scripture and then I'm going to pray... and then we'll be finished tonight. Reading from 2 Chronicles 30:15-20:

> ¹⁵Then they killed the passover on the fourteenth *day* of the second month: and the priests and the Levites were ashamed, and sanctified themselves, and brought in the burnt offerings into the house of the LORD. ¹⁶And they stood in their place after their manner, according to the law of Moses the man of God: the priests sprinkled the blood, *which they received* of the hand of the Levites. ¹⁷For *there were* many in the congregation that were not sanctified: therefore the Levites had the charge of the killing of the passovers for every one *that was* not clean, to sanctify *them* unto the LORD. ¹⁸For a multitude of the people, *even* many of Ephraim, and Manasseh, Issachar, and Zebulun, had not cleansed themselves, yet did they eat the passover otherwise than it was written.
>
> But Hezekiah prayed for them, saying, The good LORD pardon every one ¹⁹*That* prepareth his heart to seek God, the LORD God of his fathers, though *he be* not *cleansed* according to the purification of the sanctuary.
>
> ²⁰And the LORD hearkened to Hezekiah, and healed the people. 2 Chron. 30:15-20

This is a powerful scripture of God's love. Not just in the area of total sanctification but in the area of partial sanctification. God pardoned them and healed them. Those scriptures really got to me. So I'm going to pray a prayer tonight. I believe that everyone in this building is very sincere. I believe you've come with believing hearts expecting, and I'm going to ask God to meet you at whatever level it is possible for Him to do that in conjunction with Who He Is.

I'm going to ask God to meet you in your lives, spirit, soul and body, and that many of the things that you are believing for in your life, that He will make it start to come to pass. And even tonight, many of the oppressions and depressions and many of the things that you are dealing with, that you will see much of that start to change.

I have to believe that, because it's in the Word.

> Father, I stand before You and I sanctify myself before You. God I repent for my failures and my sins, and the sins of my ancestors. God, in my uncleansed state, I tell You that I love You, and by faith I accept Your provision in my life and the work of the Holy Spirit of sanctification in my life. And, God, as I stand before these people, representing You to the best of my ability, I ask that as in the days of Hezekiah, that You will hear from heaven and You will heal.
>
> Father, I come to You in the name of the Lord Jesus Christ, and I ask that You be a Father to these people. These are Your children; these are the sheep of Your pasture; these are those that have been called by Your name, sanctified and set aside for You forever. God, I know that You are on the throne. I know that You sit high above all things, that You look down to see that we do understand. God, we understand, and we seek Your face and Your mercy and

Your person in our lives, our families, and in every area of our lives. So, God, tonight I pray that as these people have come before You that You will come before them and that You will meet them, every one, according to Your good pleasure through the work of the Holy Spirit. I pray this in the Name of the Lord Jesus Christ, AMEN. And all God's people said, AMEN.

Goodnight. Adios.

The information in this book is intended for your general knowledge only. The information is presented only to give insight into disease, its problems and its possible solutions in the area of disease eradication and/or prevention. It is not a technical reference book. It should not be used as a medical tool. All information is intended for your general knowledge only and is not a substitute for medical advice or treatment for specific medical conditions.

The information in this book should not be a substitute for a visit or consultation with a medical doctor or other health care provider. We recommend you seek prompt medical care for any specific health issues.

Treatment modalities around your specific health issues are between you and your physician.

As a pastor and an individual, I am not responsible for a person's disease, nor am I responsible for their healing. All I can do is share what I see about the problem. I am not a professional, I am not a healer; I am a pastor administering the Scriptures and what they say about this subject along with what the medical and scientific community have also observed in line with this insight. There is no guarantee that any person will be healed or any disease prevented. The fruits of this teaching will come forth out of the relationship between the person and God based on the insights given and applied.

Bibliography

"Danger in the Diet Pills?" *Time*, July 21, 1997.

"Deadly Rx: Why are drugs killings so many patients?" *USA Today*, April 24, 1998.

"Greater Expectations." *Newsweek*, September 24, 1990.

"Hormonal Reaction to Stress Tied to Disease, Researchers Say." *Dallas Morning News*, November 16, 1996.

"Mysteries of Stress Probed." *Houston Chronicle*, May 28, 1998.

"The Power to Heal." *Newsweek*, September 24, 1990.

"When Drugs Do Harm." *Newsweek*, April 27, 1998.

Merck Manual. Rahway, NJ: Merck & Co., 16th edition, 1992.

McCance, Kathryn L. and Sue E. Huether. Pathophysiology: The Biologic Basis for Disease in Adults and Children. Mosby, 2nd edition, 1994.

Miller, Claudia S. and Nicholas A. Ashford. *Possible Mechanisms for Multiple Chemical Sensitivity.* www.ul.cs.cmu.edu/books/multiple_chem/mult143.htm

Physician's Desk Reference.

Strong, James. *The Exhaustive Concordance of the Bible.* Hendrickson Publishers.

Tortora, Gerard J. and Nicholas P. Anagnostakos. *Principles of Anatomy & Physiology.* Harper & Row, 2nd edition, 1978.

Notes

Index

Resources

A More Excellent Way is now available in audio book version.

Seminars

Live seminars are available worldwide. If your group or church is interested in scheduling a live seminar, please contact Pleasant Valley Church, Inc.

Annual Teaching Program

Annual teachings of Pleasant Valley Church are available. You will receive at least one tape each week for 52 weeks covering a wide range of subjects. You may subscribe to this program on a monthly, quarterly, semiannual or annual basis.

Books

Biblical Foundations of Freedom compiled by Art Mathias, is now available.

Audio Tapes

Many audio tapes on a wide range of subjects are available for purchase. To receive a list of materials available or that will be available in the near future and to be on our mailing list, please call or write Pleasant Valley Church. There is no obligation.

Here's a sample listing of popular teachings that are available now:

A More Excellent Way .... audio book
Blocks to Healing .... 1 audiocassette
Cancer Seminar .... 3 audiocassettes
Pain Seminar .... 2 audiocassettes
Fibromyalgia .... 1 audiocassette
Witchcraft/Sorcery/Pharmakeia .... 18 audiocassettes
Insight into Allergies (includes Multiple Chemical Sensitivities/Environmental Illness)
.... 2 audiocassettes
Accusing Spirits .... 11 audiocassettes
Fear, Stress and Physiology .... 3 audiocassettes
Spiritual Discernment .... 18 audiocassettes
7 Steps to Sin .... 2 audiocassettes
Unloving Spirits .... 14 audiocassettes

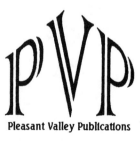

Pleasant Valley Publications

Pleasant Valley Publications
4178 Crest Highway
Thomaston, GA 30286

(800) 453-5775 – ordering and information
(706) 646-2074 – main office
fax: (706) 646-2865 ♦ pvcm3@alltel.net